# The Child with Traumatic Brain Injury or Cerebral Palsy

# The Child with Traumatic Brain Injury or Cerebral Palsy

## A Context-sensitive, Family-based Approach to Development

**Edited by**

Lúcia Willadino Braga, PhD
Neuropsychologist,
SARAH Network of Rehabilitation Hospitals, Brasilia,
Brazil

Aloysio Campos da Paz Jr, MD
Orthopaedic Surgeon,
SARAH Network of Rehabilitation Hospitals, Brasilia,
Brazil

**Forewords by**

Professor Michael Cole
and
Professor Michael Barnes

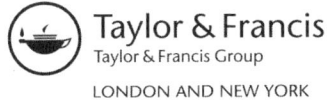

Taylor & Francis
Taylor & Francis Group

LONDON AND NEW YORK

© 2006 Taylor & Francis, an imprint of the Taylor & Francis Group. Taylor & Francis Group is the Academic Division of Informa plc

First published in the United Kingdom 2006
by Taylor & Francis, an imprint of the Taylor & Francis Group, 2 Park Square, Milton Park, Abingdon, Oxon OX14 4RN

Tel.:       +44 (0) 20 7017 6000
Fax.:      +44 (0) 20 7017 6699
Website:  http://www.tandf.co.uk/medicine
E-mail.:   info.medicine@tandf.co.uk

Although every effort has been made to ensure that all owners of copyright material have been acknowledged in this publication, we would be glad to acknowledge in subsequent reprints or editions any omissions brought to our attention.

Although every effort has been made to ensure that information is presented accurately in this publication, the ultimate responsibility rests with the prescribing physician. Neither the publishers nor the authors can be held responsible for errors or for any consequences arising from the use of information contained herein. For detailed instructions on the use of any product or procedure discussed herein, please consult the prescribing information or instructional material issued by the manufacturer.

A CIP record for this book is available from the British Library.

Library of Congress Cataloging-in-Publication Data
Data available on application

ISBN 1 84184 503 5
ISBN 978-1-84184-503-6

Distributed in North and South America by
Taylor & Francis
2000 NW Corporate Blvd
Boca Raton, FL 33431, USA
*Within Continental USA*
Tel:  800 272 7737;     Fax:  800 374 3401
*Outside Continental USA*
Tel:  561 994 0555;     Fax:  561 361 6018
E-mail:  orders @crcpress.com

Distributed in the rest of the world by
Thomson Publishing Services
Cheriton House
North Way
Andover, Hampshire SP10 5BE, UK
Tel:  +44 (0)1264 332424
E-mail:  salesorder.tandf@thomsonpublishingservices.co.uk

Composition by Wearset Ltd, Boldon, Tyne and Wear.

Printed and bound in Spain by Grafos SA

# Contents

# Contributors

Lúcia Willadino Braga, PhD, Neuropsychologist, SARAH Network of Rehabilitation Hospitals, Brasilia, Brazil

Aloysio Campos da Paz, Jr, MD, Orthopedic Surgeon, SARAH Network of Rehabilitation Hospitals, Brasilia, Brazil

Eliane G. Catanho, Physical Therapist, SARAH Network of Rehabilitation Hospitals, Brasilia, Brazil

Sheila M. Denucci, Physical Therapist, SARAH Network of Rehabilitation Hospitals, Brasilia, Brazil

Timothy Feeney, PhD, Clinical Director, School and Community Support Services, Schenectady, New York, USA

Marc A. Forman, MD, PhD, Emeritus Professor of Psychiatry and Pediatrics, Tulane University School of Medicine, New Orleans, Louisiana, USA; Senior Medical Consultant for Clinical Research, SARAH Network of Rehabilitation Hospitals, Brasilia, Brazil

Ingrid L. Gil, MS, Psychologist, SARAH Network of Rehabilitation Hospitals, Brasilia, Brazil

David A. Johnson, PhD, Clinical Psychologist, University of Edinburgh, Scotland, UK

Katia S. Pinto, MS, Occupational Therapist, SARAH Network of Rehabilitation Hospitals, Brasilia, Brazil

David Rose, PhD, Professor of Psychology, University of East London, England, UK

Luciana Rossi, MS, Psychologist, SARAH Network of Rehabilitation Hospitals, Brasilia, Brazil

Flávia Y. Shikida, Speech Therapist, SARAH Network of Rehabilitation Hospitals, Brasilia, Brazil

Ligia N. Souza, PhD, Psychologist, SARAH Network of Rehabilitation Hospitals, Brasilia, Brazil

Mark Ylvisaker, PhD, Professor, School of Education, College of Saint Rose Albany, New York, USA

# Foreword

Recent decades have witnessed an unprecedented increase in knowledge about the brain and its development. Advances in brain imaging have made it possible to identify, with great accuracy, the location of cortical lesions, and in many cases the brain structures that implement a variety of essential cognitive, motor, and emotional functions. Neurosurgery, benefiting from a wide range of technological innovations, has made it possible to remove diseased brain tissue in a minimally invasive way or to minimize the damage of traumatic injury to a particular part of the brain that threatens to result in secondary damage of nearby structures. Remarkable achievements in computer science have not only extended the range of diagnostic and surgical procedures, but have made possible the construction of prosthetic devices that were literally unimaginable in the middle of the twentieth century.

But despite all of these impressive gains in knowledge and the ability to support children who have suffered from brain injuries arising either from external causes such as a blow to the head or infarction resulting from congenital factors or events accompanying otherwise normal birth, many children and youths never fully recover from such brain injuries. A distressingly large percentage do not recover fundamental behavioral capacities sufficient to allow them to live with their families as members of their community. Not only does the inability of such children to acquire skills necessary to find a niche in society devastate their lives, it forces them to live in hospital facilities adequate to keep them alive, but not to afford them any semblance of normal adulthood. Such failures to find means to incorporate brain-injured children are ruinous for their parents and family members, whose lives are forever affected, whether by the burden of submitting their kin to the semi-human conditions of inadequate caretaking facilities, or of subordinating themselves to the often crushing burdens of home care.

Obviously, it is in the interests of everyone concerned that the possibilities of rehabilitation following traumatic brain injury, from whatever cause, at whatever age, be optimized. Yet, for reasons that are, ironically, linked in some measure to the scientific progress that has taken place in the diagnosis and surgical treatment of brain injury – the high levels of specialization that are characteristic of the medical sciences – it is rare to find systems of rehabilitative treatment that optimize the potential for recovery, not only by providing optimal regimes of rehabilitative therapy within the medical and behavioral science professions, but by forging links with the families who will have primary responsibility for the integration of the child into the community once he or she is released from the hospital. After all, surgeons specialize in surgery and pediatricians focus on children with more or less acute, treatable diseases. Rehabilitation specialists may synthesize knowledge from many different areas of sensory, motor, and cognitive development, but by and large they are expected to work with recovering children in settings specially organized for that purpose. Given the need to see many children in the course of a normal work day, they naturally cannot be expected to be making house calls as it is far more efficient for children to come to them. Consequently, for perfectly understandable reasons, while injured children receive the best care that society can routinely provide, they do not receive the best care possible, except in cases where the parents are both exceedingly wealthy, well educated, and willing to devote their own time to the optimal rehabilitation and integration of their child back into their families and society.

Yet, without giving in to the illusion that all children can more-or-less fully recover from severe brain injury, we know, from cases where well informed and pervasive care has been provided for children who, under normal circumstances, could be expected to suffer devastating long-term effects of brain injury, that the potential plasticity of the brain, *provided the right circumstances*, is far greater than common sense, even well educated common sense, would suggest. This is especially true of young children, but there is ample evidence to indicate that functional reorganization of brain-behavior functions can be achieved well after the period when the brain is assumed to be optimally plastic.

From the classic work of Alexander Luria, we came to appreciate that even an adult for whom no modern computer prosthetics was available, a deep understanding of the functional organization of cortical functions can, in some circumstances, mitigate the effects of traumatic brain injury sufficiently for the patient, who in this case was an active accomplice in his own therapeutic regime, to return to life in his rural village and to enjoy some of the simple pleasures that life affords.[1] A sufficiently strong neuropsychological theory is an essential element in any program of rehabilitation.

We also know from recent research such as Antonio Battro's study of Nico, a boy who underwent a right hemispherectomy at the age of 5, that well informed neuropsychological theory implemented with the full cooperation of parents who did not need to spare costs, and the potentials afforded by computer technologies that enabled high levels of dense and relevant environment stimulation can result in remarkable recovery of function.[2]

But these are individual cases. They are exceptional. What, in principle, does it require to create regimes of rehabilitation that make heretofore unthinkable levels of recovery possible? What does it require that parents without great economic means, and children who will never recover normal motor functions, can still be able to learn to communicate and live within a regime of care that is supportable by their families without superhuman sacrifices?

It is to answer these questions that this book is dedicated. The approach to the medical care and rehabilitation of brain-injured children described in the following pages takes its inspiration from an approach to integrating state of the art medical care in a specialized hospital, with an ongoing regime of parental education and involvement that integrates the work of hospital staff with the caregiving practices of the children's families as a long term partnership.

For almost 30 years, a remarkable team of surgeons, doctors, psychologists, and rehabilitative therapists from the SARAH Network of Rehabilitation Hospitals have taken it as their basic task to work with parents and family members to make it possible for brain-injured children to return to their homes where they can live among family and friends as part of their local communities. By adopting the ability of such children to live in their homes and communities as the criterion for successful medical intervention, the SARAH team has created optimal conditions for children's recovery. Rehabilitative therapy is no longer restricted to the hospital grounds where it must be carefully coordinated with the schedules of busy hospital personnel. Such experiences are of course essential, but they are not sufficient. To approach sufficiency, it is necessary to take as an ideal the goal that every moment of the child's waking day will be organized to optimize the child's development.

Since children are living with their families, the only way to create a maximally therapeutic environment is to make the family members a part of the rehabilitation team. This goal at first glance seems utopian. Even in industrially advanced societies such as those found in Europe, North America, and parts of Asia, it seems outrageously implausible to think that it would be possible to provide parents with the knowledge, motivation, and ongoing support that a fully implemented professional therapist-family circle therapeutic environment would require. But the SARAH group has shown that this goal is, in fact, realizable. Even families whose members are not well educated and who have modest fiscal means can be, and in the SARAH regime of care, are, integrated into a wholistic system of care for children that optimizes their life experiences.

Such an undertaking requires a great deal: strong theory (not only of the brain and its relationship to development and behavior, but of the sociology of professional work and its relationship to the lives of everyday working people); strong desire (none of the work is easy for any of the participants, it spills outside of normal work hours on the one hand and on the other it stretches the boundaries of family life beyond normal bounds); strong support, not only from hospital administrators and family members but from society as a whole, as represented by their legislators and government officials. But, as the reader will discover in the pages to follow, such an undertaking *is* possible. It is even possible to develop it into the norm of medical care and rehabilitation for thousands of children in a country where many struggle in poverty and resources are, relative to wealthy neighbors to the north, scarce and often fragile.

This is a book worth reading not only for its practical lessons, but for its deep lesson about the possibilities of institutionalizing an effective, human form of medical treatment that should provide a standard for the world. Who dares to say they are doing enough, when they are not meeting up to the standard of science and care that is the daily experiences of the SARAH Network and its community?

*Michael Cole*
*Distinguished Professor*
*Communication, Psychology, and Human Development*
*Stanford Berman Chair of Language, Thought, and Communication*
*Director, Laboratory of Comparative Human Cognition*
*UC San Diego*

# References

1.      Luria AR. *The Making of Mind*. Cambridge, MA: Harvard University, 1979.

2.      Battro AM. *Half a Brain is Enough: The Story of Nico*. New York: Cambridge University, 2000.

# Foreword

It is a pleasure to write a Foreword to this wonderful book that Lúcia Willadino Braga and Aloysio Campos da Paz, Jr have put together. With their team at the SARAH Network, they have developed their own methods and style of rehabilitation for children with brain injury over many years. The principles and practice have been slowly refined and developed and this book is the culmination of their work. Their methodology of rehabilitation has been tried and tested on more than 15,000 children – both with cerebral palsy and traumatic brain injury. Although the results of their approach have been published in many articles and book chapters in the last few years, this book provides an invaluable summary.

Although each chapter is self-contained, the book is best approached by reading it in its entirety, as only then does the whole ethos of the SARAH rehabilitation approach become clear. In my view, the two essential components of the SARAH methodology are the major emphasis on multidisciplinary teamwork, and the key emphasis on the involvement of the parents and family in the whole rehabilitation process. The SARAH team have clearly demonstrated the benefits of family-supported treatment over and above treatment exclusively by professionals. It is very clear from their work that better outcomes can be obtained for disabled children by the direct involvement of the families in the rehabilitation process.

This book will be of great interest to a wide range of health professionals working in the field. However, it is also an invaluable source of reference for families with disabled children. It is written in an easy and comprehensive style and is free of the jargon that usually makes clinical textbooks relatively inaccessible to the lay reader. The book itself mirrors the philosophy of the SARAH Network in that it is a textbook for the whole team – the child, the family and the professionals.

If the reader wishes to take the subject further then each chapter also has a good range of key references. Each chapter is well illustrated with clear and helpful drawings of the difficult therapeutic approaches, which breaks up the text to make the whole book a pleasure to read. All aspects of child development are covered. Motor developments, unlike in many textbooks, do not take precedent over the equally important cognitive and neuropsychological developments in the child. It is the development of the whole child which is so important.

One of the keys to the success of the SARAH approach is not only the involvement of the family but also the provision of accurate and meaningful information to the family in order to prevent misunderstanding and misinformation. This book is sensible, practical and provides clear, unambiguous information not only to clinicians, but also to the families of children with cerebral palsy and traumatic brain injury. I hope and believe this book will go some way to improving our knowledge, and thus provide a brigher future for children with disabilities.

*Michael Barnes*
*Professor of Neurological Rehabilitation*
*Newcastle upon Tyne, UK*
*President, World Federation for NeuroRehabilitation*

# Acknowledgments

The editors would like to thank: Paulo Roberto de Freitas Guimarães MD, who drew all illustrations in this book while carrying on with his work as pediatrician; Olinda Paula Costa Azevedo, who translated into English the chapters originally written in Portuguese; Luciana Rossi, psychologist, who organized the drawings in Chapters 2 through 6; and Luciana Sollaci, librarian, who reviewed the bibliographic references for all the chapters.

Lúcia Willadino Braga, PhD
Alysio Campos da Paz Jr, MD

**Note on the text**

Please note that for consistency, throughout the book, all children will be referred to as 'he' or 'his'.

# 1

# The Context-sensitive Family-based Approach: Basic Principles

*Lúcia Willadino Braga*

Children begin life with a view of the world that is filtered through the prism of their families. Their development is mediated, stimulated and strengthened through interaction with those closest to them. It is, indeed, the natural role of every family to stimulate the development of their child; they teach the child to explore objects, eat independently, to talk, walk unassisted and socially interact.

Once the diagnosis of brain injury has been established, both in cerebral palsy (CP) and traumatic brain injury (TBI), the mediation of the subsequent development or rehabilitation process is, in large measure, transferred to health care professionals.

The child is a whole person and the treatment depends on the participation of diverse professionals. Nevertheless, this group of sometimes wide-ranging specialists does not always work in a unified manner within a multidisciplinary perspective that understands the child as both a unique individual and a member of a family that has a profound interest in his development.

This book presents an approach that integrates the multidisciplinary team and the family, so that they can closely work together at finding ways to facilitate the learning and specific developmental processes of each child and adolescent based on their motivations, capacities and interests, within the familial and socio-cultural context.

At the core of this methodology is a program that is continually updated to accommodate the stages of the child's development and progress, and is guided by a focus on combining the activity of professionals from various fields of specialization with the family's effective, hands-on participation.

The concept and practice of "family-centered" rehabilitation has been amply discussed in the literature.[1-5] The approach proposed in this book is founded on a family-based process. It is the family who will bring the relevant information and act alongside a team of professionals in all stages of the child's rehabilitation and development.

1

This book contains a CD-ROM with a series of illustrated activities, to be carried out by the family, that facilitate motor, cognitive and neuropsychological development, and foster communication skills, visuo-motor coordination and independence in activities of daily life – the Illustrated Manual. The team of professionals, together with the family, can choose the stimulation activities that are most appropriate for each child. However, the objective is not to transform family members into therapists. The professionals will simply, based on their specific body of knowledge, help the parents continue their natural role of teaching the child and stimulating his development.

This methodology has been tested over the course of 27 years on more than 15,000 children with CP and TBI at the SARAH Network of Rehabilitation Hospitals. The results and the description of this approach have been published in articles and book chapters since 1983.[6-13] In 2005 we published a randomized controlled trial,[14] which studied 72 children with history of moderate to severe TBI for twelve months to test the efficacy of this family-based approach. The children were randomized into two groups, the Direct Clinician Delivered (DCD) and the Indirect Family-Supported Treatment (IFS). The children in both samples were submitted to intensive rehabilitation services for one year. Physical and functional outcomes were measured by the SARAH motor scale[15] and the cognitive outcomes by the WISC III[16] before and after the intervention. The DCD group was treated exclusively by professionals for two hours a day, five days a week, in a clinical setting, working in relative isolation. The IFS group was submitted to the SARAH family-based rehabilitation methodology described in this book. At the end of year, the results confirmed that the parents in the family-supported intervention sample had developed the necessary skills for effectively delivering physical and cognitive intervention within the context of everyday routines of the child's life at home; family education level was not a factor. Although both groups demonstrated improvement, only the children in the family-supported intervention group demonstrated statistically significant improvements in both outcome measures twelve months after starting treatment.

This randomized controlled trial study provides evidence for organizing cognitive and physical interventions and supports for children with TBI around the everyday routines of their lives, with intensive supports for their families. The results of this approach had already been observed in studies with children with cerebral palsy.[6-9]

Although TBI and CP are conditions with very different characteristics, as we discuss more comprehensively in the following chapters, the family's involvement in all of the stages of the child's neurodevelopment has been shown to be equally important and effective in both conditions. The principles of the methodology are similar for both TBI and CP, although the application may vary, depending on the needs of the child and family within their particular socio-cultural context. The main focus of this approach is on the child and his family, and not on his pathology.

# Basic Principles: How to put this Methodology into Practice

This context-sensitive, family-based approach is structured on five basic, integrated principles that serve as the foundation for the rehabilitation program. These principles, consolidated and tested over the course of almost three decades (since the late 1970s), were co-constructed by the team of professionals and the families. The following section of this chapter will discuss these principles and provide examples that describe how to put them into practice within the daily life context of the child, family and rehabilitation team.

**Principle 1: Create an individualized program appropriate to the child's specific developmental stage in a manner that is playful, uses simple materials and integrates activities of different specialties into the same task to facilitate learning.**

This approach aims at targeting the entire treatment to the specific needs of each child, with the team and the family working in a highly integrated manner. Children with brain injury manifest, in non-uniform ways, problems in different aspects of development (motor, neuropsychological, communication, visuo-motor coordination, independence, and so on). Some children with TBI or CP have more motor problems while others experience predominantly neuropsychological or communication difficulties. Consequently, various professionals are needed to work alongside the family to assess and propose activities that facilitate development.

Numerous rehabilitation centers and hospitals embrace the concept of multi-disciplinary teamwork; however, these team members must often work in a relatively isolated manner. They exchange information about the child only periodically and post patient data relative to their specialty in medical charts that are accessed by all the professionals involved in that child's rehabilitation process. The concept behind our development and rehabilitation approach differs in that it is based on a group program that integrates knowledge and experience from the professionals of various specialties. For example, if the physical therapist feels the child needs training in standing balance and the cognitive psychologist recommends exercising the mental function of classification, these two stimulation tasks can be integrated into one playful activity: while standing with front support (Figure 1.1, Activity 26), the child can play at grouping objects by two physical characteristics (Figure 1.2, Activity 71).

In one simple activity, the child can work different objectives for distinct functions, thereby constructing his development through games that target

**Figure 1.1    Activity 26**
Standing with front
support

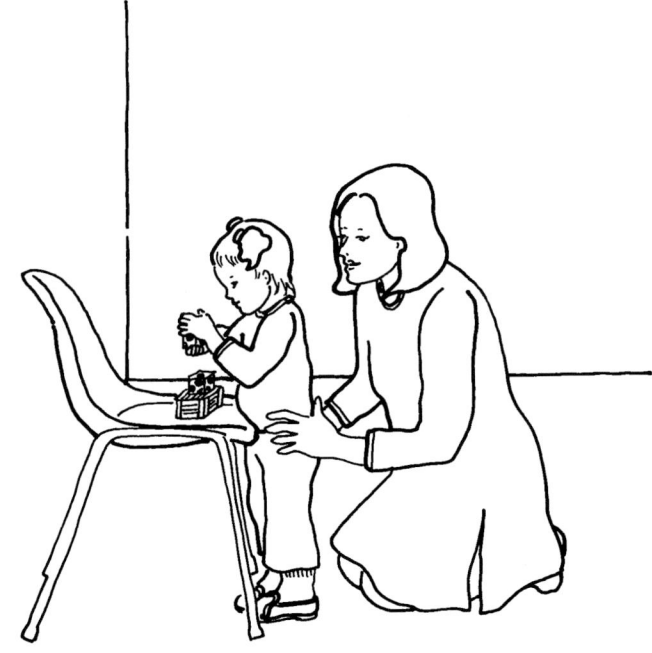

**Figure 1.2    Activity 71**
Grouping by two
physical characteristics

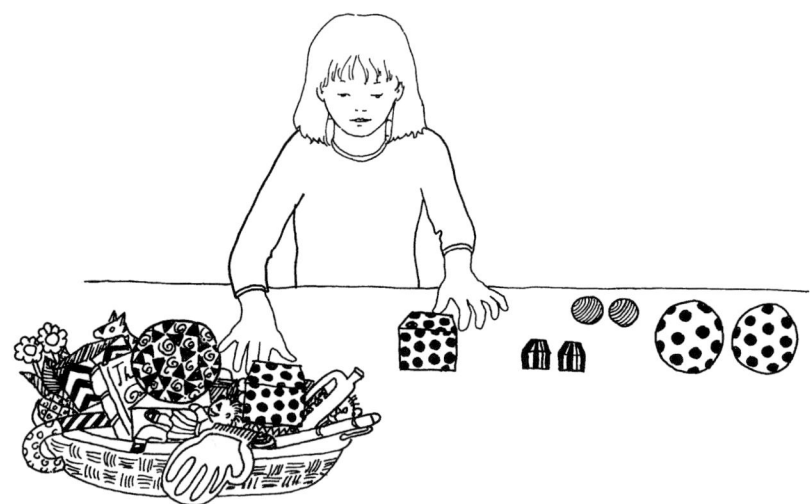

his specific needs. When a given activity is proposed by professionals based on their knowledge of a specific area, this does not mean that the family is relegated to mere observation and passive listening; on the contrary, the family will provide important feedback about the child's context, his capacities and interests, helping to hone each task into a targeted exercise uniquely tailored to that specific child. The idea here is that the team discuss with the family the child's developmental stage, why they are proposing that specific activity, and listen to the family's views on what materials would most pique their child's interest and the ways to help make the activity more engaging and pleasurable for him.

The family is also free to give their opinion about the inappropriateness of a specific activity for their child. As the parents' understanding about the goals of each activity grows, it becomes increasingly important to listen to their suggestions; they may have ideas about how to better perform the activity, how to make it more fun and meaningful for their child, which will lead to better results.[17–19] To this end, instead of having each professional independently assess and propose an activities program, the team can make an evaluation together with the family and create the activities in conjunction with the various areas of specialization for each individual child. The illustrated exercises in the manual are then used as a group: the program is comprised of activities that integrate different areas and is adapted to each child's reality, with the family serving as mediators of this highly individualized process.

This program uses simple household materials found in most homes and schools. This is very important, because a foundation of this methodology is the use of activities that make sense to the child's life, are meaningful to him, and applicable to his daily reality.

The development or rehabilitation program is periodically revised. Activities that stimulate skills already acquired by the child are removed, and in their place enter new exercises that will foster the attainment of new functional or cognitive abilities and promote learning.

**Principle 2: Design a program founded on realistic, viable objectives that are based on each child's motor, neuropsychological and communication prognosis.**

The neurodevelopment program is designed to include short-term goals that the child can easily attain. Development is a step-by-step co-construction process. Establishing simple objectives that are easy to achieve will help motivate the child or adolescent, the family and the team. Observing and valuing each small gain, then defining the next step helps facilitate development and promote integration of all the individuals involved in the process.

It is also important to have long-term goals and to be attentive to the coherence between these and short-term goals. This integration and consistency demands a detailed assessment of the child's prognosis in each area (see further discussion in the following chapters). For example, if after the evaluation of a child with CP the team concludes that he does not have prognosis for walking,[20–22] then extra emphasis must be placed on communication, cognition and schooling from the very beginning. In the case of the child who will not walk, it is beneficial to place a greater emphasis on cognitive gains, for his future and autonomy will depend on these skills. Naturally, motor functions are also worked on, and assistance from bioengineering technology to facilitate movement through mobility aids is introduced. We occasionally observe that in some rehabilitation centers, as well as in some families, there is a tendency to place more emphasis on the area in which the child is struggling most. While it is essential to work intensively on the functions that are impaired, the areas in which the child is more capable should also be stressed for it is in these areas that he will acquire skills more rapidly and easily, increasing his self-esteem while preparing him for the future.

**Principle 3: Ensure integration of the family, child and members of the rehabilitation team.**

Since brain injury in both CP and TBI often affects many areas of development, the number of professionals involved in rehabilitation is usually large. Consequently, their integration and relationship with the family are sometimes difficult. The case manager is a clinician who has the role of overseeing, organizing, and integrating the team, family and entire rehabilitation process. Case managers can help establish a consensus within the team so that they can conduct a rehabilitation program in conjunction with the family. Our methodology works with two case managers to integrate all of the information and act as liaisons between the team and the family. Some centers work with one case manager. However, experience has shown us that the participation of two is significantly more effective because it permits an ongoing dialogue about the child and creates a situation that promotes reflection and discussion about the case by both the family and the team. This also has a practical function in that it permits the family access to at least one of the two managers should the other be unavailable (e.g. attendance at scientific events, vacation, illness, and so forth).

The case managers can be from among any of the team members (physical therapist, neuropsychologist, speech therapist, physician, educator, occupational therapist, psychologist, social worker, nurse, nutritionist, or other professionals). It is beneficial to choose the case managers based on the child's greatest difficulties and potentials; for example, if the child's main problems after TBI are with language but he has good cognitive potential, then a speech therapist and an educator from the team can be chosen.

The pair of managers will accompany the entire rehabilitation process, the consultations at the rehabilitation center, and periodic visits to the child's school and home, and will call on specific professionals to lend added assistance when the situation requires it. Over time, as the child's needs change, the team may wish to make changes in the pairing of the case managers. However, continuity of care is essential and changes should be made only after examination and consultation with the child and family.

**Principle 4: Contextualize the development program and integrate the child or adolescent into the community.**

In this family-based approach, the activities that facilitate neurodevelopment are conducted in an ecological manner within the framework of the child's daily life. This approach creates a context-sensitive rehabilitation program based on the child's or adolescent's life. Each activity selected from the illustrated manual is functional and relates to a task that has meaning for the child. When choosing these activities, the family and team considers not only the child's present developmental stage, which is fundamental, but also the relationship between this activity and the child's daily life, the family's day-to-day reality, the child's interests and motivations, and the objects and materials available at home and in school.

The acquisition of knowledge and skills, in the context of the settings, activities, and content to which the knowledge and skill apply, is more effective than the acquisitions made outside of the routines of everyday academic, social and family life.[23] Limited transfer of cognitive training is highlighted in several cognition theories, dating back to the classic works of Vygotsky[24] and Luria[25] as well as contemporary situated cognition theories,[26–27] situated theories of learning[28] and standard information processing theories.[29] Various studies[17–19;30–31] have shown that when cognitive and behavioral interventions are performed within the daily routine of the child and adolescent with TBI, and when they involve the training of adults that are significant to the child's life, the results are better. Cognitive functioning and the performance of any given task should be sensitive to the individual's specific contexts of application and domains of relevant content.[32–36] In motor development and restoration, the neuronal group selection theory also emphasizes the environmental and action-context factors as a critical factor in motor learning.[37]

The concept behind this methodology is integration of the activities into the child's daily life. They should be playful and enjoyable, performed by the parents, siblings, grandparents, and teachers along with other activities that are part of the same setting. The aim is not to have a specific time and place for doing the exercises with the child, but rather that the stimulation activities be distributed throughout the day, incorporated into daily routines and habits, which will facilitate the integration and participation of the child or adolescent into the home and school environment.

The visits to the home and school by the case managers can yield much important information for the whole team and help point to the activities that are most meaningful to the child, based on the context of his life. At school, the rehabilitation professionals help the teachers by bringing them information about their assessments and suggestions about how to facilitate the child's performance; for example, how to best position the child for writing or using the computer, the best place for an adolescent with hemineglicence to sit in the classroom, etc. On the other hand, the teachers often have much to teach the rehabilitation professionals about the learning capacity, socialization skills, and behavior of the child or adolescent. The parents' visits to the school are also of fundamental importance to the process of sharing knowledge and accompanying their child's development, which helps promote a context-sensitive rehabilitation.

**Principle 5: Lend assistance to the family by means of family support groups and meetings that provide information about their child's problems.**

This family-based rehabilitation approach requires that the family be as well informed as possible about the pathology and all of the accompanying aspects of the problems faced by their child or adolescent; for this reason, information groups for family members were created. The rehabilitation professionals conduct classes on various topics such as brain injury, its causes, diagnosis, prognosis, motor development, cognition, communication, independence, nutrition, nursing care, schooling processes, and many more. Didactic materials are used to illustrate each issue and the families are given the opportunity to express their doubts, pose questions, and also contribute with their experiences in this open exchange of information.

These group meetings are important because there are times when one family will have information that can help other families understand their child's problems. The team also benefits from listening to the parents, for there are very few professionals who have experienced what the family of a brain-injured child has lived with daily, for 24 hours a day. The meetings constitute a process of empowerment for both the professionals and the families; they are a process of co-construction of knowledge. In this setting, the professionals pass on what they have learned in simple, accessible language, avoiding excessive use of medical terminology and explaining the technical words that the family will probably hear frequently. The family's need for information about the pathology, development, rehabilitation process, results, and what can be expected from the future has been discussed in the literature.[38-42] The information groups stimulate the participation of not only the parents, but of all those who interact with the child or adolescent. Naturally, because of the family's other daily life commitments, inescapable in today's hectic society, not all members are able to participate in all of the encounters. Therefore, the team provides a chronogram of the topics that will be addressed in each of the meetings to allow the family time to organize their schedules so that they can at least be present for the meetings that address the issues that are most relevant to them.

In addition to information groups, this program includes emotional support groups for family members. The stress experienced by the family, their ways of coping and other emotional aspects need to be addressed.[41] These groups are conducted by specially trained psychologists and aim at creating a propitious setting for the family to discuss their feelings and coping mechanisms during the various stages of rehabilitation, while being able to count on the assistance of a psychologist. This exchange is the chance for the parents to meet other families facing similar problems, and to share their feelings with them.

Although this methodology is applicable to both traumatic brain injury and cerebral palsy, the support and information groups are usually comprised of families whose children have the same pathology. This is because the most relevant medical information differs between CP and TBI, as do the emotional aspects of coping with each condition. Families whose child has CP must learn to deal with the brain injury since birth or within the first twelve months, because the child begins life with specific developmental disorders. Meanwhile, the families with children who sustained a TBI had previously lived with a child who had no neurological deficits; their challenge, then, is to face the fact that an injury has interrupted his development and ways of dealing with the world around him.

# Assessment

This book is about an approach to development and rehabilitation based on the child's life, and the joint participation of the family and the multidisciplinary team. However, it is not possible to design an individualized rehabilitation and development program without a thorough, correct and periodic assessment of each child. Every specialty has evaluation instruments that are standardized in each country. We will not address those instruments in this book, since the professionals from each field already have this information and are prepared to make the necessary evaluations. We will discuss only some aspects relevant to the assessment of the child within the framework of this context-sensitive, family-based approach.

The child's performance is strongly dependent on environment.[43] It is very common for families to comment that their child does not have the same skills in different contexts; for example, he may have one performance level at home and a different one at the rehabilitation center. This is not simply a matter of familiarity with and adaptation to the setting; it is also due to how different developing skills are dependent on and supported by a given context. To obtain valid data on the child's development, it is important to consider development's context-dependent nature and understand the natural variability of child behavior. Deficits in one or another area of development or the severity of the child's difficulties are also determined by the moment at which the skill is measured.[39] Information about development can combine observation of the child's performance in diverse, carefully organized settings that involve the use of videotaping, as well as visits to the home and school, in a combined effort between family, teachers and rehabilitation professionals.

In this approach, the family actively participates in the evaluation process by sharing their observations about the child's development, and the difficulties and strengths that they observe in their daily interactions. The parents' physical presence usually makes the child feel more secure in demonstrating his abilities. While the team is observing the child's behavior, they discuss their impressions with the family, listen to their experiences with daily caregiving, and look for ways to resolve the difficulties that are present. This allows the family and team to participate in an educative, gradual, bidirectional process.

Of course, not all assessments can be made as a group, such as psychometric tests or other evaluations, that demand specific settings so as to avoid attentional problems, or examinations that require specialized equipment, as in the case of audiometries. However, these assessments, done exclusively by one professional, are conducted at separate times and locations, and serve to complement the team's overall evaluation.

In the case of TBI, there may be an increase in natural variations in behavior and the child may be more vulnerable to stress factors in his environment. The type of behavior and reactions after the injury are oftentimes informed by the child's individual characteristics prior to the trauma.[44] It is important to talk to the family about the child's previous development, his behavior before the TBI, types of interests, motivational factors, and preferred activities. A brain injury in the child can affect the acquisition of new skills or damage skills that were developing at the time of the accident. For example, if an injury occurs before the prescribed age for reading and writing, systematic, continuous evaluations should be conducted to determine whether he will have problems acquiring these skill when he begins this phase of the educational process.[10]

In both TBI and CP, qualitative evaluation and observation are of great benefit. Spontaneous observation provides important references about different areas of development such as interest and motivation, spontaneous verbalizations, cognitive strategies, independence, forms of locomotion, manual function, and more. An assessment process is usually begun with simple exercises whose degree of complexity will increase in step with the child's performance in previous activities. The team gradually adjusts their behavior as they become more familiar with the child and, when necessary, will propose, with the help of the family, tasks of varying complexity. During the observation process, the team makes associations between the different behavioral domains and can select more specific, targeted activities for a given area.[45]

Spontaneous observation can be done in conjunction with directed evaluation activities. These two techniques often produce different results. The child may exhibit skill when he is being instructed to perform a given task or when the setting is structured to facilitate the task's performance.[25] For example, a situation for evaluating the reaching capacity of a hemiplegic child can be organized by placing two cubes in front of him and asking him to hold one in each hand. He may be able to do it, and it is expected that he will have varying levels of difficulty, but this does not mean that in daily life, or in situations in which he is engaged in unstructured leisure time, he will spontaneously use the hand with which he is having problems. Another example is a child with attention deficits who is able to concentrate on a specific task because other stimuli that vie for his attention have been removed from the setting: a situation from which the stimuli have been eliminated is not a realistic condition in daily life and does not represent a setting in which the child will act similarly.

Fatigue, limits in attention span, variations in motivation and engagement in the tasks should all be considered during an evaluation of the child. If he is not engaged and motivated to perform a given exercise, his performance will be significantly compromised.

Quantifying a specific skill through guided activity or organized settings may not be a sensitive measure of the child's day-to-day performance,[46] although we cannot deny the validity and importance of quantitative instruments as references and auxiliary tools.

## Further Methodological Aspects and the Illustrated Manual

This family-based approach is context-sensitive; as such, it is adaptable not only to the reality of each individual child and family, but also to diverse settings, cultures and countries. We will present some practical aspects of this methodology, which has been used at the SARAH Network of Rehabilitation Hospitals since the late 1970s, and which can serve as reference for the elaboration of programs in other rehabilitation centers.

The program begins with a consultation with the child or adolescent and his family, conducted by a pediatric neurologist or a developmental pediatrician and at least one multidisciplinary team professional from each area of specialization. The first evaluation is performed, complementary exams are scheduled and the initial bases for the rehabilitation plan are defined.

Next, each child and his family are individually seen by one group of different rehabilitation professionals, who conduct both structured and spontaneous observations and assessments. Whenever possible, they observe and evaluate together, which enables several professionals to collect diverse information and data relevant to their area of specialization while another conducts his assessment. This increases the team's contact with the family and child, reduces the likelihood of repetitive questions, and initiates the child–family–team integration process. At this point in the evaluation stage the two case managers are selected.

The rehabilitation program is then created, using all of the information gathered from the observations, evaluations, complementary tests, home visits, and the family's and child's input. Activities to stimulate development are selected and worked into simple, fun exercises for each child, based on his motivation and interests. During this process, the parent support and information groups also begin. One of the basic tenets of this methodology consists in adapting what would otherwise feel laborious for the child into playful, game-like exercises without losing any of the goal-oriented and developmentally necessary aspects of the activities.

The multidisciplinary nature of this approach is not limited to the composition of the team; it also extends to the elaboration of each activity. Whenever possible, each one addresses more than one area of development, integrating objectives identified by the family and different professionals. For example, as mentioned earlier, an activity suggested by the physical therapist is incorporated into another from the speech therapist; or an occupational therapy task is integrated into a pedagogical exercise. When defining the program of activities, the team relies on their evaluations of the child's or adolescent's developmental stage, the family's suggestions, and the child's response to each proposed task. Short-term goals and prognosis are also significant considerations in this process.

To provide mnemonic support of the developmental activities for the families, we created, between 1983 and 2005, the Illustrated Manual. This manual is in the accompanying CD-ROM and contains 185 drawings of activities related to different areas of development (motor, visuo-motor, cognitive, communication, neuropsychological rehabilitation, and independence in activities of daily life). Each drawing in the CD is accompanied by a description of the activity's specific goal and an explanation on how to perform it. These drawings can be printed out and copied. In general, when we design a development program for a child with CP or TBI, the family and the entire team gather to discuss and select a group of activities, print them out, and mount a small, individualized illustrated manual that the family then takes home. As the child or adolescent progresses, the drawings relating to the activities that the child no longer needs to perform are removed and new illustrated exercises are chosen, printed out, and inserted into the small manual to be performed at home. Occasionally during the school visits conducted by the case managers, some illustrated activities are proposed and given to the teachers for inclusion in the child's routine scholastic activities.

An individual manual usually contains between eight and fifteen drawings from the Illustrated Manual, comprising activities from the diverse developmental areas, which are changed and updated according to the child's progress. No two children have the same program.

During the initial period, when the basic evaluations are conducted and the first program of activities established, the family attends the rehabilitation center on a daily basis. The family then begins to conduct the rehabilitation and stimulation at home with the child, returning to the rehabilitation center weekly or every two weeks to meet with the team. These periodic meetings between the family and the professionals help ensure that the child's every change, progress or acquisition, however small, is incorporated into the program.

This approach sees the child as a whole that cannot be compartmentalized. However, for the purpose of clarity and explanation, the various components of development are broken down into chapters for optimum understanding. To this effect different areas of development are discussed, as are their relation to impairments resultant from neurological damage and their ramifications on the child's development. As such, Chapters 2 through 6 deal with specific developmental areas correlating the explanations with the use of appropriate activities in the Illustrated Manual: motor development, cognitive development and neuropsychological disorders, speech, language and communication, visuo-motor coordination, and activities of daily life. Next, Chapter 7 discusses the orthopaedic approach and participation of the family, while Chapter 8 delves into issues about the family and the child with brain injury. Chapter 9 addresses aspects related to the child's success after the brain injury, such as behavioral, social, and academic issues. Chapter 10 focuses on needs, beliefs and prognosis.

This book presents a way of sharing, with the family, the process of stimulating the development of a child or adolescent after brain injury in an individualized, humanistic, ecological, context-sensitive approach. The goal is to give the family back its natural role, which is to teach and stimulate the development of the child. And, in turn, to give the child back his childhood, naturally, without having to be constantly surrounded by professionals and required to engage in activities that are not related to his daily life, simply because he sustained a brain injury.

# References

1.  Aitken ME, Mele N, Barrett KW. Recovery of injured children: parent perspectives on family needs. Arch Phys Med Rehabil 2004; 85(4):567–573.

2.  Alexander J, Moore D. Primary care for children with brain injury. N C Med J 2001; 62(6):344–348.

3.  Hinojosa J, Sproat CT, Mankhetwit S, Anderson J. Shifts in parent–therapist partnerships: twelve years of change. Am J Occup Ther 2002; 56(5):556–563.

4.  King S, Teplicky R, King G, Rosenbaum P. Family-centered service for children with cerebral palsy and their families: a review of the literature. Semin Pediatr Neurol 2004; 11(1):78–86.

5.  Palisano RJ, Snider LM, Orlin MN. Recent advances in physical and occupational therapy for children with cerebral palsy. Semin Pediatr Neurol 2004; 11(1):66–77.

6.  Braga LW. O desenvolvimento cognitivo na paralisia cerebral: um estudo exploratorio (dissertation). Brasilia: University of Brasilia, 1983.

7.  Campos da Paz Jr A, Nomura A, Braga LW, Burnett SM. Speculations on cerebral palsy. J Bone Joint Surg Br 1984; 66(2):283.

8.  Braga LW. Efeitos do processo de ensino/aprendizagem dos pais no desenvolvimento da crianca com paralisia cerebral. Brasilia: Proceedings of the Seminario A pesquisa em educacao no Distrito Federal, 1986.

9. Campos da Paz Jr A, Burnett SM, Nomura A. Cerebral palsy. In: Duthie RB, editor. Mercer's orthopedic surgery. London: Arnold, 1996: 444–468.

10. Braga LW, Campos da Paz Jr A. Neuropsychological pediatric rehabilitation. In: Christensen AL, Uzzell BP, editors. International handbook of neurological rehabilitation. New York: Kluwer Academic/Plenum, 2000: 283–295.

11. Braga LW. Family participation in the rehabilitation of the child with traumatic brain injury. J Neuropsychol Soc 2000; 6:388.

12. Mogren L. Foraldrar, barn och larande. Sluta skolan: en larares tankar och rad till unga foraldrar. Trycheri books-on-demand, 2003.

13. Ylvisaker M, Adelson PD, Braga LW et al. Rehabilitation and ongoing support after pediatric TBI: twenty years of progress. J Head Trauma Rehabil 2005; 20(1):95–109.

14. Braga LW, Campos da Paz Jr A, Ylvisaker M. Direct clinician-delivered versus indirect family-supported rehabilitation of children with traumatic brain injury: a randomized controlled trial. Brain Inj 2005; 19(10):819–831.

15. SARAH Network of Rehabilitation Hospitals. SARAH scale of motor development. Brasilia: SarahLetras, 1989.

16. Wechsler D. WISC III: Escala de inteligencia Wechsler para criancas. Adaptacao e padronizacao de uma amostra brasileira. 3rd ed. São Paulo: Casa do Psicologo, 2002.

17. Feeney TJ, Ylvisaker M. Choice and routine: antecedent behavioral interventions for adolescents with severe traumatic brain injury. J Head Trauma Rehabil 1995; 10:67–82.

18. Feeney TJ, Ylvisaker M. Context-sensitive behavioral supports for young children with TBI: short-term effects and long-term outcome. J Head Trauma Rehabil 2003; 18(1):33–51.

19. Ylvisaker M, Feeney T. Collaborative brain injury intervention: positive everyday routines. San Diego, CA: Singular, 1998.

20. Campos da Paz Jr A, Burnett SM, Braga LW. Walking prognosis in cerebral palsy: a 22-year retrospective analysis. Dev Med Child Neurol 1994; 36(2):130–134.

21. Molnar GE. Cerebral palsy: prognosis and how to judge it. Pediatr Ann 1979; 8(10):596–605.

22. Bleck EE. Locomotor prognosis in cerebral palsy. Dev Med Child Neurol 1975; 17(1):18–25.

23. Mann L. On the trail of process: a historical perspective on cognitive processes and their training. New York: Grune and Stratton, 1979.

24. Vygotsky LS. Thought and language. Cambridge, MA: MIT Press, 1934.

25. Luria AR. The making of mind. Cambridge, MA: Harvard University, 1979.

26. Lave J. The practice of learning. In: Chaiklin S, Lave J, editors. Understanding practice: perspectives on activity and context. New York: Cambridge University Press, 1996: 3–32.

27. Rogoff B. Apprenticeship in thinking: cognitive development in social context. New York: Oxford University Press, 1990.

28. Butterfield E, Slocum T, Nelson G. Cognitive and behavioral analyses of teaching and transfer: are they different? In: Detterman DK, Sternberg RJ, editors. Transfer on trial: intelligence, cognition, and instruction. Westport, CT: Ablex, 1993: 192–257.

29. Singley M, Anderson JR. Transfer of cognitive skill. Cambridge, MA: Harvard University Press, 1989.

30. Ylvisaker M. Context-sensitive cognitive rehabilitation: theory and practice. Brain Impair 2003; 4:1–16.

31. Ylvisaker M, Jacobs HE, Feeney T. Positive supports for people who experience behavioral and cognitive disability after brain injury: a review. J Head Trauma Rehabil 2003; 18(1):7–32.

32. Gersten R, Fuchs LS, Williams JP, Baker S. Teaching reading comprehension strategies to students with learning disabilities: a review of research. Rev Educ Res 2001; 71:279–320.

33. Swanson HL, Hoskyn M. Instructing adolescents with learning disabilities: a component and composite analysis. Learn Disabil Res Pract 2001; 16:109–119.

34. Pressley M. Cognitive strategy instruction that really improves children's academic performance. Cambridge, MA: Brookline Books, 1995.

35. Sweet AP, Snow C. Reconceptualizing reading comprehension. In: Block CC, Gambrell LB, Pressley M, editors. Improving comprehension instruction: rethinking, research, theory, and classroom practice. San Francisco, CA: John Wiley & Sons, 2002: 17–53.

36. Gresham FH, Sugau G, Horner RH. Interpreting outcomes of social skills training for students with high-incidence disabilities. Except Child 2001; 67:331–344.

37. Howle J. Neuro-developmental treatment approaches: theoretical foundations and principles of clinical practice. Laguna Beach, CA: Neuro-Developmental Treatment Association, 2003.

38. Armstrong K, Kerns KA. The assessment of parent needs following paediatric traumatic brain injury. Pediatr Rehabil 2002; 5(3):149–160.

39. Johnson DA, Rose D. Prognosis, rehabilitation and outcome after inflicted brain injury in children – a case of professional developmental delay. Pediatr Rehabil 2004; 7(3):185–193.

40. McPherson KM, McNaughton H, Pentland B. Information needs of families when one member has a severe brain injury. Int J Rehabil Res 2000; 23(4):295–301.

41. Savage R, DePompei R, Tyler J, Lave J. Paediatric traumatic brain injury: a review of pertinent issues. Pediatr Rehabil 2005; 8(2):92–103.

42. Waaland PK, Burns C, Cockrell J. Evaluation of needs of high- and low-income families following paediatric traumatic brain injury. Brain Inj 1993; 7(2):135–146.

43. Ylvisaker M. Traumatic brain injury rehabilitation: children and adolescents. Woburn, MA: Butterworth-Heinemann, 1998.

44. Anderson VA, Morse SA, Catroppa C, Haritou F, Rosenfeld JV. Thirty month outcome from early childhood head injury: a prospective analysis of neurobehavioural recovery. Brain 2004; 127(Pt 12):2608–2620.

45.    Ylvisaker M, Feeney T. Executive functions, self-regulation, and learned optimism in paediatric rehabilitation: a review and implications for intervention. Pediatr Rehabil 2002; 5(2):51–70.

46.    Fedrizzi E, Pagliano E, Andreucci E, Oleari G. Hand function in children with hemiplegic cerebral palsy: prospective follow-up and functional outcome in adolescence. Dev Med Child Neurol 2003; 45(2):85–91.

# 2 Motor Development

*Sheila M Denucci and Eliane G Catanho*

Sensorimotor experiences during children's first years of life help develop motor skills by establishing and reorganizing synapses, and forming new neuronal networks. Despite the many variations, children's motor development follows a sequence of events; for example, children's ability to balance the head and, subsequently, the trunk, makes it possible for them to stand, which in turn sets the groundwork for walking in the future. Some children may have different sequences, developing the ability to walk before they are able to crawl.[1]

When an injury occurs, the brain is able to alter its structure and function through mechanisms of neuroplasticity and motor learning, and forge alternative pathways to more efficient movements.[2] Environmental experiences play an important role in the formation of neural networks. This process, however, is defined by the neurological potential of each child. Children with brain injury can find alternative means of performing motor functions, in accordance with their potential.[3] Different postures and adapted movements may afford greater stability and functionality with less energy expenditure. Therefore, treatment should not focus on the disability, but rather on the attainment of functionality. Intervention should aim at improving the child's performance in daily life activities.

The motor development of children with cerebral palsy (CP) differs from that of children or adolescents who have sustained a traumatic brain injury (TBI). All children with CP have motor deficits and, in most cases, they will exhibit motor delays, develop adaptive forms of motor expression and may not attain all the developmental milestones. Some children with CP will not walk. Establishing the motor prognosis will inform the process of creating, together with the family, a treatment program that takes into account the child's potential; one that, for example, includes discovering alternative forms of locomotion when gait is impossible. In CP, the persistence of primitive reflexes and the age at which milestones such as head balance, sitting and crawling are attained all have a bearing on gait prognosis.[4-7]

In children with TBI, the level of motor acquisition prior to the trauma and the pace at which motor function is recovered are important factors that help guide the rehabilitation program. After the injury, these children may reacquire motor skills in their own way and at their own pace, bypassing stages that are common to child development.[8] Even in children with severe TBI, most will walk again, usually within the first six months after the injury, and will continue to make progress with balance, postural control and movement coordination during the two to three subsequent years. The persistence of mild motor impairments, such as balance and coordination deficits, may compromise activities that demand greater motor skills, especially in sports, or when in groups with other children.

Movement disorders in TBI are different from those in CP. Weakness, ataxia, apraxia and perceptual disorders are more prevalent in children with TBI than in children with CP.[9] It is common for the child with TBI to present two or more movement disorders that affect pace, speed and coordination of motor skills, resulting in fragmented, uncoordinated, slow movements; this condition may also be due to difficulties planning and executing the motor functions required for performing a given task.

## Program of Activities

The stimulation of motor abilities helps children develop their potential while helping them reach each milestone and discover adaptive movement patterns that can serve as alternative solutions to achieving better functional results. Activities that take into account children's interests, and are integrated into their context and daily life, facilitate learning.

The attainment of each new motor milestone should be valued because progress contributes to children's participation in tasks and activities. For example, head balance allows children to orient themselves and visually explore their surroundings; sitting balance may facilitate use of their hands; and crawling or creeping can help them explore their home, reserving wheelchair use for outside excursions. The family's participation can help motivate the child and help him discover different pathways for adapting and improving his motor functions.

This chapter will present and discuss the activities in the Illustrated Manual related to the different stages of motor development, which the family can perform with the child at home and in different settings to promote his learning processes and motor development. These activities are specifically indicated to assist children with cerebral palsy, or, when noted, children with TBI. Many of the activities described for children with TBI may also be used, or adapted, for adolescents with TBI, depending on the individualized treatment plan.

## Head Balance

During the first few months of life, children develop body alignment responses. These reactions permit the necessary adjustments for movement and head balance. Head balance is fully attained when children are able to maintain head alignment in the prone, supine and sitting positions. This milestone increases their visual range, allows better exploration of their surroundings, and facilitates transporting and feeding.

Children with CP may have delayed development of head balance and, in some cases, may never attain it. Those who do not achieve head balance will require adapted carriage or wheelchair seating. Head and trunk support permit better trunk alignment and stability during transporting, and facilitate the children's care as well as their participation in playful activities.

A number of activities that foster development of head balance can be incorporated into the child's daily routine. Changing the child's positioning during games and encouraging him to move his head in different directions can help him attain this milestone.

### Lifting head in tummy-lying position

The prone position contributes to the development of head balance, aids control of shoulder and upper trunk movements, and allows the child to experiment with some of the first forms of moving about, such as rolling or creeping. During the initial stages of head balance training, placing rolls or small ramp-type inclines under the child's chest while he is in the prone position permits greater transference of body weight to the hips and lower limbs, making it easier for him to raise his head (Figure 2.1, Activity 1). Visual stimuli or toys that make sounds capture the child's attention and motivate him to move his head in search of the object.

**Figure 2.1  Activity 1**
Lifting head in tummy lying position

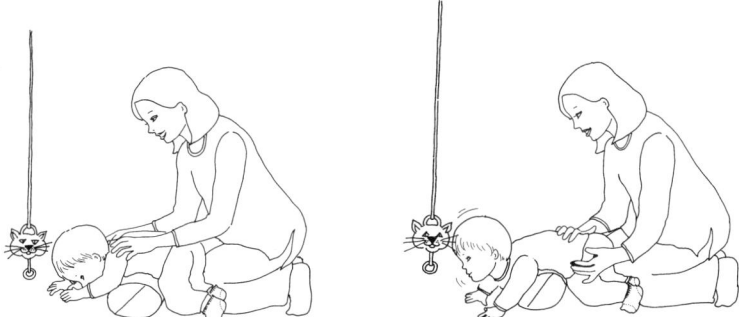

As children achieve greater control of head movements in the prone position, they begin to use their arms to raise their body by supporting themselves on their forearms. Supporting the body on one forearm frees up the other hand for playing with objects. Proprioceptive information derived from this support helps the child maintain stability while in the prone position.

### Lifting head with additional support

A child with hydrocephaly and macrocrania or axial hypotonia may have problems raising his head from the prone position. You can help him sustain part of the weight of his head by holding his forehead with one of your hands (Figure 2.2, Activity 2).

**Figure 2.2   Activity 2**
Lifting head with additional support

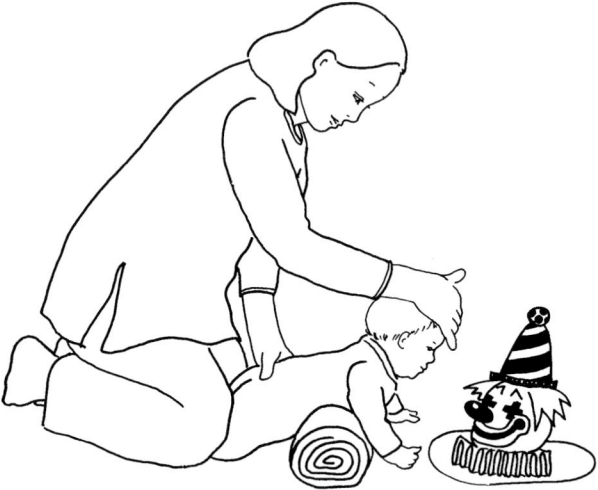

Children with TBI in the early stages of recovery may also be uncomfortable in the prone position, especially those who are tracheotomized and have deformities and hypotonia of the lower limbs. In these cases, head balance training begins in the sitting position and gradually progresses to the prone position.

### Lifting head with shoulder support

To stimulate head balance in the sitting position, it is important that the child's trunk be stabilized. Position the child in front of your body, resting your hands on the child's shoulders, back of the neck, and chin in a manner that keeps his head from falling but does not restrict his movements (Figure 2.3, Activity 3). Gradually decrease your support until he is able to keep his head well aligned.

**Figure 2.3   Activity 3**
Lifting head with shoulder support

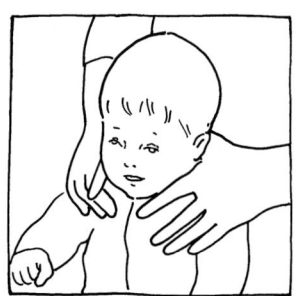
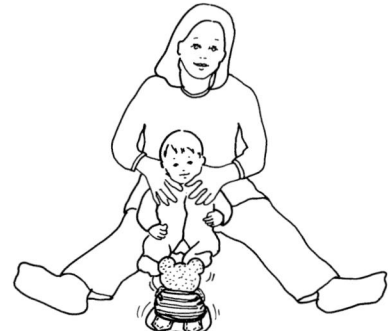

**Lifting head on back position**

Children without head balance tend to drop their head back when pulled up from the supine position. This posture is caused by both lack of head balance and the gravitational pull. The slow, repeated motion of pulling the child into a seated position fosters the acquisition of head balance (Figure 2.4, Activity 4). Initially, you can use one of your hands to support the child's neck and prevent abrupt extension, but as he learns to partially control his head in this position, shift your support from the head to the shoulders. Sing to the child during this activity to help motivate him.

**Figure 2.4    Activity 4**
Lifting head in back
position

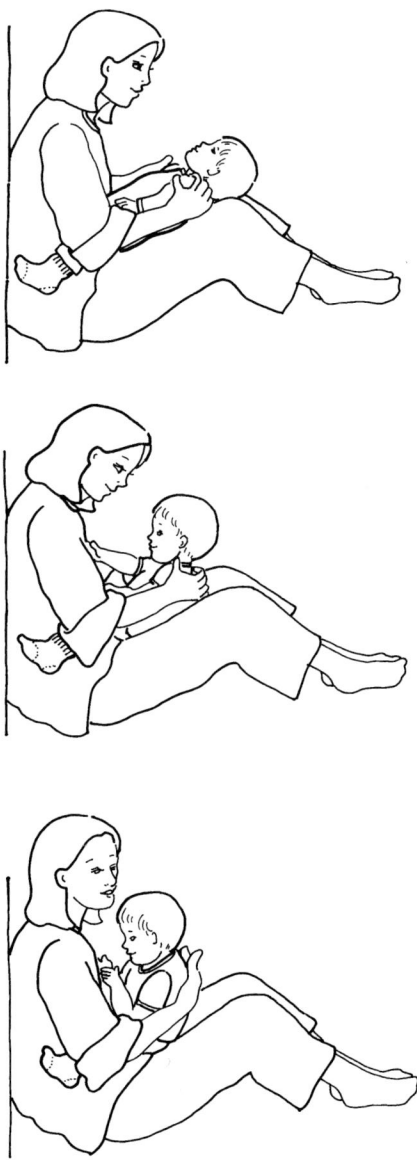

**Pull to sit**

Pillows or small ramps can help stimulate head balance in the supine position in children with TBI (Figure 2.5, Activity 5). This recourse may be transitory, used mostly to help the child raise his head, for it reduces the gravitational pull when placing him in as close to vertical alignment as possible.

**Figure 2.5   Activity 5**
Pull to sit

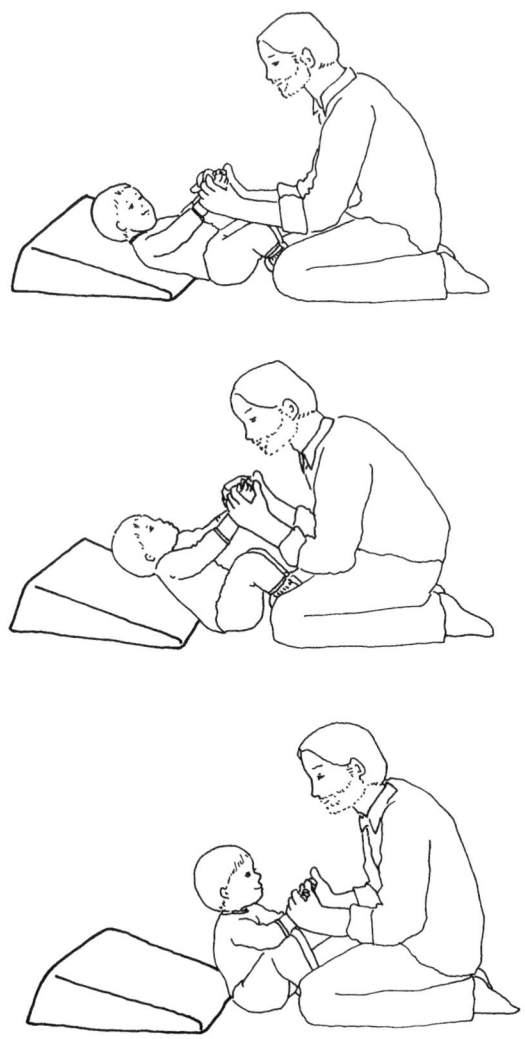

**Balancing head with trunk movement, face to face**

When the child has attained partial head balance in the prone, seated, and supine positions, allow him to experiment with more complex head-adjusting movements (Figure 2.6, Activity 6). Seat the child on the floor either facing you or with his back to you, depending on the type of game, and gently rock his trunk back-and-forth and side-to-side while holding his shoulders. This motion will disrupt his balance and trigger straightening-up reactions while promoting correction of head positioning. An added benefit of this activity is that it affords the child a chance to experience his first reactions to trunk balance, as well as his protective responses in sitting, to the extent that he is able to occasionally support his hands on the floor for balance.

**Figure 2.6  Activity 6**
Balancing head with trunk movement, face to face

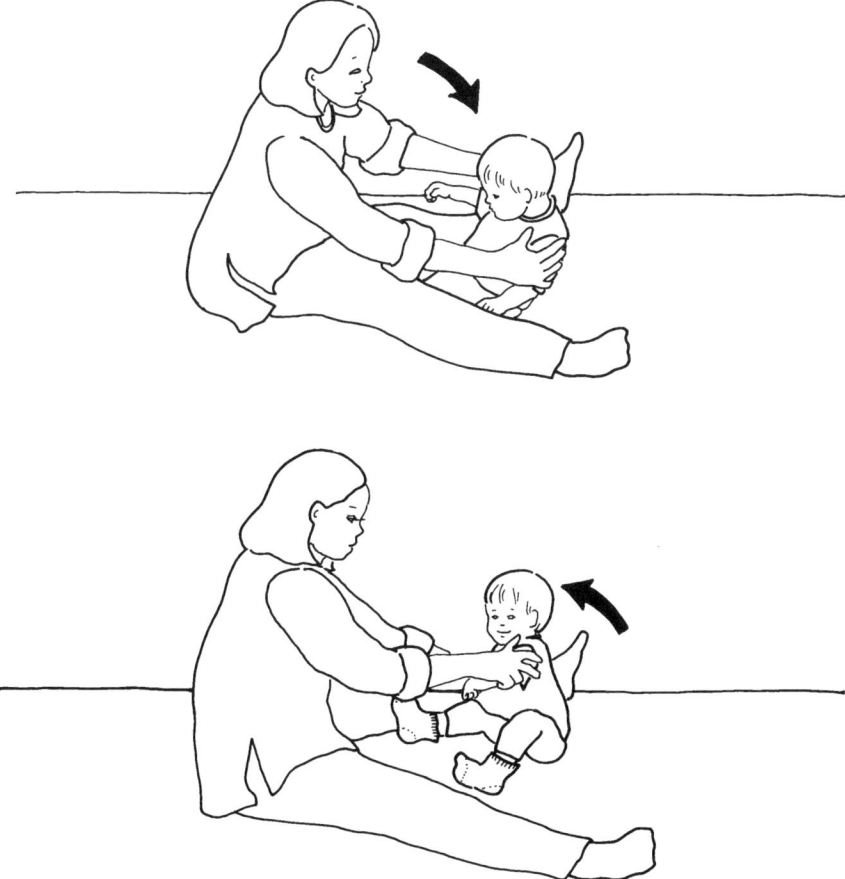

## *Rolling*

**Rolling over using the legs**

The child learns to roll over motivated by visual and auditory stimuli as well as proprioceptive and kinesthetic experiences. Spasticity and uncoordinated or involuntary movements may impair the child's ability to roll. You can take advantage of day-to-day situations, such as changing his diaper or playing floor games, to help him practice rolling over, at first by rotating his body from side to side. With the child in the supine position, help him begin to roll by flexing one of his legs and gently propelling it over the other (Figure 2.7, Activity 7). Remember to engage him in the act of pushing his body from one side to another.

**Figure 2.7    Activity 7**
Rolling over using the legs

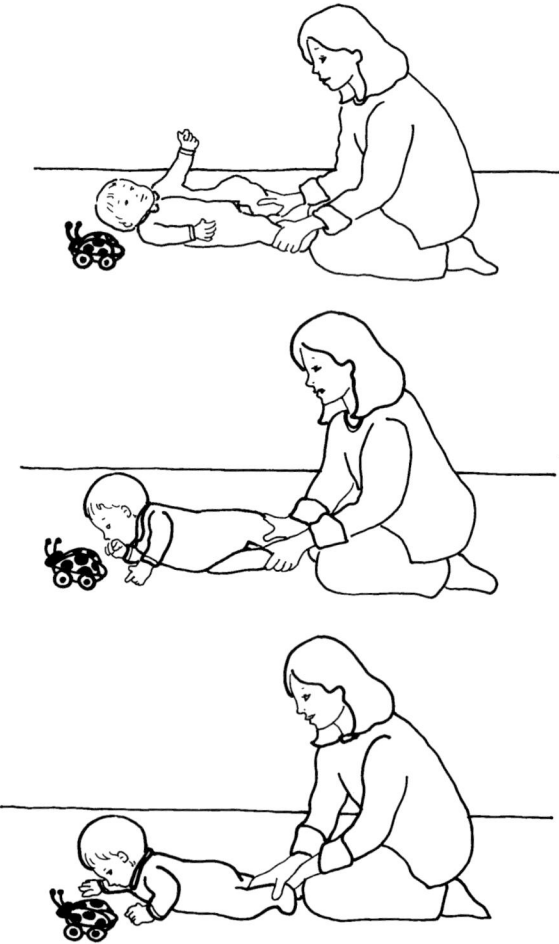

**Rolling over using the arms**

When the child has attained better control of his shoulder and arm muscles, you can help him use his upper limbs to push his body (Figure 2.8, Activity 8). Each child should be assessed to determine whether he is able to perform this movement, so as to devise the best way to help him. Some children will have different ways of rolling over.

**Figure 2.8    Activity 8**
Rolling over using the arms

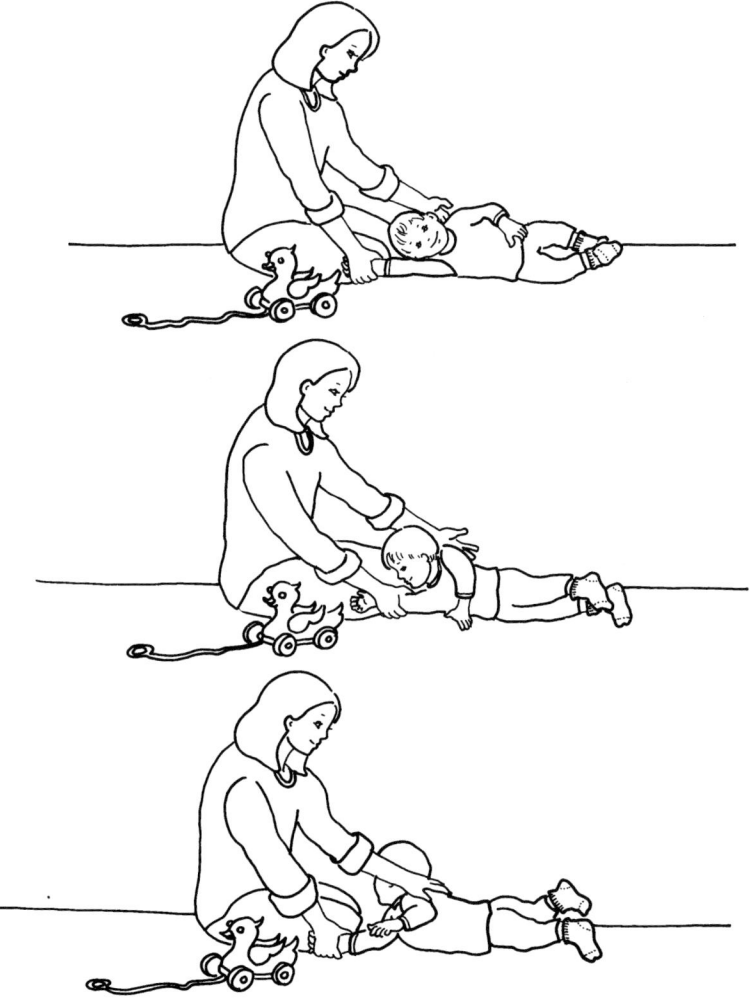

Hemiplegic children usually roll to the impaired side, pushing with the opposite side of their bodies. Many of those with very pronounced involuntary movements do not get around by rolling, mostly due to difficulties using their arms and keeping their heads extended while prone.

In children with TBI during the early stages of recovery, the rolling motion can help promote the first changes of position in bed, the use of the arms for support, the training of transfers, and the shift from the lying-down to the sitting-up positions. Furthermore, stimulating the rolling over movement fosters body awareness and exploration of kinesthetic sensations through the gradual shifting of weight.

## Creeping

Creeping permits a child to go longer distances at a faster pace and with more efficient changes in direction than rolling. To pull himself along, the child must move his arms and legs in a symmetrical and coordinated manner. This movement pattern may be more difficult for children with brain injury because of selective movement disorders and lack of coordination between the arms and legs.

---

**Creeping**

You can help the child learn to creep in a prone position by flexing one of his legs; this provides the necessary support for him to pull his body forward by extending the flexed leg. This movement is completed by using the arms to pull the body along (Figure 2.9, Activity 9).

**Figure 2.9    Activity 9**
Creeping

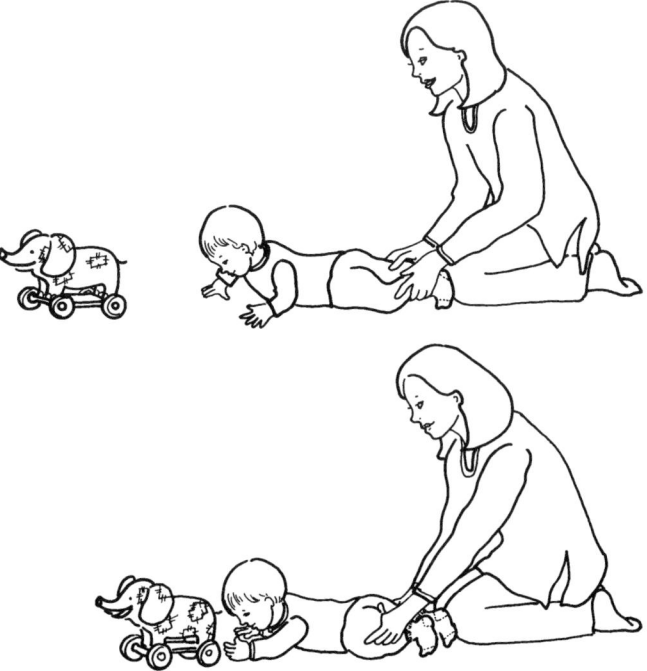

Children with CP exhibit varied forms of creeping. Moving while in the supine position is common in children with involuntary movement disorders, while those with diplegia predominantly use their arms. In cases of hemiplegia, frequent in children with TBI, creeping may be asymmetrical or done in the sitting position.

## *Sitting*

The sitting position increases the child's visual range, permitting greater exploration of his surroundings. Furthermore, attaining sitting balance helps improve manual skills because the child no longer needs to use his hands for support. Children who do not have a prognosis for independent sitting may benefit from the use of chairs and modified carriages, which permit better trunk balance and alignment, thereby simulating the same opportunities afforded by independent sitting.

Postural adjustment mechanisms are prerequisites for acquiring sitting balance. Straightening-up reactions, incorporated into balance responses, allow the child to perform body adjustments to sustain the sitting position. These mechanisms may be impaired in children with brain injury.[10] Slow, incomplete or delayed responses are often present and hinder sitting acquisition. Many times these children need more time and encouragement to reach this milestone.

### Protective reaction

The child has attained control of his body in the sitting position when he is able to keep his head and trunk aligned, even while moving. During this process, the child employs mechanisms of protection against falling. When a child loses his balance, he responds with a parachute reaction: his arms extend outwards and his hands reach out for support.

You can help the child develop more agile motor responses in his arms by quickly leaning his trunk forward, simulating a fall. This can be done during games or playtime (Figure 2.10, Activity 10).

**Figure 2.10    Activity 10**
Protective reaction

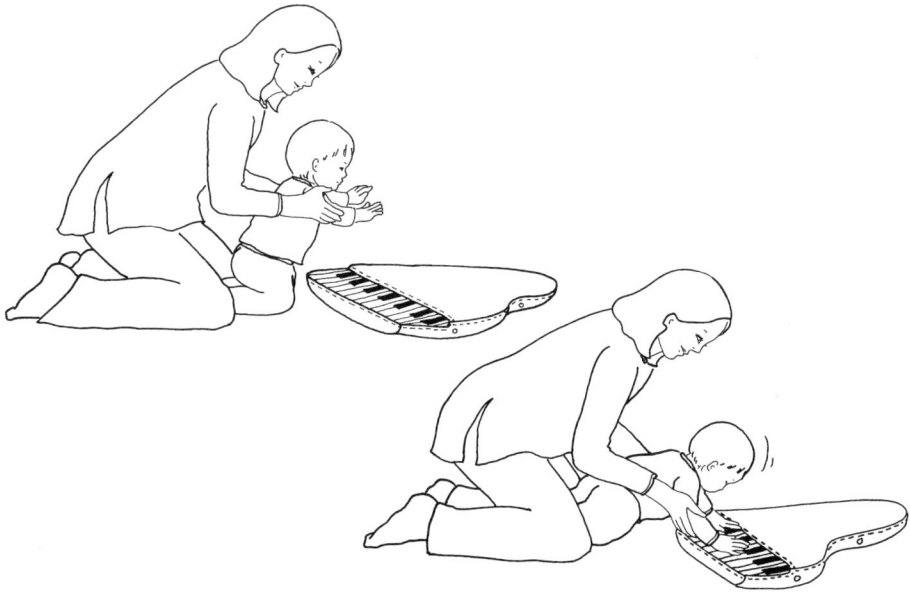

**Balancing on the lap**

During daily life activities, you can encourage the child to experiment with the body adjustment mechanisms that will help him develop sitting balance. With the child on your lap, perform the slow, reciprocal motions of raising and lowering his legs enough to displace his center of gravity and tilt his trunk sideways (Figure 2.11, Activity 11).

**Figure 2.11   Activity 11**
Balancing on the lap

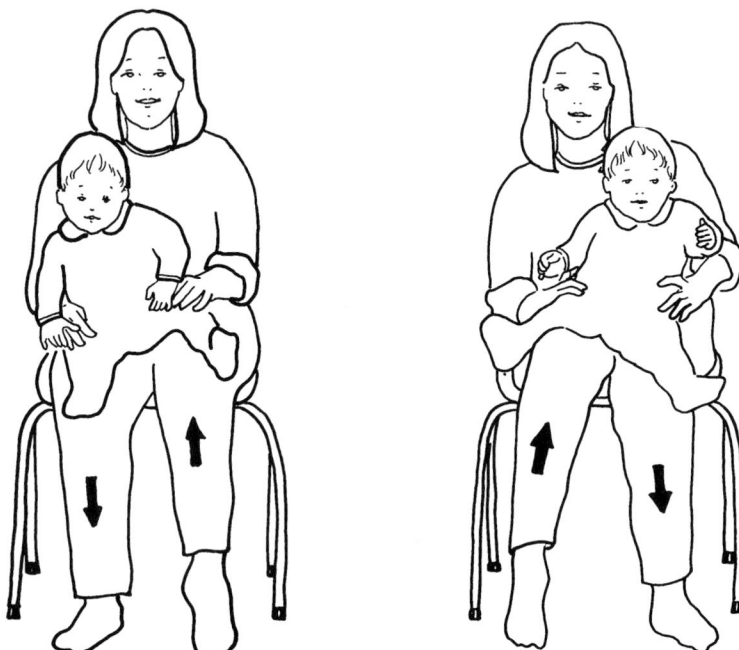

**Sitting balance on the lap, face to face**

The moments that the child is playing in your lap can be used to invent new ways of practicing sitting balance. With the child on your lap facing you, play at swaying his trunk to the side, forward and backward while singing or talking to him and varying the intensity of the movements. This enables the child to better interact with you and perhaps even learn to respond with greater self-assurance when faced with loss of balance (Figure 2.12, Activity 12).

**Figure 2.12   Activity 12**
Sitting balance on the lap, face to face

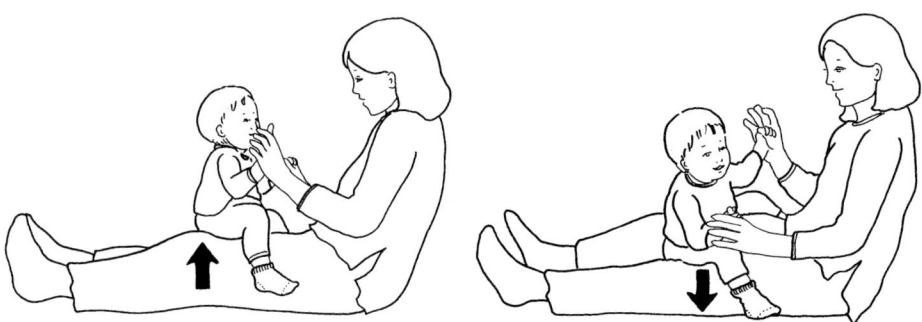

## Sitting with arm support

When the child begins to sit, he keeps his balance by using his hands for support, developing forward prop reactions and, subsequently, lateral prop reactions. With the child positioned on the floor, help him practice forward support with the hands while he plays (Figure 2.13, Activity 13). As his balance improves, offer him a favorite toy that he can reach only if he releases one of his hands, thereby making him practice balance reactions.

**Figure 2.13    Activity 13**
Sitting with arm support

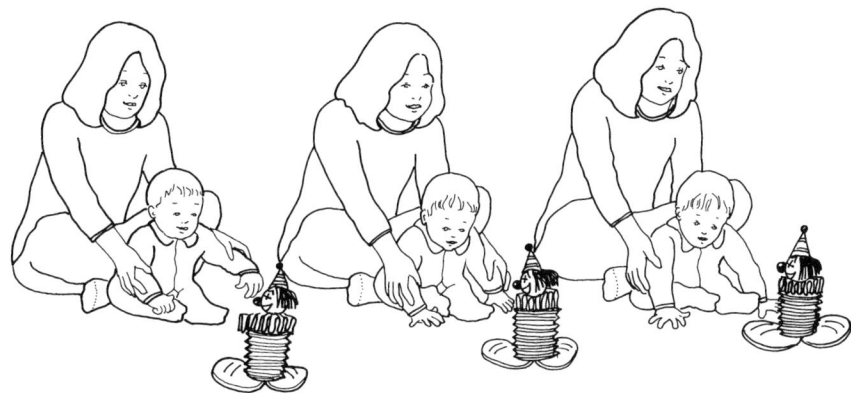

## Lateral balance reaction

After the child has achieved sitting balance with front support, lateral protection reactions can be promoted by playing games that include gently rocking his body to the side. Show him how to stabilize his body by supporting himself with one hand, leaving the other free for reaching toys (Figure 2.14, Activity14). Children with brain injury, with hemiplegia and sensory deficits, can benefit from this activity for it provides proprioceptive information and helps them control the muscles of the arm during weight bearing. Once a child has attained trunk balance, he is able to correct his posture when faced with changes in head, trunk and arm positioning without using his upper limbs for support, freeing up his hands for bimanual activities.

**Figure 2.14    Activity 14**
Lateral balance reaction

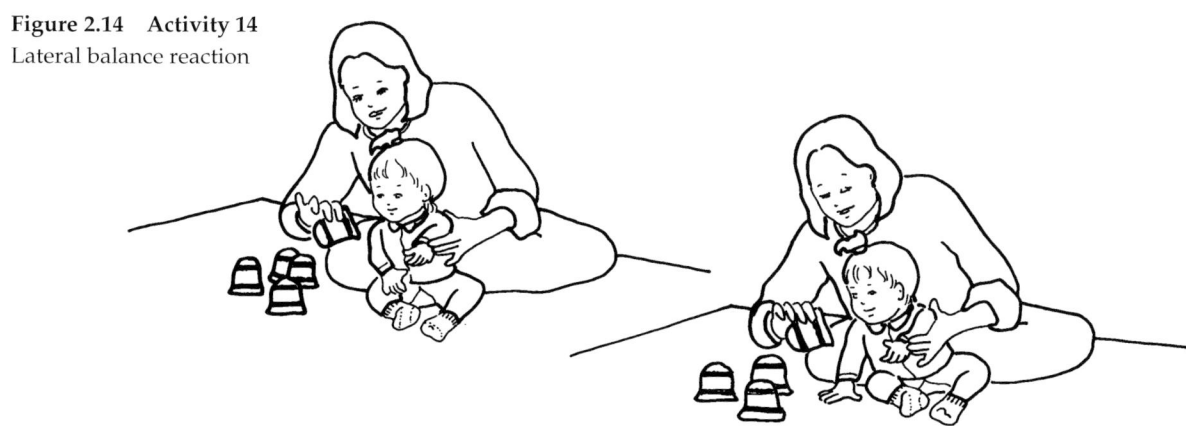

**Moving from lying down to sitting position**

After attaining trunk control, children begin to sit up from the lying down position. Motivate the child to learn this movement by helping him rotate his body with one hand on the floor. Next, encourage him to extend the supported arm and push up until he is sitting (Figure 2.15, Activity 15).

**Figure 2.15   Activity 15**
Moving from lying down
to sitting position

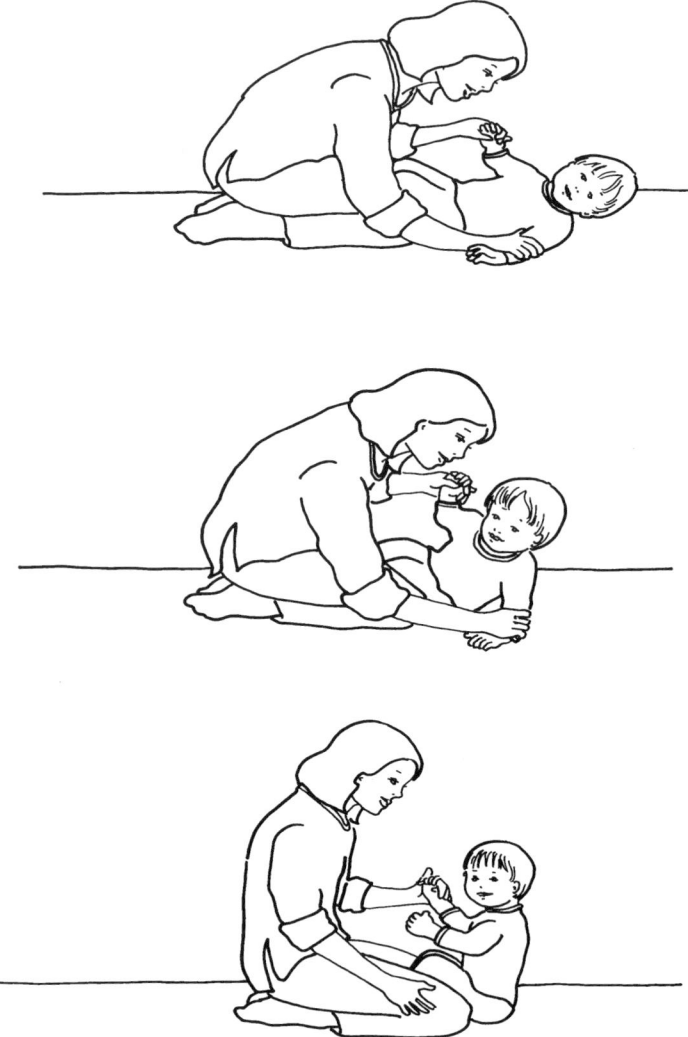

**Sitting on floor and turning**

Once the child is able to sit without using his hands for support, you can encourage rotational movements of the trunk during games to improve his sitting balance. Place toys to the side of the child, encouraging him to move them from one side to another (Figure 2.16, Activity 16).

**Figure 2.16    Activity 16**
Sitting on floor and
turning

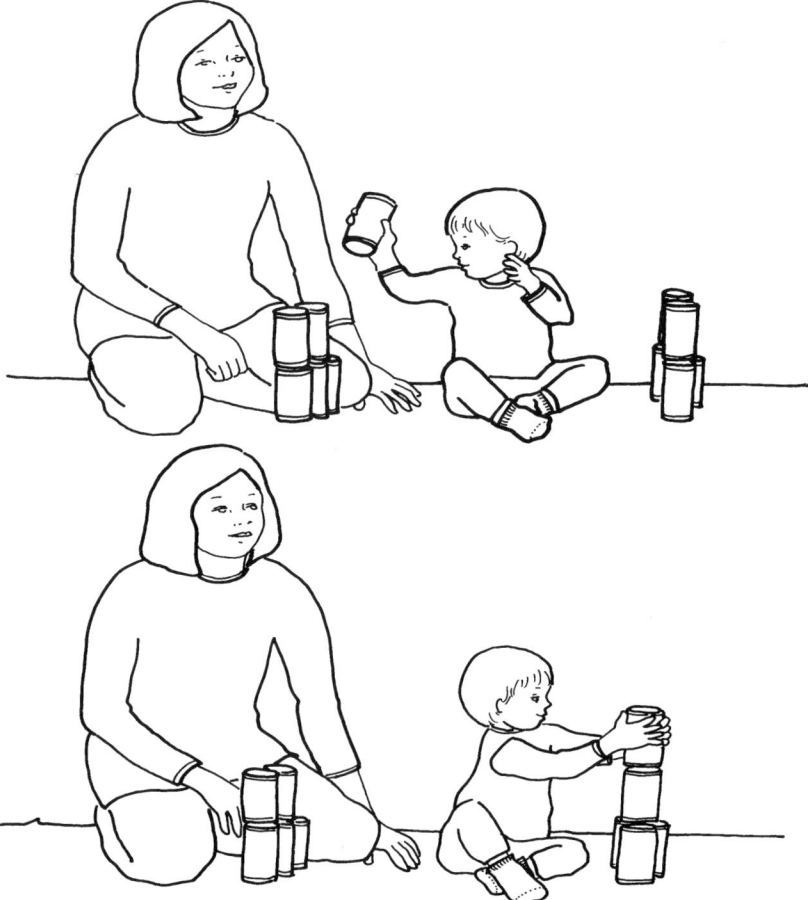

**Sitting on bench and turning**

Some children with brain injury and spasticity may benefit from sitting on small benches or stools to practice trunk rotation. This technique promotes alignment of the pelvis by relaxing the posterior muscles of the thigh. It is important to support the child's feet to aid trunk stability (Figure 2.17, Activity 17). While the child is in this position, you can initiate games or playful activities that include shifting an object from one side of his body to another so that he follows its movement and, finally, reaches out for it with one of his hands. Try to remain close to the child and supervise his actions in case he loses his balance.

**Figure 2.17    Activity 17**
Sitting on bench and turning

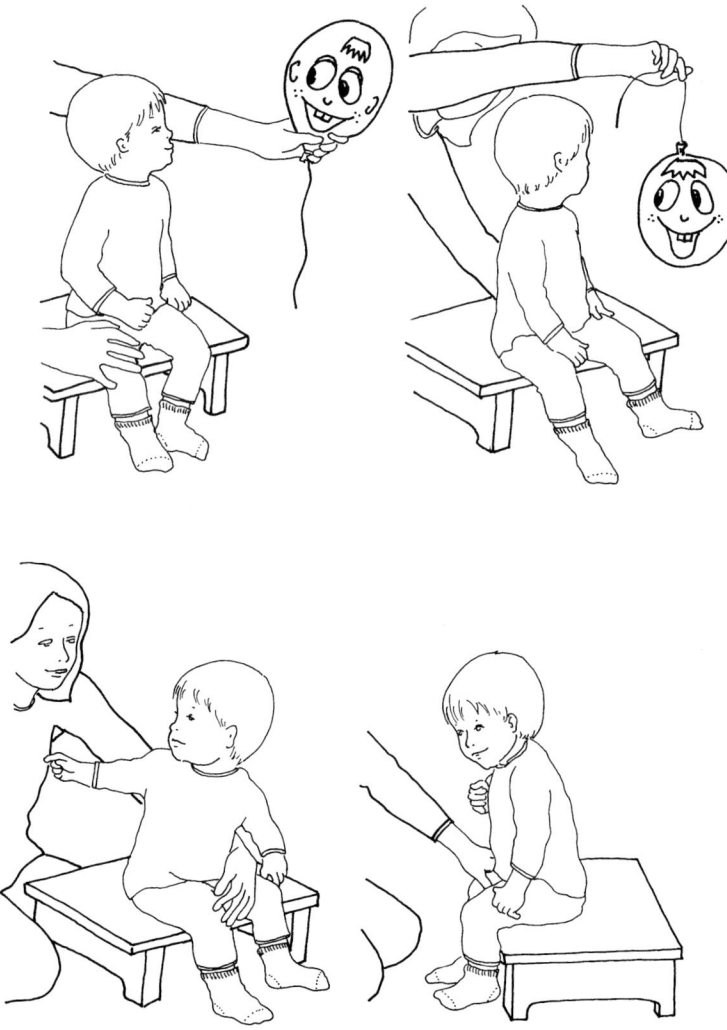

### Body balance sitting on a round object

The use of rolls also fosters trunk balance. The size of the roll should be adjusted so that the child has his feet off the ground. Children with TBI, especially those with ataxic disorders, may require more intensive exercises for improving adjustment and control of their posture (Figure 2.18, Activity 18). The amplitude and velocity of the rolling movements should be in accordance with the child's ability to respond; at first, you may have to support him with your hands. Placing a mirror in front of him can help him control his body when it is thrown off balance because it provides additional sensory information.

**Figure 2.18  Activity 18**
Body balance sitting on a round object

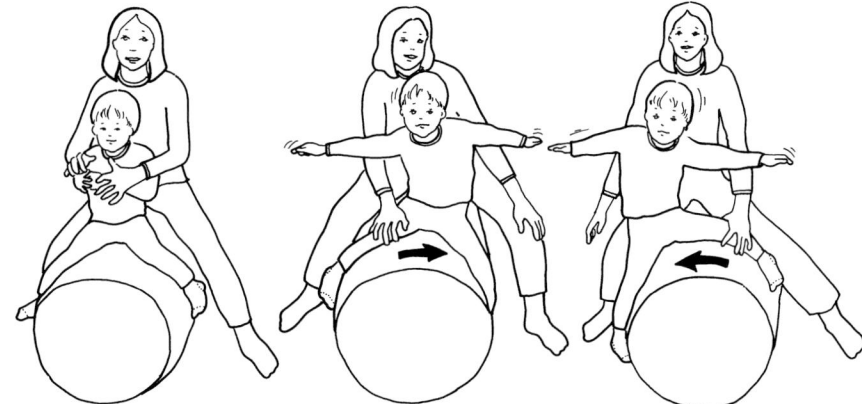

In many cases, children or adolescents with TBI regain the ability to sit in the early stages of recovery; however, they may, at times, be insecure or apprehensive when doing so. In the beginning, it is important for the activities to be performed on firm surfaces with close adult supervision to prevent very expansive or abrupt movements. Initially, the child should be seated with support; at the same time, he should be encouraged to use his arms for front and lateral support reactions until he has regained trunk balance. The amount of time the child remains seated should be gradually increased. In the early stages of recovery, children with TBI have little tolerance for repeated movements and static postures. They tire easily, due to prolonged periods of hospitalization and time spent in intensive care units.

## *Crawling*

### Balancing on hands and knees

Some children may crawl for only a short time before they start walking, or may bypass crawling altogether, neither of which negatively affects the attainment of subsequent motor milestones. On the other hand, achieving balance in this position is important for it helps with transfers, especially in children with TBI.

Children with brain injury may have problems balancing on their hands and knees. You can encourage this position while playing with the child because during play he is able to learn adapting to the position, to the weight bearing and learns to balance himself (Figure 2.19, Activity 19). In children with diplegic-type CP, this position can involve marked adduction and internal rotation of the hips and excessive knee flexion while balance is maintained.

**Figure 2.19   Activity 19**
Balancing on hands and knees

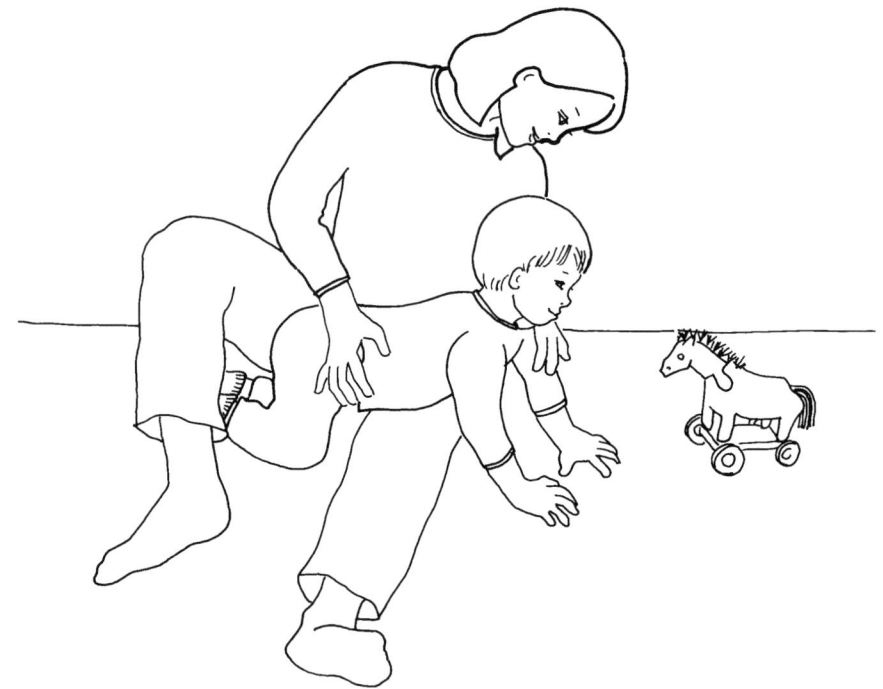

**Moving from prone to hands and knees**

As the child acquires the ability to balance himself on his hands and knees, you can begin teaching him how to move from this position to sitting. Initially, while the child is lying down in prone position, you should help him raise his hips and extend his arms to achieve balance on his hands and knees (Figure 2.20, Activity 20).

**Figure 2.20    Activity 20**
Moving from prone to
hands and knees

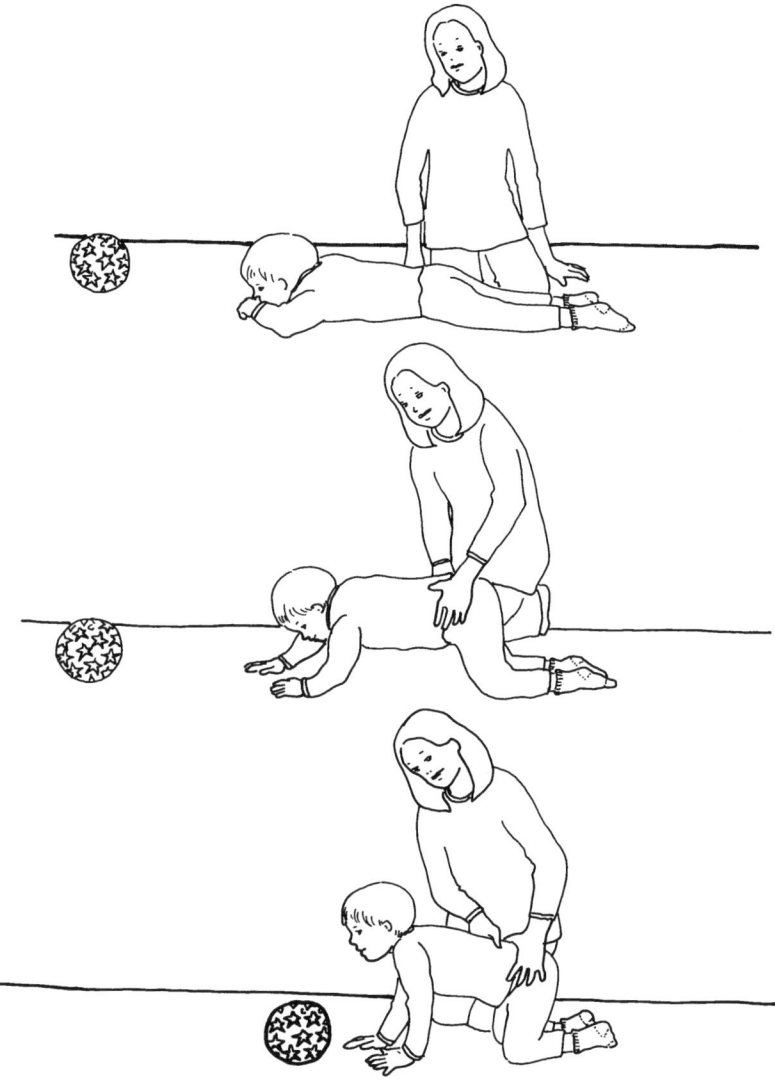

**Moving from hands and knees to sitting position**

Next, try helping the child to shift his body weight and rotate his pelvis to sit down (Figure 2.21, Activity 21). This change in position gives him greater independence when he is playing on the floor.

**Figure 2.21   Activity 21**
Moving from hands and knees to sitting position

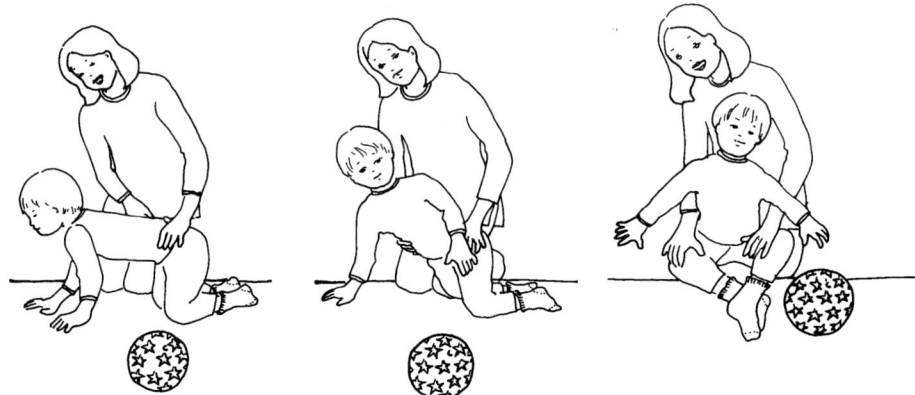

**Crawling with support**

Once a child has mastered static balance, you may begin introducing strategies that promote crawling. Toys that move away when he touches them may encourage him to crawl after them (Figure 2.22, Activity 22).

**Figure 2.22   Activity 22**
Crawling with support

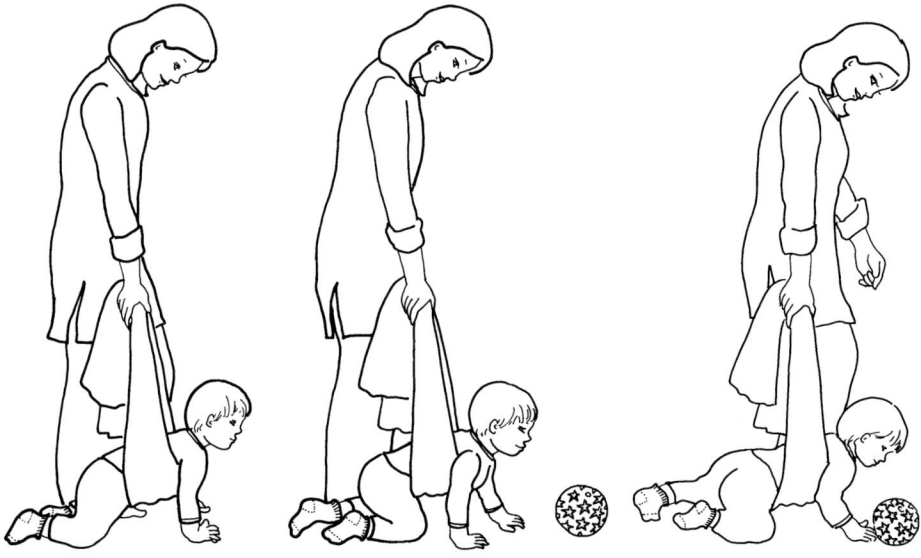

Children with hemiplegia, who present greater impairment at the brachial level, may not be able to crawl due to difficulties transferring and supporting body weight on the affected side, and may prefer to creep in the sitting position. Those with severe diplegia or quadriplegia frequently crawl in a homologous manner, without dissociating leg movements.

## *Standing up*

Moving along the floor and shifting and changing positions help the child to develop the skills for improving movement coordination and acquiring the postural control needed to stand up. When standing, the child will keep his balance by making anticipatory and/or compensatory postural adjustments during movement, with occasional loss of balance.[11] This entire dynamic allows the child to integrate perceptual information and corresponding motor responses, thereby acquiring greater confidence and independence.

### Balance in kneeling position

Balance in the kneeling position helps a child exercise control over his pelvic muscles and may assist in transfers and standing (Figure 2.23, Activity 23). While the child is learning balance, you can encourage him to play games that will aid his communication or cognitive development; these games should consist of context-sensitive activities based on his interests, age, developmental stage and lifestyle.

**Figure 2.23  Activity 23**
Balance in kneeling
position

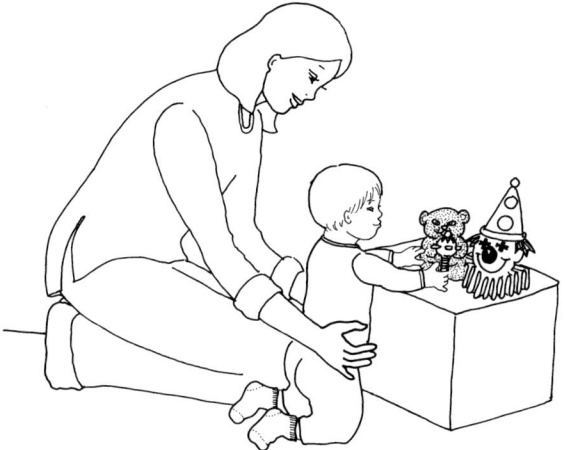

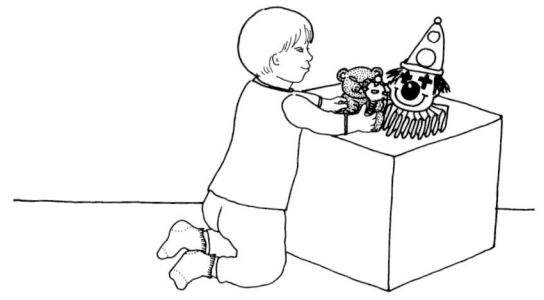

**Moving from hands and knees to standing position**

If a child is able to remain in the hands and knees position, you can try motivating him to kneel, first by supporting his hands on a firm surface in front of him and then helping him move one of his legs forward until his foot is on the floor. Once he is in this position, encourage him to raise his body (Figure 2.24, Activity 24).

**Figure 2.24 Activity 24**
Moving from hands and knees to standing position

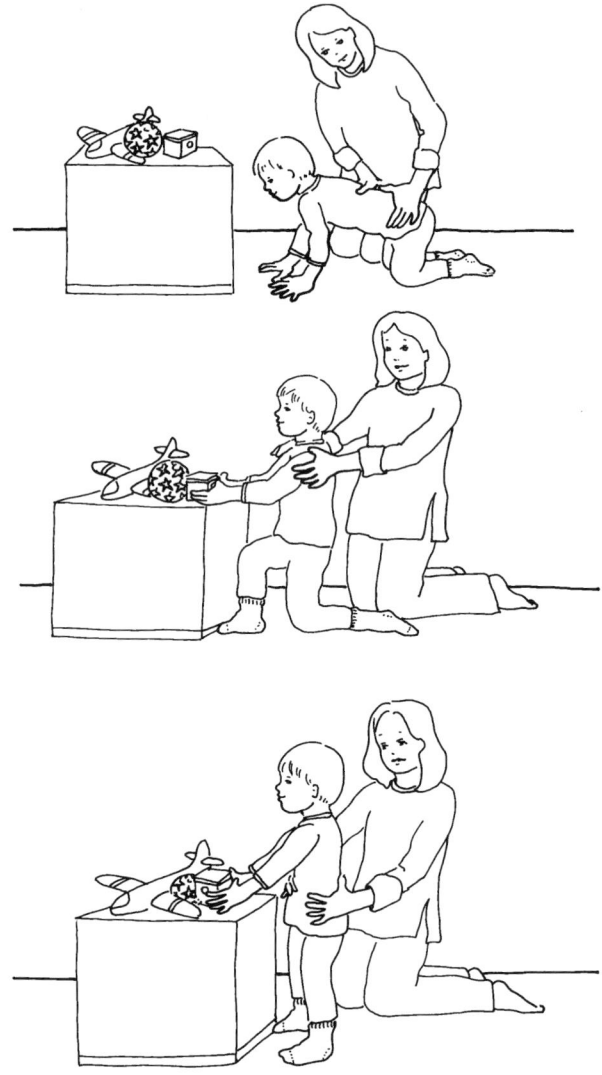

Children with TBI are generally able to dissociate leg movements during transfer to the standing position. This movement is more difficult for children with CP and spasticity, and they may need to support their arms and trunk on a nearby surface in order to lift their body. In cases of hemiplegia, it is advisable to begin the movement with the non-impaired leg.

**Moving from sitting to standing**

Another way the child can stand up, especially if he has difficulties dissociating leg movements, is from a sitting position on a bench or an adult's lap, with both feet planted on the floor. In order to get him to move, you should place toys in front of him at a level where he can reach them (Figure 2.25, Activity 25).

**Figure 2.25   Activity 25**
Moving from sitting to standing

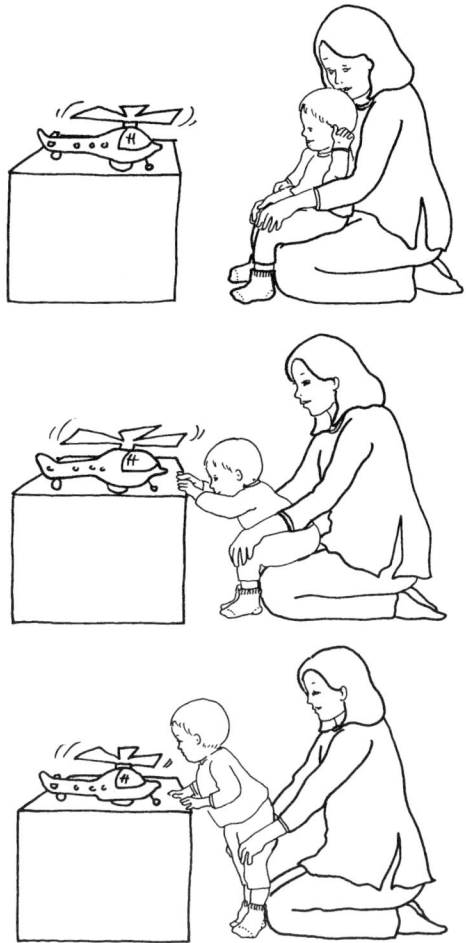

Children with TBI can begin transferring to standing even though they did not attain prior motor milestones such as crawling. While performing these movements the child may initially require support around the pelvis, which provides more proprioceptive information and pelvic control.

Independently transferring from the floor to the standing position helps the child develop lower limb function, balance, and overall postural control, necessary for walking upright. It is important that children with a poor motor prognosis perform these movements for they contribute to their ability to transfer to the wheelchair and participate in activities of daily life.

## *Standing*

In order to remain standing, children must first adopt compensatory positions that foster balance. Initially they will use a wide support base to remain standing, with abduction and external rotation of the hips, and the feet turned outwards. In addition, semiflexion of the hips and knees lowers the center of gravity, facilitating postural control in the standing position.[12] Frequently, children with brain injury have impaired compensatory mechanisms for control of standing balance. Spasticity of the lower limbs can narrow the base of support and result in slow motor responses to bodily adjustments; alterations and delayed development of the balance reaction can impair the motor responses necessary for realigning the body. Defining the rehabilitation exercises and the need for parental assistance and/or supervision during the activities should be analyzed.

### Standing with front support

You can encourage the child to play in the standing position, with front and back support and, next, persuade him to let go of the support with his hands. Placing toys in elevated places, on a chair or small table facing the child, may contribute to the effectiveness of this activity (Figure 2.26, Activity 26). Children with hemiplegia or triplegia due to CP or TBI may need more help stabilizing the pelvis to compensate for the difficulties they have supporting themselves on one of their hands.

**Figure 2.26  Activity 26**
Standing with front
support

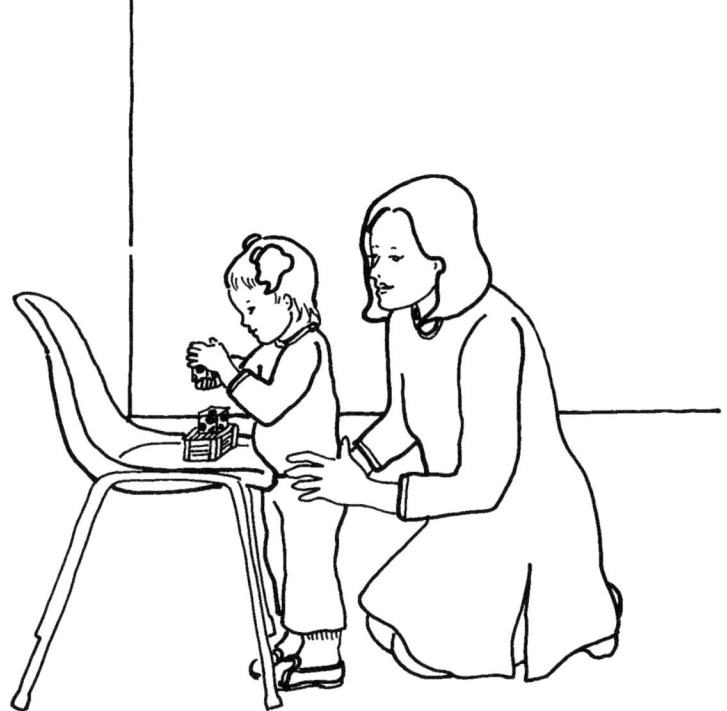

**Standing with lateral trunk movement**

While the child plays in the standing position with front support, there are a number of strategies that you can use to help him practice his postural control reactions. For instance place yourself behind the child and gently push his trunk from side to side with just enough intensity to generate an imbalance that he will be able to correct. If he loses his balance, remember to hold him and help him regain it. He must feel safe and confident during this game (Figure 2.27, Activity 27). Also in this position, you can involve him in the appropriate activities that stimulate his cognition and language; this helps make the exercises a playful, integrated, contextualized part of his daily life and rehabilitation process.

**Figure 2.27    Activity 27**
Standing with lateral
trunk movement

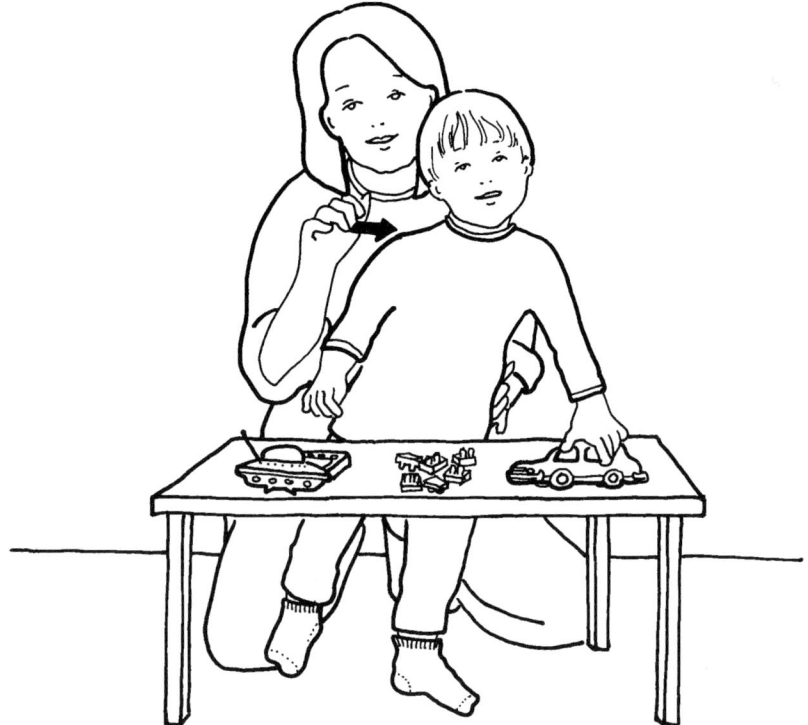

### Independent standing

Once the child has improved balance, he will need less support to remain standing. You can then include other forms of practicing his postural adjustment reactions during play. For example, chalk boards or sheets of paper taped to a wall will allow him to draw with one hand while he supports himself against the wall with the other. Holding him around the waist may keep him from losing his balance and falling backwards (Figure 2.28, Activity 28).

**Figure 2.28   Activity 28**
Independent standing

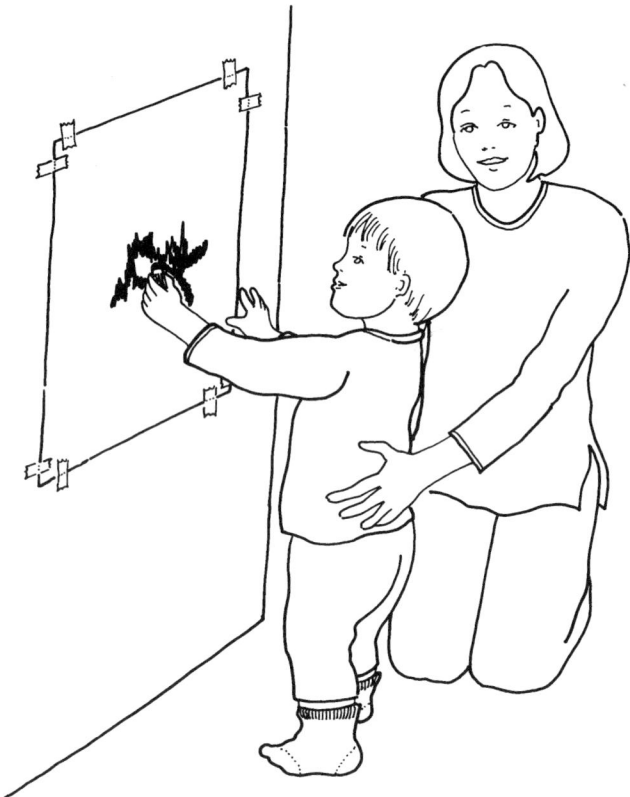

**Standing with back support**

You can explore different ways of stimulating the child to remain standing. There are a number of positions that will help him exercise balance reactions and postural adjustments using varied movements with different intensities. For example, help him stand with his back propped against the wall and engage him in a contextualized activity, such as tossing a ball back and forth (Figure 2.29, Activity 29). If back support alone leaves him insecure, try substituting it with pelvic support.

**Figure 2.29   Activity 29**
Standing with back support

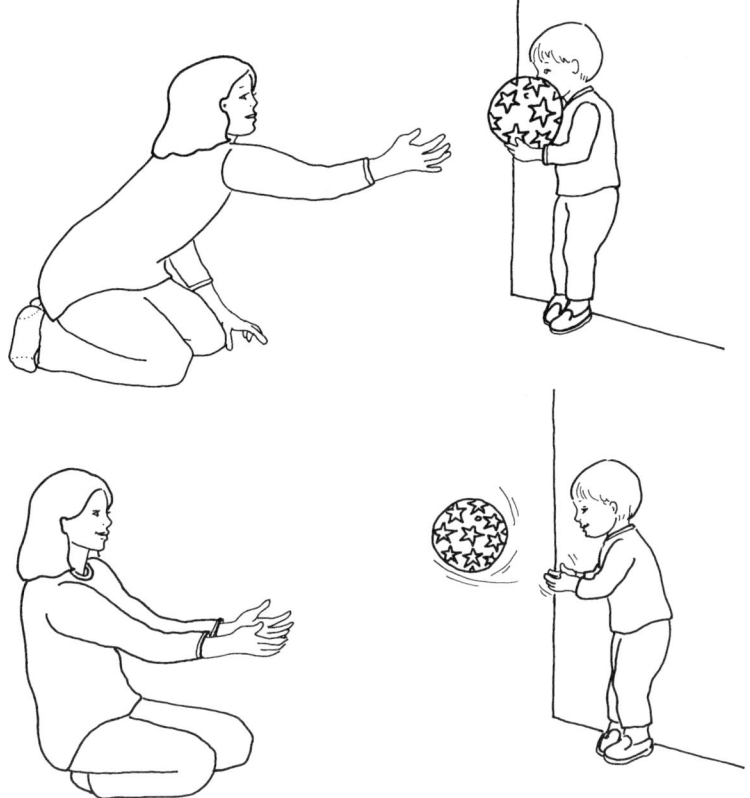

**Standing with waist support**

Children with spasticity of the lower limbs may have problems standing because of a narrow support base, and can benefit from placing their feet as far apart as possible for better balance. Help the child feel more secure by holding him around the waist while another adult, positioned in front of him, holds his attention by playing ball with him, for example (Figure 2.30, Activity 30).

**Figure 2.30   Activity 30**
Standing with waist support

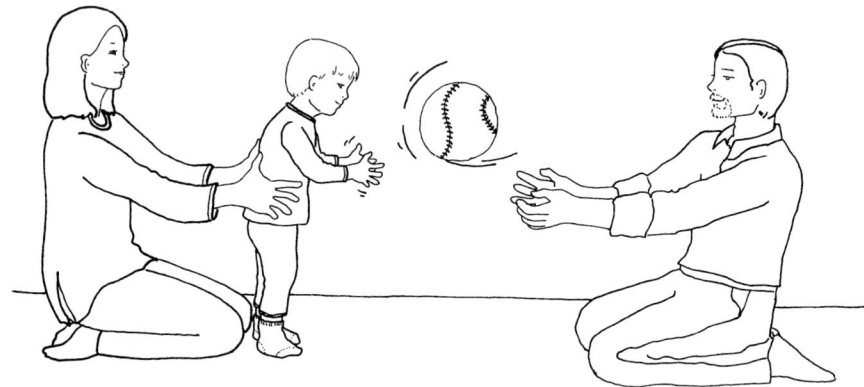

**Back and forth rocking in the standing position**

Gently rocking the child back and forth while standing can help him develop bodily adjustment mechanisms since they generate loss of backward and forward balance. By experiencing these imbalances, he can learn to use postural control strategies not unlike the ones he will eventually need when he begins walking. This activity helps teach him to perform compensatory mechanisms such as leaning his body forward or making a quick step (Figure 2.31, Activity 31).

**Figure 2.31   Activity 31**
Back and forth rocking in the standing position

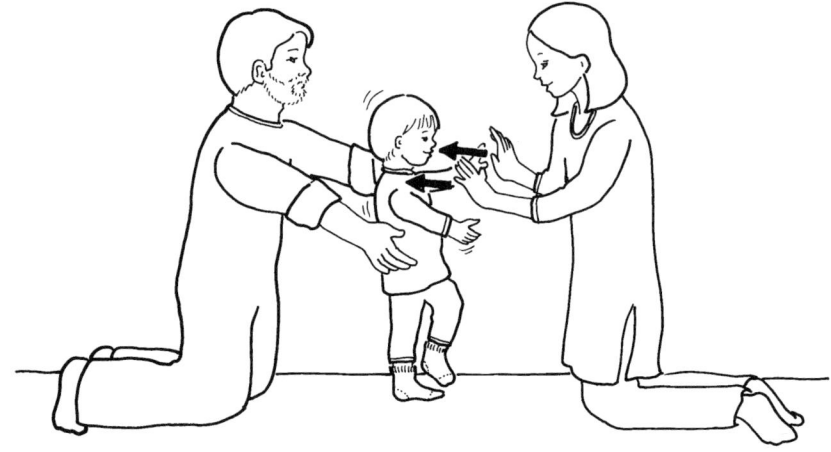

## *Walking*

When children start to walk, their gait pattern is characterized by a broad support base, increased cadence with short steps, semiflexed knees and feet turned outwards; this pattern is the result of still immature balance development and postural control. At this stage, they have not yet developed the reciprocal movements between arms and legs.

Children with brain injury and spasticity usually have reduced selective muscle activity, with simultaneous contraction between the antagonistic muscles, which causes joint restriction and postural control deficits. From the first moment they start walking, these children may exhibit peculiar gait characteristics such as a restricted support base, adduction and rotation of the hips, and equinus feet, depending on the extent of their motor disorder. Despite their impaired motor patterns, they find ways of adapting their positioning and movement to permit greater stability, improved performance, and reduced energy expenditures during gait.

However, children with brain injury and involuntary movements may not have the motor control needed to develop mechanisms to compensate for movement impairments. They may have guarded gait prognoses, or walk in an atypical manner, with inconsistent movements and lack of stability. These adaptive gait patterns can serve to improve the child's function and help them move about better.

Children with CP and good walking prognosis usually have delayed walking and may require the temporary or definitive support of mobility aids such as walkers or canes. Gait prognosis varies depending on the type of CP: while all children with hemiplegia walk, a few children with quadriplegia may develop some form of walking. Severe cognitive impairments, attentional deficits, and behavioral disturbances may delay or interfere with the child's ability to walk, especially when mobility aids are needed. Cases in which the child is able to develop nonfunctional gait, with significant slowness and increased energy expenditures, walking potential may be limited to the home. It is important for the family and rehabilitation team to consider the child's gait prognosis, and to evaluate and discuss the benefits of using a wheelchair for transporting the child who, if well positioned, may be able to participate in social and educational activities. Most children with TBI regain independent gait, but often continue to have impaired balance and speed.[13]

### Walking with parallel supports

There are several strategies that you can use to help the child begin walking. Parallel bars can be used for gait training once he is able to take steps by holding onto surfaces and no longer requires trunk support. Materials such as lightweight wood or bamboo, which provide adequate support for the child's hands, can be used as parallel bars at home. The benefits of this activity can be enhanced by incorporating motivational games that stimulate the child to repeatedly walk back and forth and from one side to the other; for example, pose fun challenges, sing familiar folksongs or employ other artifices to encourage the child (Figure 2.32, Activity 32).

**Figure 2.32   Activity 32**
Walking with parallel supports

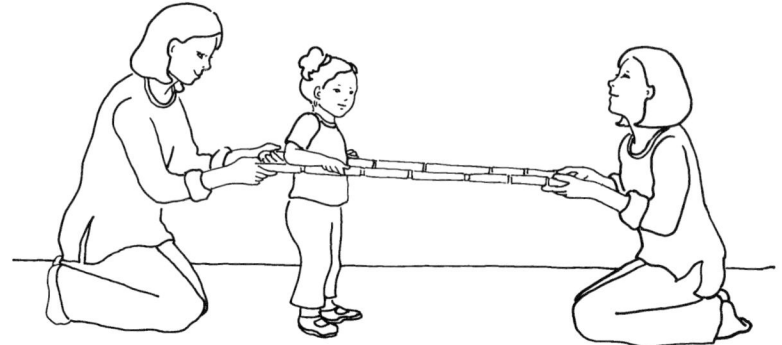

## Walking with chest support

During the stages in which the child is still developing his dynamic balance responses, you can help stimulate him to walk by holding up his trunk. Using a bed sheet around the child's waist can help you control and gradually reduce the amount of support; eventually, when he is ready, you can remove this type of support and allow him to exercise independent postural control. Remember to allow him to practice whatever forms of compensatory movements he may need to keep his standing balance, such as raising and abducting his arms or experimenting with ways to protect himself from falling (Figure 2.33, Activity 33).

**Figure 2.33   Activity 33**
Walking with chest support

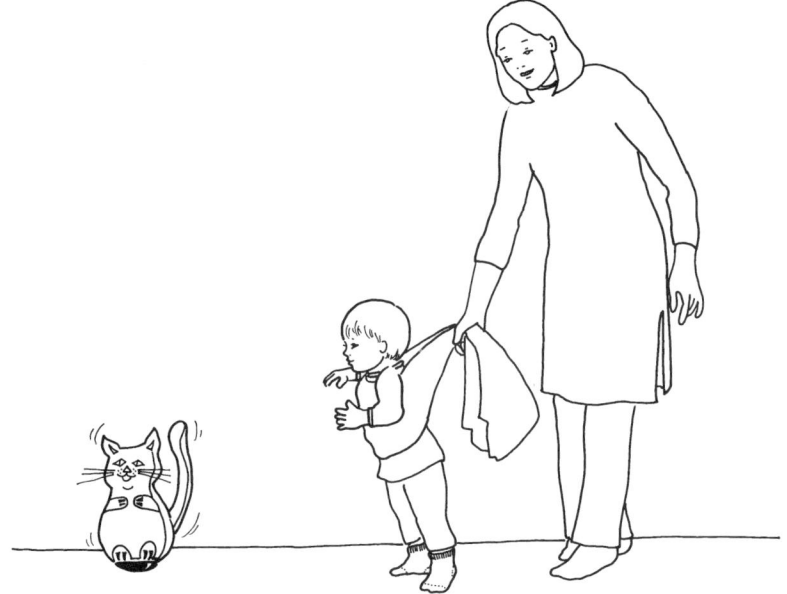

**Walking with hula-hoop**

Small children who have not yet mastered standing balance reactions may benefit from the playful use of hula-hoops. Hold the hula-hoop firmly. Allow the child to move his hands around the rim of the hoop to keep his balance while he safely rocks his trunk back and forth, and side to side. Take advantage of his natural need to move about by incorporating this type of assisted gait into his daily routine (Figure 2.34, Activity 34).

**Figure 2.34 Activity 34**
Walking with a hula-hoop

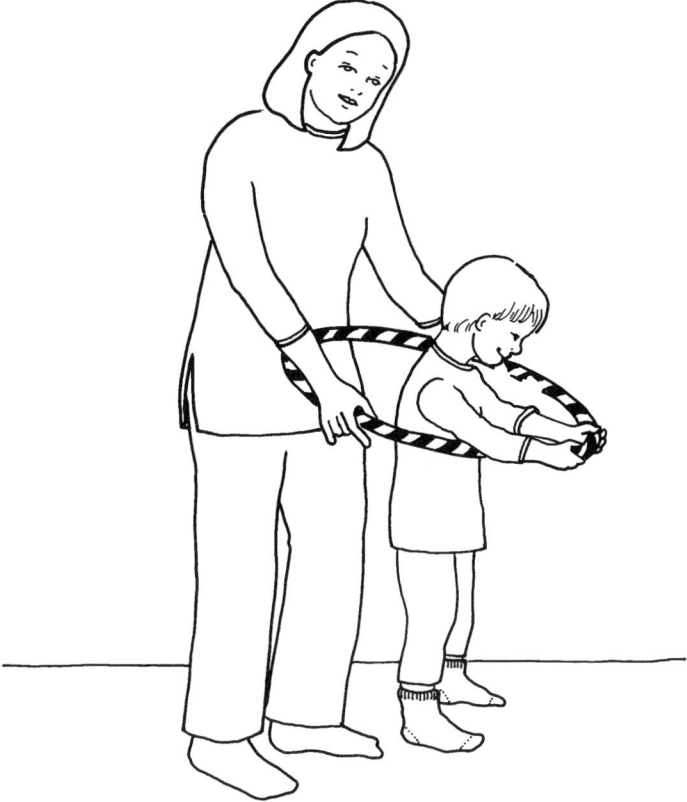

**Walking by pushing toys**

If the child is not able to take unassisted steps, use forward-moving supports, such as shopping carts or baby carriages, to help him practice walking. Smaller children may prefer this type of support over walkers; they are smaller and more fun. If he needs sturdier support, place weighty toys inside the carriages or carts, adjusting the load and the stability it provides until you have attained the ideal steadiness (Figure 2.35, Activity 35).

**Figure 2.35   Activity 35**
Walking by pushing toys

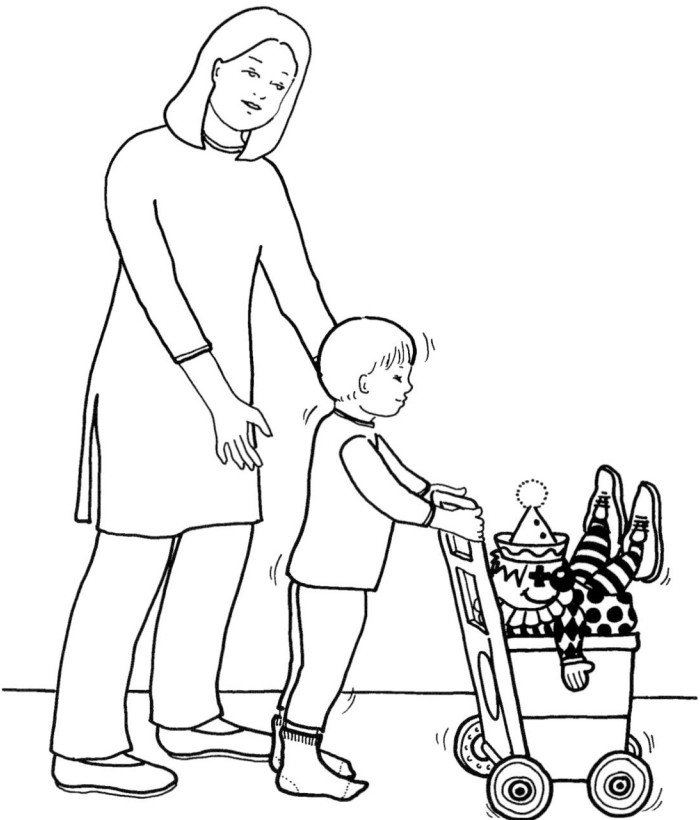

Some children with TBI may need the support of mobility devices, usually walkers, when they begin to walk again after the injury. The type of support can vary, depending on the gains they have made, especially those related to balance; however, most of these children are able to walk unassisted a few months after the injury.

**Walking with sticks**

Children with brain injury and good motor prognosis, with side-to-side balance deficits in the standing position, may need canes for walking. Small children can begin training with colored sticks, simulating the use of crutches. In addition to being lightweight, the sticks allow you to contribute to his learning process (Figure 2.36, Activity 36).

**Figure 2.36   Activity 36**
Walking with sticks

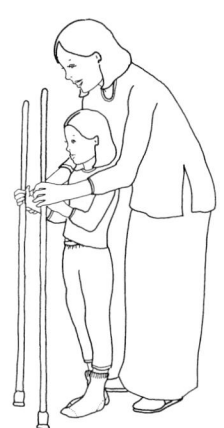
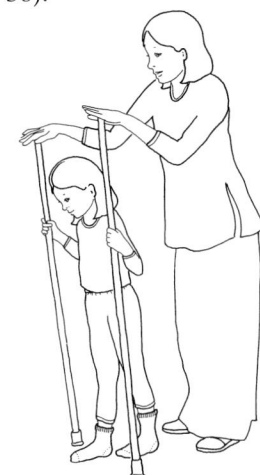

**Walking on irregular surfaces**

Whenever possible, it is advisable to allow the child to experiment with different settings when he is learning to walk. This will help him gradually learn to deal with common obstacles such as steps, uneven or rocky terrains, sand and dirt. Children with brain injury, balance deficits or limited movement of the lower limbs may initially require assistance to overcome these difficulties. Nevertheless, it is by experiencing different situations and obstacles that he will acquire independence (Figure 2.37, Activity 37).

**Figure 2.37   Activity 37**
Walking on irregular surfaces

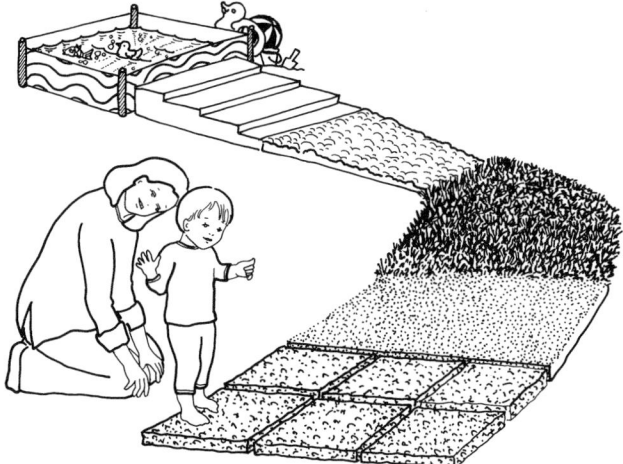

**Playground activities**

Playground activities are part of childhood. Various motor skills can be exercised and perfected while the child enjoys himself. Children with brain injury, with balance deficits and uncoordinated movements, can also benefit from playground activities, irrespective of their level of motor development (Figure 2.38, Activity 38). Specially adapted tricycles or bikes, in addition to being fun, can contribute to the child's independence in the playground. Toys that encourage rapid body movements, such as swings and carrousels, may help him develop greater postural control through labyrinthic stimulation. Children with hemiplegia can benefit from playground activities that exercise the coordinated use of their arms and legs, and promote muscle strength by climbing or hanging from fixtures such as monkey bars.

**Figure 2.38   Activity 38**
Playground activities

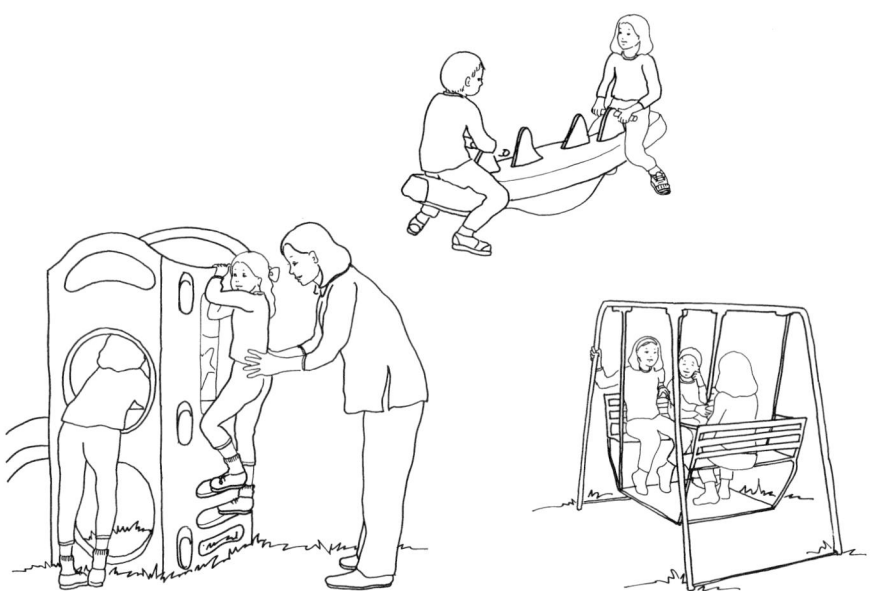

The performance of already acquired motor skills in school-aged children can be improved by physical activities, either leisure or sports. Choose an activity that the child enjoys and adapt it to his capacities and potential; this process entails joint efforts from the team and the family, as well as the child's input.

There are a number of sports activities, such as basketball and table tennis, which can be played in a wheelchair; they have been specially adapted for children who cannot walk but are able to grasp and have enough strength in their arms to manipulate accessories, rackets and balls. When well organized, these activities can improve the child's motor performance, increase his feelings of well-being, and boost social interactions.

# School-aged Children and Adolescents with TBI

Post-TBI motor impairment varies depending on the neuronal damage. Moderate to severe injuries usually affect motor skills, resulting in initial loss of function.[14] In most cases, however, there is positive motor progress with good prognosis for gait recovery, which generally occurs during the first few months post-injury.

Neuropsychological disorders, particularly deficits of attention, memory and executive functions, as well as cognitive impairment can affect the motor recovery of children and adolescents with TBI. It is important that the family and treatment team be aware of the child's or adolescent's difficulties, especially those related to their understanding of motor commands, to ensure that the interventions and activities are targeted to their specific needs and potential.

When planning and establishing goals for motor rehabilitation programs of school-aged children and adolescents with TBI, it is important to take their cognitive potential and chronological age into account.

Once a child or adolescent with TBI has passed the acute post-injury stage, an accelerated recovery of motor functions frequently occurs, unlike the case of congenital lesions. Motor stages are usually recovered in unique ways, with the bypassing of milestones that are normally observed in child development. The child may recover head balance simultaneously with sitting balance, and both can be stimulated at the same time.

The goals of a motor stimulation program in TBI vary among school-aged children and adolescents. Smaller children can derive greater benefit from stimulation of developmental stages such as moving along the floor by creeping or crawling. It is essential that this stimulation be done in a playful manner. On the other hand, programs for recovery of motor function in school-aged children and adolescents should exclude activities that cause them to regress to infantile situations.

When the child or adolescent returns home or to the school, the parents and teachers should incorporate the motor exercises into his daily life activities to facilitate his reintegration in the family and school contexts while respecting his abilities and present needs. Some adjustments in the activities of the school-aged and adolescent's routine should be planned together. For example, the teacher can promote the child's or adolescent's involvement in the group by telling the other students what happened to him and explaining what he is going through, emphasizing that their help and understanding will be important contributions to their classmate's recovery. Participation in extracurricular activities or sports can help school-aged children and adolescents with TBI refine their motor skills and experiment with movements that require greater balance, speed and coordination.[15–17]

Motor improvement primarily occurs during the first twelve months after the TBI. In the two to three subsequent years, changes in motor performance can still be expected and, generally, are associated with improvement of motor abilities that have already been recovered, such as speed, precision, greater movement coordination, and balance.[8]

Throughout the rehabilitation process, a close relationship between the treatment team, family and schoolteachers is essential. This connection allows for the exchange of information and provides a source of support in defining the approaches and attitudes that will most benefit the child or adolescent with TBI throughout the various stages of his development and progress.

# References

1.  Hadders-Algra M. The neuronal group selection theory: promising principles for understanding and treating developmental motor disorders. Dev Med Child Neurol 2000; 42(10):707–715.

2.  Lent R. Cem bilhoes de neuronios: conceitos fundamentais de neurociencia. São Paulo: Atheneu, 2002.

3.  Latash ML, Anson JG. What are "normal movements" in atypical populations? Behav Brain Sci 1996; 19:55–106.

4.  Bax M. A diagnosis/a natural history. Dev Med Child Neurol 1996; 38(10):871–872.

5.  Farmer SE. Key factors in the development of lower limb co-ordination: implications for the acquisition of walking in children with cerebral palsy. Disabil Rehabil 2003; 25(14):807–816.

6.  Campos da Paz Jr A, Burnett SM, Braga LW. Walking prognosis in cerebral palsy: a 22-year retrospective analysis. Dev Med Child Neurol 1994; 36(2):130–134.

7.  Molnar GE. Cerebral palsy: prognosis and how to judge it. Pediatr Ann 1979; 8(10):596–605.

8.  Swaine BR, Sullivan SJ. Longitudinal profile of early motor recovery following severe traumatic brain injury. Brain Inj 1996; 10(5):347–366.

9.  O'Suilleabhain P, Dewey RB, Jr. Movement disorders after head injury: diagnosis and management. J Head Trauma Rehabil 2004; 19(4):305–313.

10. Brogren E, Hadders-Algra M, Forssberg H. Postural control in sitting children with cerebral palsy. Neurosci Biobehav Rev 1998; 22(4):591–596.

11. Adolph KE, Vereijken B, Shrout PE. What changes in infant walking and why. Child Dev 2003; 74(2):475–497.

12. Sutherland DH, Olshen R, Cooper L, Woo SL. The development of mature gait. J Bone Joint Surg Am 1980; 62(3):336–353.

13. Kuhtz-Buschbeck JP, Hoppe B, Golge M, Dreesmann M, Damm-Stunitz U, Ritz A. Sensorimotor recovery in children after traumatic brain injury: analyses of gait, gross motor, and fine motor skills. Dev Med Child Neurol 2003; 45(12):821–828.

14. Ylvisaker M, Feeney TJ. Traumatic brain injury in adolescence: assessment and reintegration. Semin Speech Lang 1995; 16(1):32–44.

15. Gagnon I, Friedman D, Swaine B, Forget R. Balance findings in a child before and after a mild head injury. J Head Trauma Rehabil 2001; 16(6):595–602.

16. Kuhtz-Buschbeck JP, Stolze H, Golge M, Ritz A. Analyses of gait, reaching, and grasping in children after traumatic brain injury. Arch Phys Med Rehabil 2003; 84(3):424–430.

17. Gagnon I, Swaine B, Friedman D, Forget R. Children show decreased dynamic balance after mild traumatic brain injury. Arch Phys Med Rehabil 2004; 85(3):444–452.

# 3

# Cognitive Development and Neuropsychological Disorders

*Lúcia Willadino Braga, Mark Ylvisaker, Luciana Rossi and Ligia N Souza*

As human nature is fundamentally variable, so too is the ultimate cognitive functioning of children and adolescents with brain injury.[1] Generalizations about cognitive function should be analyzed with caution; the concept of cognition is very broad and is given various definitions by the numerous schools of thought in neuropsychology.[2-3] Success in many aspects of life depends perhaps more on how individuals effectively understand their potential and needs, and how they strategically use their skills and strengths to attain their goals, than on the abilities themselves.[4]

This chapter will discuss elements of cognitive development and the main neuropsychological problems faced by children with cerebral palsy (CP) or traumatic brain injury (TBI).

Children construct and guide their cognitive development process through motivation, attention and action; this action can be internal, in other words, it does not necessarily require tactile contact with an object. Nevertheless, mediation is part of children's entire developmental process because it is through others that they will interact with culture and, gradually, learn and acquire knowledge. The higher mental functions originate in and are mediated by social interactions.[5] Affective interaction also plays a crucial role in socio-cognitive development.

## Program of Activities

The first half of this chapter will describe activities for the cognitive development of children during the first few years of life. These activities may be more appropriate for children who suffered injuries at birth, during early childhood or at preschool age. Nevertheless, many school-aged children and adolescents who sustain a brain injury can benefit from some of these activities during the early stages of recovery. Specific activities for school-aged children and adolescents with TBI are described in the second half of this chapter.

## Sensory and Perceptive Processes

Sensory and perceptive processes develop at different rates during children's maturation. Early sensorial experiences have a significant impact on the development of brain structures and cognitive functions.[6] By using their sensory, visual, auditory and tactile abilities and social skills, small children begin to experience and, gradually, interact with others and with their surroundings.[7]

### Horizontal gaze

Children with CP may have delayed visual development.[8] Infants with CP caused by prematurity have a greater likelihood of developing visual disorders because their immature visual system is vulnerable to injury.[9] By being attentive to the child's visual responses you can help him, if necessary, by playing at staring at and following objects, particularly high-contrast objects. Once the child has fixed his gaze on an object, make short horizontal movements while observing and waiting for his reactions to these movements (Figure 3.1, Activity 39).

**Figure 3.1    Activity 39**
Horizontal gaze

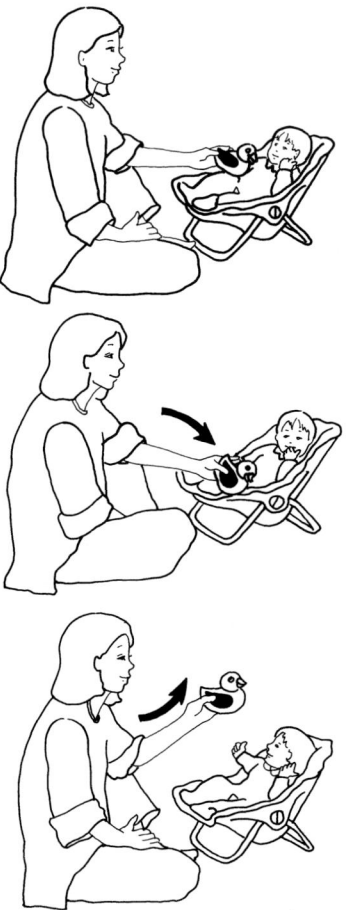

**Vertical gaze**

Next, make additional horizontal, vertical and diagonal movements, but keep the object within the child's visual field. If he is able to hold an object, it is important to give him a toy so that he can explore it with his hands after he has visually inspected it (Figure 3.2, Activity 40).

**Figure 3.2   Activity 40**
Vertical gaze

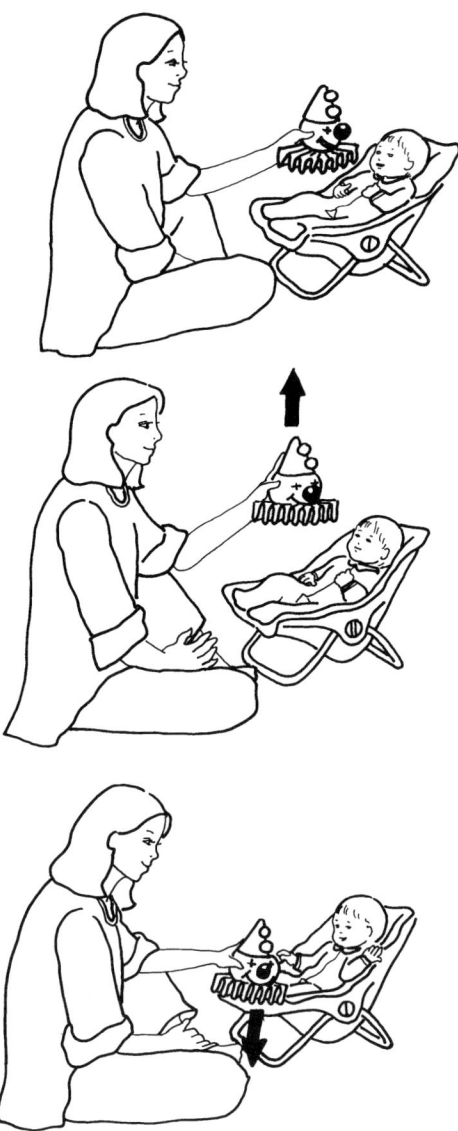

When you perceive that the child is having difficulties visually fixating on or following an object, change the type of object that you are using and the manner in which you are presenting it to him. The intensity of the stimulus can be enhanced by showing him objects with vibrant colors, contrasts and patterns, or novel items that stand out from other stimuli in his surroundings.

**Depth perception**

By attempting to reach for a toy or locate a sound or object, the child begins to develop a relative sense of an object's positioning. Slow head movements can give him clues about the relative depth of his visual field.[10] You can help broaden the child's visual field by using contextualized tactics, such as the natural act of drawing close to him and then moving away, or bringing objects closer that are distant but still within his sight (Figure 3.3, Activity 41).

**Figure 3.3   Activity 41**
Depth perception

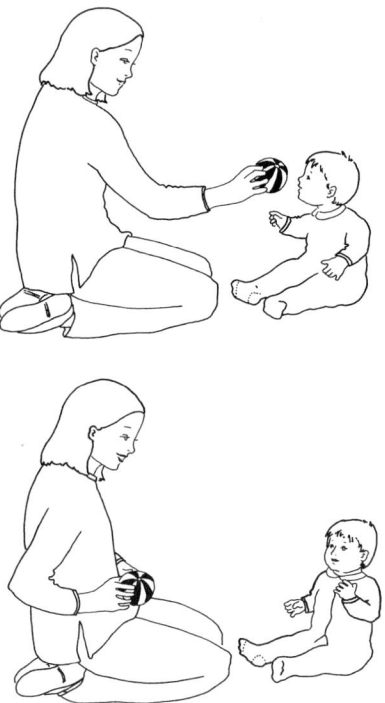

Gazing at and visually searching for an object, locating the origins of a sound, and following instructions, even if done in an inconsistent manner, are some of the signs that indicate the child is coming out of post-TBI coma.[11] To help during this early stage, attempt face-to-face contact with the child or adolescent and, later, present him with familiar toys or objects. Based on his response, move the object about slightly, always keeping it within his visual field. It is very likely that the child or even the adolescent will no longer need this activity after a short period of time.

Newborns react to sound stimuli and are able to perceive variations in sound frequency; they also exhibit a heightened sensitivity for certain aspects of basic human language.[7] The human voice and its melody catch the child's attention, as do other sounds in the home. Initially, the child will manifest reactions to auditory stimuli through behavioral changes, such as staring, blinking, or a pause in sucking.

**Sound identification**

You can get the child's attention at an early age by using toys and objects that make varied sounds (loudness, pitch, etc.) and provide visual stimuli at the same time. Place a sound-making object out of the child's sight and watch his reactions while encouraging him to find the object, or you can simply observe the changes in his behavior in response to his perception of the sound (Figure 3.4, Activity 42).

**Figure 3.4   Activity 42**
Sound identification

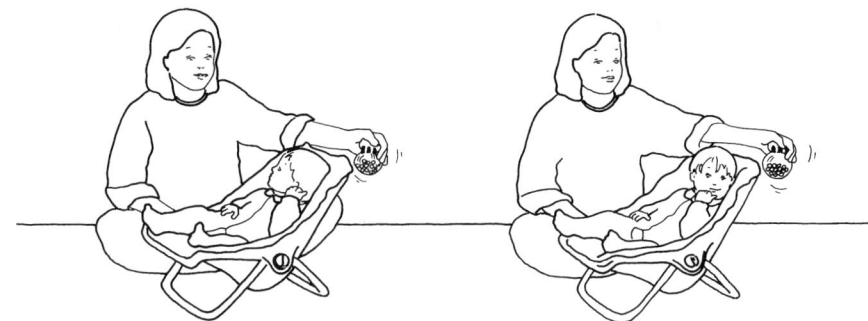

## Object Permanence, Imitation and Intentionality

Initially, infants do not seem to know that objects that are not present continue to exist; later,[12] some experiences indicate that babies understand that an object exists even if they cannot see (object permanence)[3,13] or act on the object.[7]

The infant's repeated attempts at finding an object that has been hidden reveal information about his capacity to inhibit and control his behavior; attempts to retrieve objects that are out of reach give us insight into his ability to solve problems.[14] Memory is also continuously developing during this same period; for example, depending on the child's age, he may recall, after a short time, a sequence of events that involves a toy he is not familiar with and that does not belong in the context of his daily life.[15]

During the first months of life, the infant's visual system undergoes significant evolution.[16] The visual capacity that results from these biological changes permits the small child to fixate his gaze on people. The child, involved in the family's daily routine, begins to develop an anticipatory perception of occurrences such as, for example, looking toward the locus of a predictable event. Later, he begins to demonstrate the ability to perceive and react to people in ways that differ from his interactions with an inanimate object.[3]

**Peek-a-boo**

Being attentive to the child's preference for the human face and his interested response, and expressions of surprise, when in the presence or absence of this stimulus, will lead you to naturally play at hiding, then showing your face; this allows the child to develop anticipation and build notions of object permanence (Figure 3.5, Activity 43).

**Figure 3.5    Activity 43**
Peek-a-boo

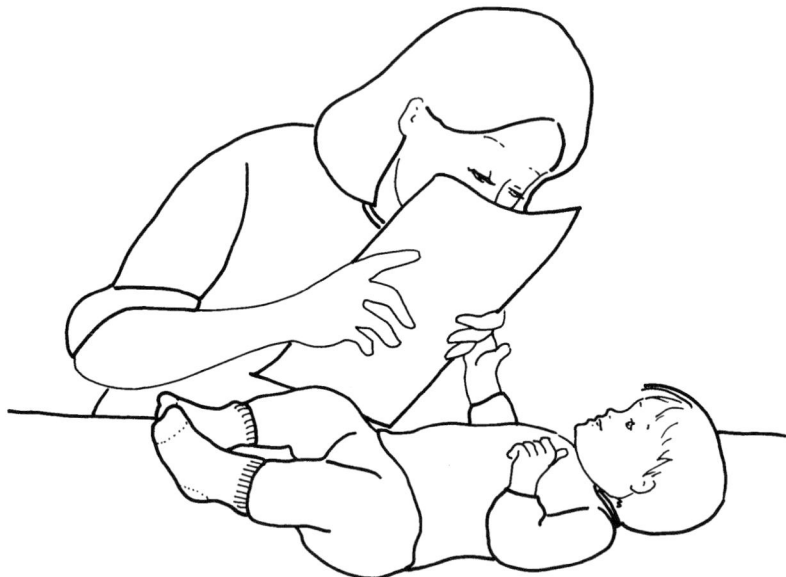

At home, the repetition of daily events, the natural flow of people who go in and out of the house, and the placement and removal of items in the child's visual field are day-to-day situations that help him begin to perceive the physical properties of objects. They help him understand that objects and people remain the same even when they move from one place to another, and that they usually continue to exist even when he cannot see them.[17]

### Hiding part of the toy and hiding the entire toy

Partially hiding toys and then removing them from the child's sight helps him retain a good deal of information about the property of objects, and may begin to help him direct his attention (Figure 3.6, Activity 44) and (Figure 3.7, Activity 45). If the child has motor limitations, play at partially covering toys and then "rediscovering" them so that he can observe the effects of the game. The child is capable of remembering an action that he has observed, even if he does not perform it himself.[15]

**Figure 3.6    Activity 44**
Hiding part of the toy

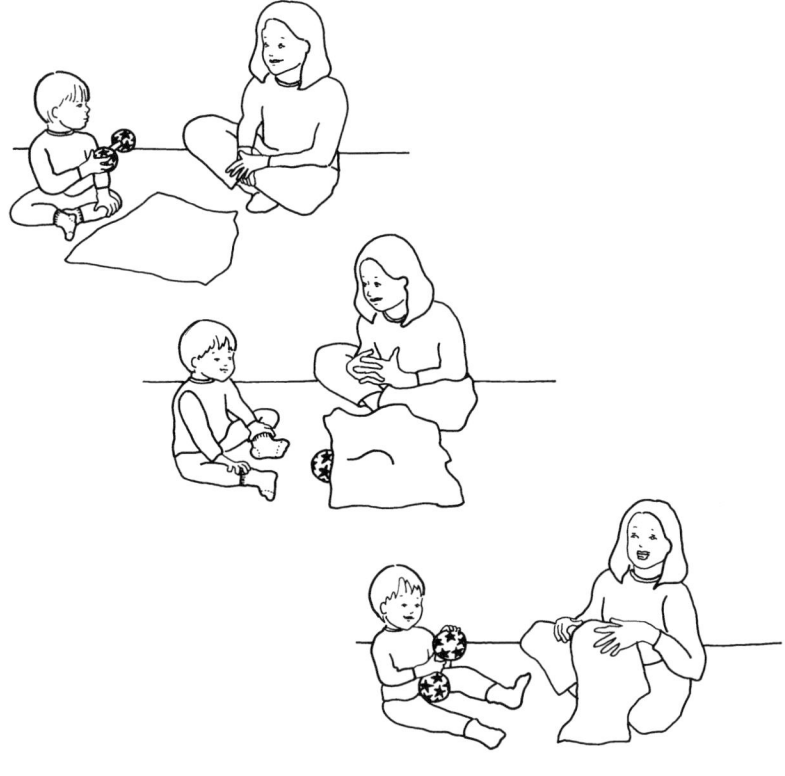

**Figure 3.7    Activity 45**
Hiding the entire toy

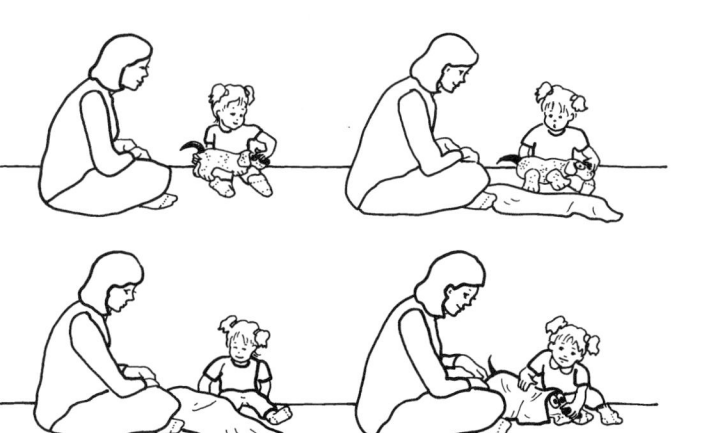

**Action imitation**

The child's mimicking behavior affects his cognitive development and social learning.[18] It is a behavior that can be observed early in the child's life and constitutes an important learning mechanism throughout development. Encourage the child to participate in games that involve mimicking and imitating, at first using examples and successive repetitions. After some time, he will be able to perform the activity without having to follow an example; this signals his understanding of the specific use of gestures in daily life situations (Figure 3.8, Activity 46).

**Figure 3.8    Activity 46**
Action imitation

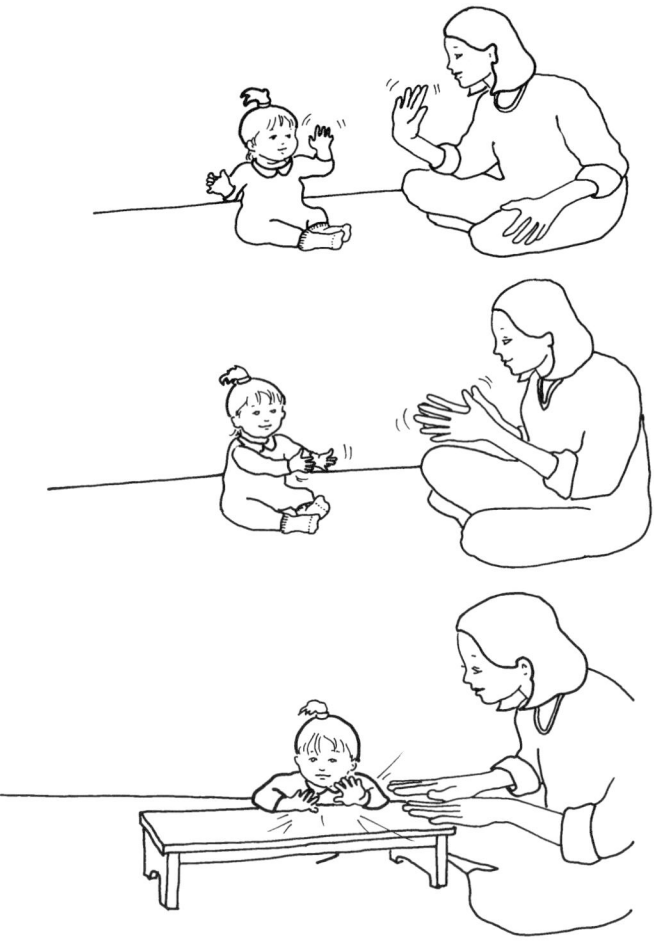

Gradually, based on experimentation, observation, and acquired notions of object permanence, the child begins to consolidate the effects of his actions on the external world. At first, he shows an interest not only in the end itself, but also in the way something is done. He may repeatedly perform a given action simply to see its results. For example, he may turn on a light switch and stare at the lamp, or pick up a remote control for the television, press its buttons, and look at the screen in anticipation of the moving images.

## Action and reaction

The child can discover these associations by engaging in playful activities that pose certain challenges. These may include playing with boxes that contain sound-making objects, or with toys that react when played with (such as a jack-in-the box), and drawing his attention to other simple situations of daily life that help him perceive and formulate these associations, making him aware of his effect on his environment (Figure 3.9, Activity 47).

**Figure 3.9   Activity 47**
Action and reaction

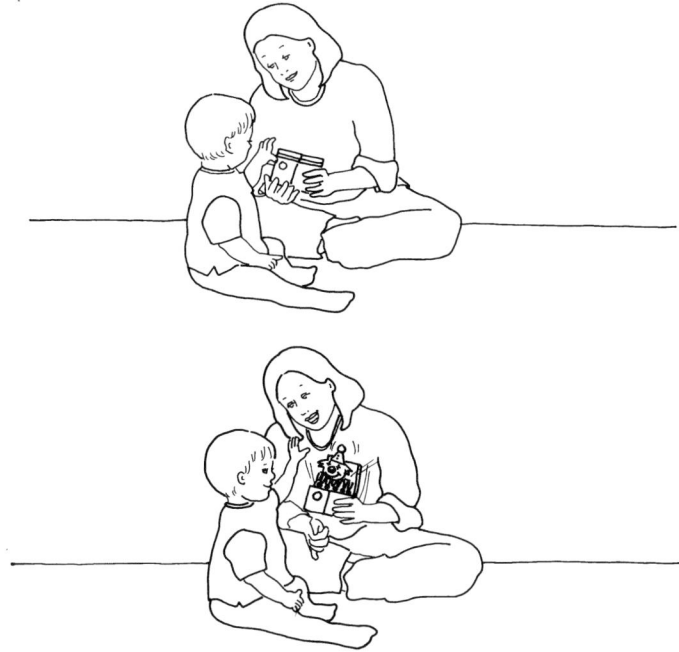

## Simple problem solving

Gradually, you can help the child plan a solution for object acquisition problems. For example, to retrieve a toy that is out of his manual reach, he may use another object as a mediating tool or even invent other ways of reaching it (Figure 3.10, Activity 48).

**Figure 3.10   Activity 48**
Simple problem solving

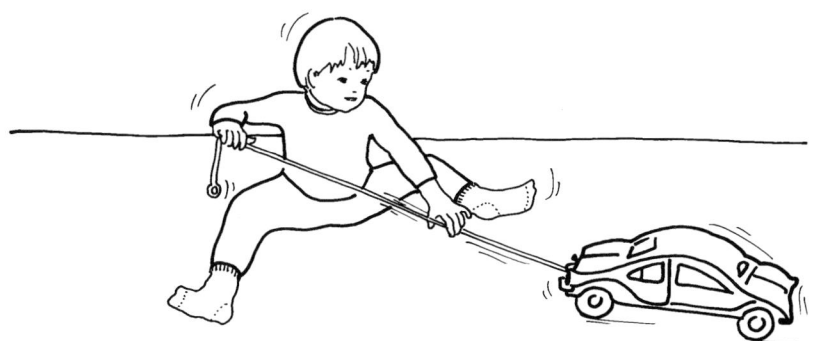

## Body Perception and Self-awareness

Interpersonal, sensory, motor and kinesthetic experiences help the child develop notions of his body and self-awareness. Through these experiences and in his social interactions, the child may construct not only images and feelings about himself but also internalize patterns or ideas about people. Notions of self-awareness are also associated with maturation and individual and sociocultural experiences.

### Pointing to body parts

During daily caregiving, bath-time, dressing, or even game playing, you can name and point to parts of the child's body, guiding his attention to what you are referring. Naming confirms what the child perceives and experiences. Initially, try naming parts of the body that are visible to the child, such as his feet, hands, or tummy (Figure 3.11, Activity 49).

**Figure 3.11    Activity 49**
Pointing to body parts

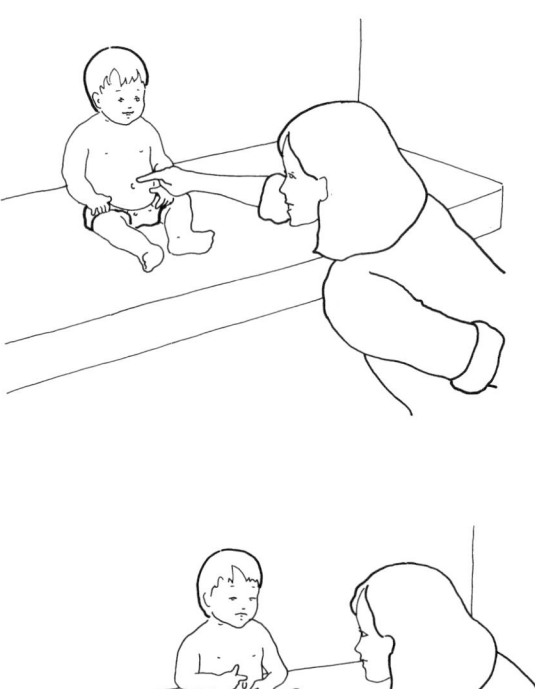

## Detailed identification of body parts

You can also gradually begin naming other parts of the body that the child cannot readily see, such as eyes, mouth, and nose (Figure 3.12, Activity 50).

**Figure 3.12   Activity 50**
Detailed identification of body parts

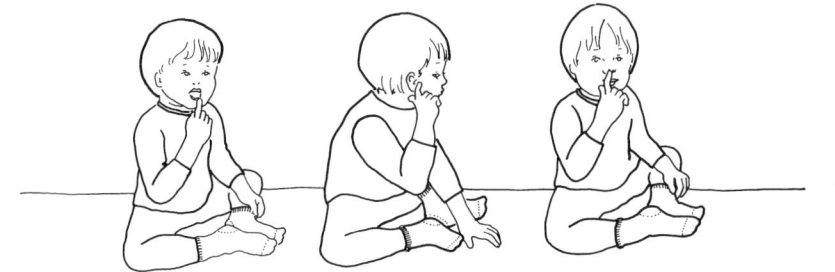

## Pointing to body parts in other people

Depending on his level of response, encourage him to identify parts of other people's bodies (Figure 3.13, Activity 51).

**Figure 3.13   Activity 51**
Pointing to body parts in other people

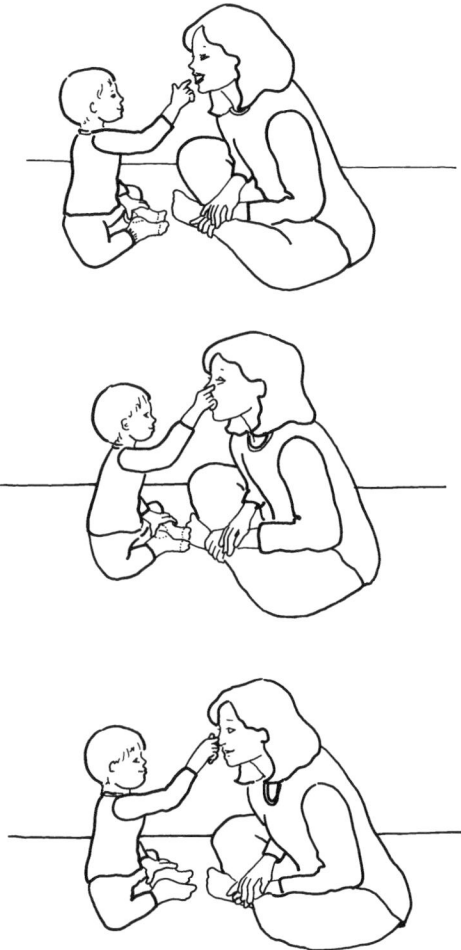

**Mirror play**

Children usually make movements, try out facial expressions and explore their bodies when they are in front of a mirror. The child will progressively associate movements of his own body with what he sees reflected in the mirror. In the child with CP these experiences may begin during the first year of life. The use of mirrors also provides feedback on movements, such as postural adjustments, thereby motivating him to participate in activities that foster motor development (Figure 3.14, Activity 52).

**Figure 3.14    Activity 52**
Mirror play

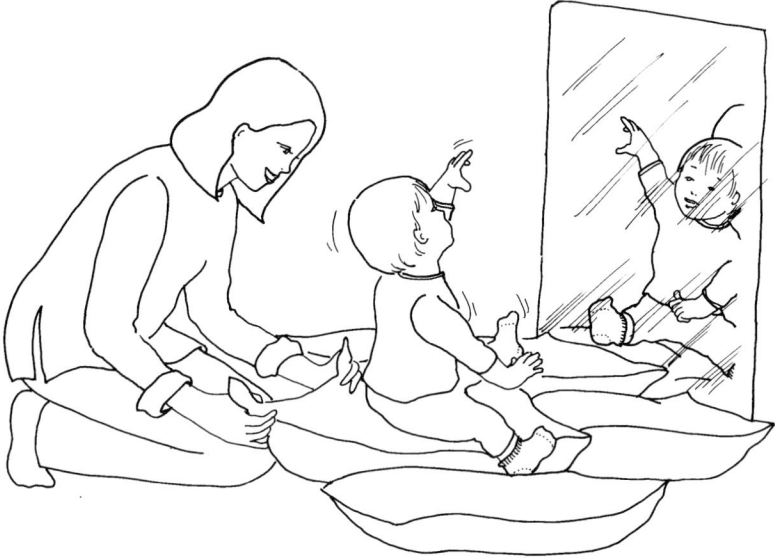

From the early stages of recovery, children and adolescents with TBI can be stimulated to identify and feel different parts of their bodies. Interactive games that associate tactile sensations with changes in positioning and verbal comprehension can help the child become aware of movement and different parts of his body.

**Balancing on a swing**

Kinesthetic perception and vestibular stimulation are important for children with brain injury. Vestibular dysfunction often persists in children after TBI and is a severe handicap for a growing child.[19] Frequently, children with TBI initially spend prolonged periods in hospital beds and this also interferes with kinesthetic information. As balance improves, some activities may help the child perceive different bodily positions and, above all, foster acceptance of postural changes and movement (Figure 3.15, Activity 53).

**Figure 3.15    Activity 53**
Balancing on a swing

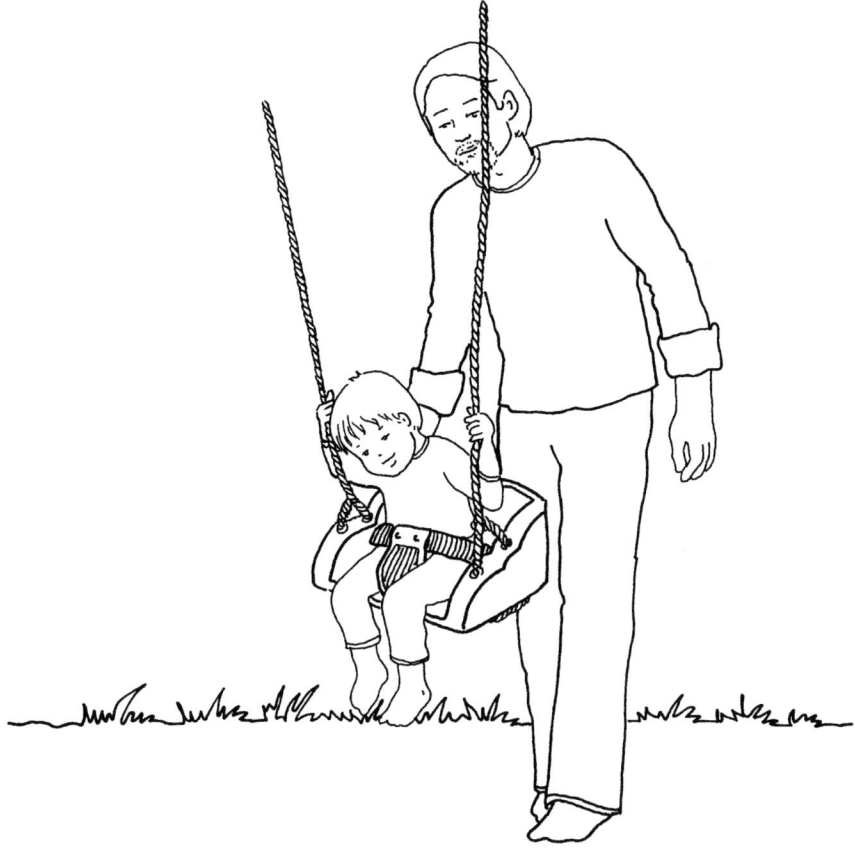

## Water play

When the child returns home, other alternatives can be explored. For example, playing in the water allows the child to integrate gentle movements with proprioceptive sensations. This activity can be performed either outdoors in a pool, or in the bath during cold weather, so long as the child is allowed to play during this time (Figure 3.16, Activity 54).

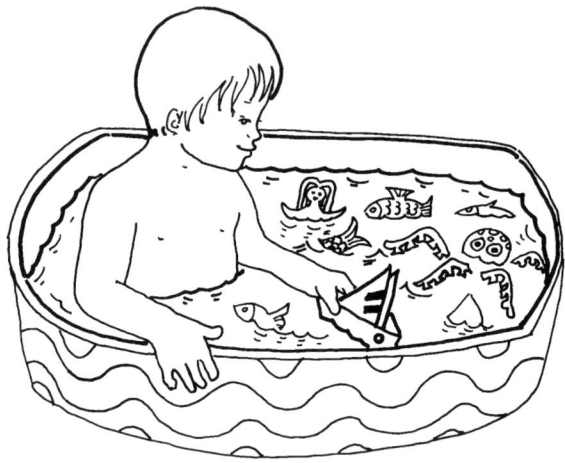

**Figure 3.16    Activity 54**
Water play

## Sand play

Playing in the sand is another activity that can be integrated into the child's daily and school life. Children usually enjoy this activity, which gives them a chance to explore tactile perception using different parts of their body and experience the feeling that their body is a unit (Figure 3.17, Activity 55). By bringing the child to the playground, you will be giving him the opportunity to have social interactions outside the family environment. These activities are also important for children with diplegic and hemiplegic types of CP, who have impaired perception of the location of the affected body parts.[20]

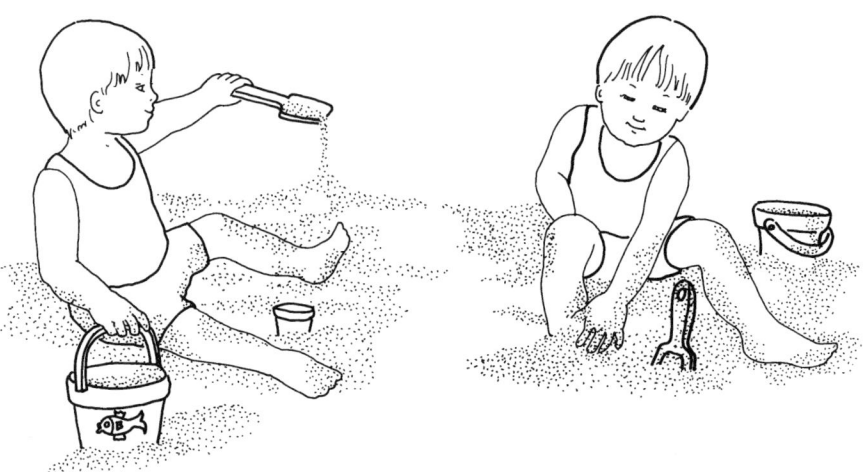

**Figure 3.17    Activity 55**
Sand play

## *Representations*

Symbolic thought in the child is the mental capacity to conceptualize an object, person or event in its absence. Children demonstrate the ability to imagine things that are not present (manifested in the search for hidden objects), solve problems, engage in symbolic play, and imitate events long after they have taken place.[7;18] Symbolic thought also allows children to use one object, event, or person to represent another. Developing this capacity gives children new ways of participating in and dealing with his surroundings.

### Hide-and-seek

Tasks that involve hiding an object and encouraging the child to search for it will help him formulate suppositions and inferences based on experience and observation. Draw the child's attention to where toys and household objects are placed and help him reach for an object that is outside his visual field, but be sure he saw it being put away (Figure 3.18, Activity 56).

**Figure 3.18   Activity 56**
Hide-and-seek

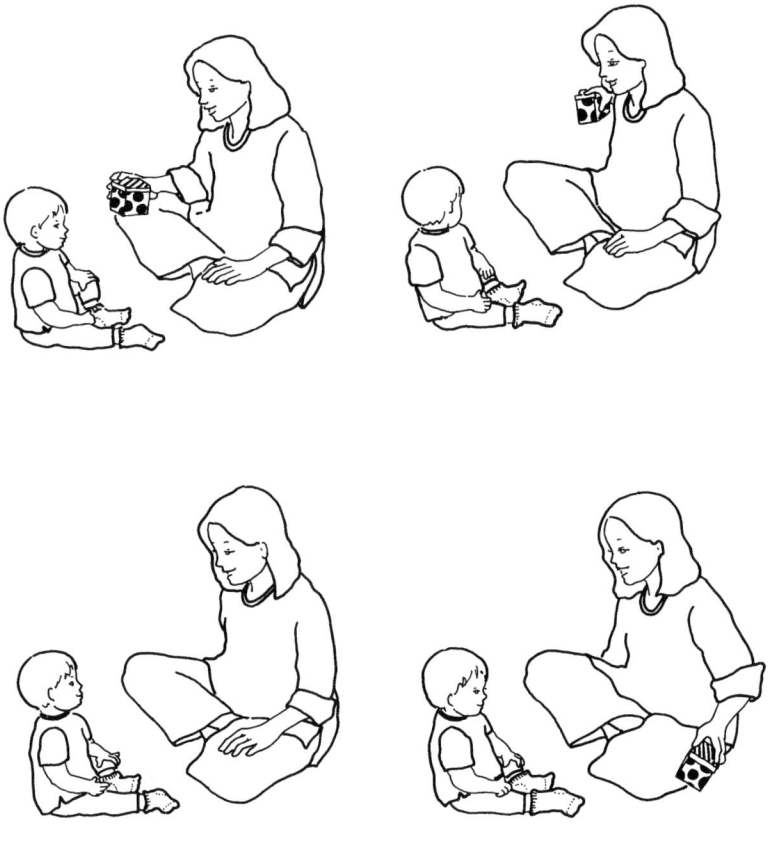

**Looking for objects that have been moved**

Another option is to simply play hide-and-seek. It is important to give the child verbal clues that enable him to formulate his own suppositions and, at the same time, encourage him in his search[21] (Figure 3.19, Activity 57).

**Figure 3.19    Activity 57**
Looking for objects that have been moved

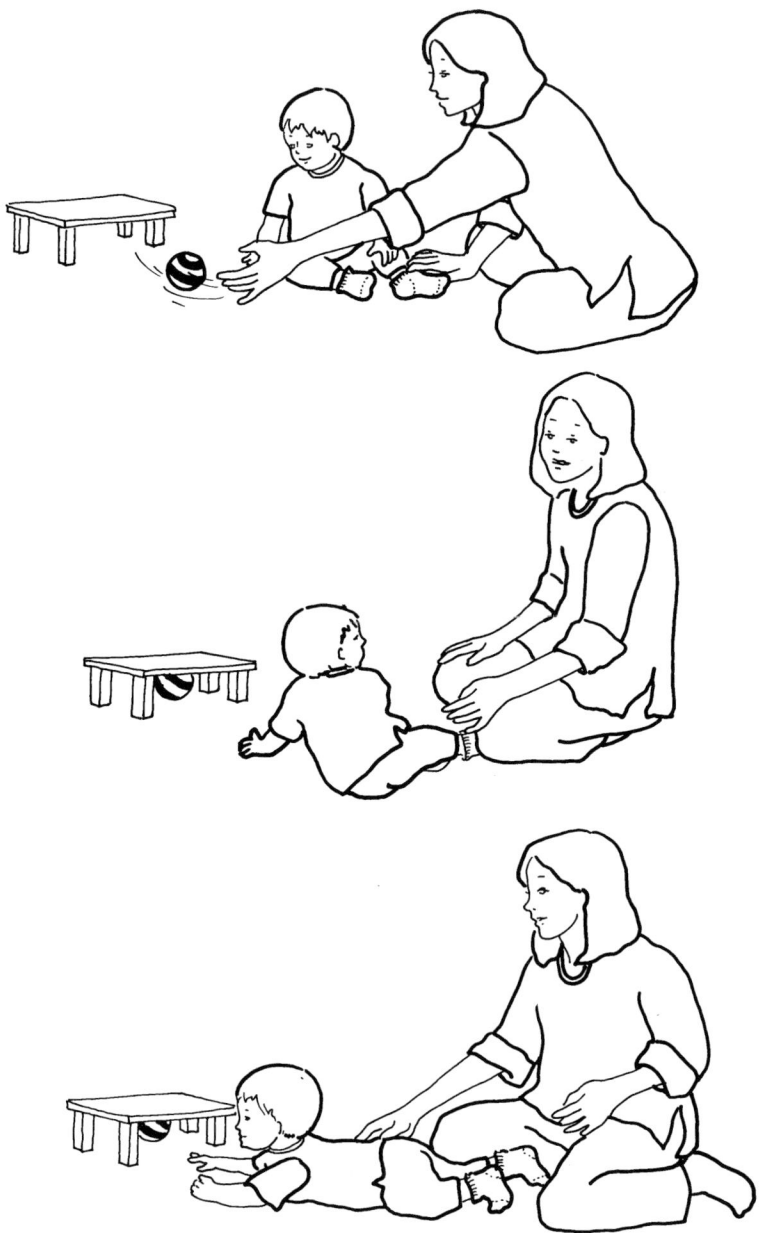

**Simple role playing**

In his day-to-day life, the child observes the way people act and how objects work. He may then play out events and invent his own variations of them. The child tends at first to repeat daily experiences, such as feeding a doll and putting it to sleep. Through symbolic thought, he engages in make-believe activities. For example, encourage the child to engage in symbolic play, such as getting him to talk on a toy telephone and then offering him a real phone so he can continue the pretend conversation (Figure 3.20, Activity 58).

**Figure 3.20    Activity 58**
Simple role playing

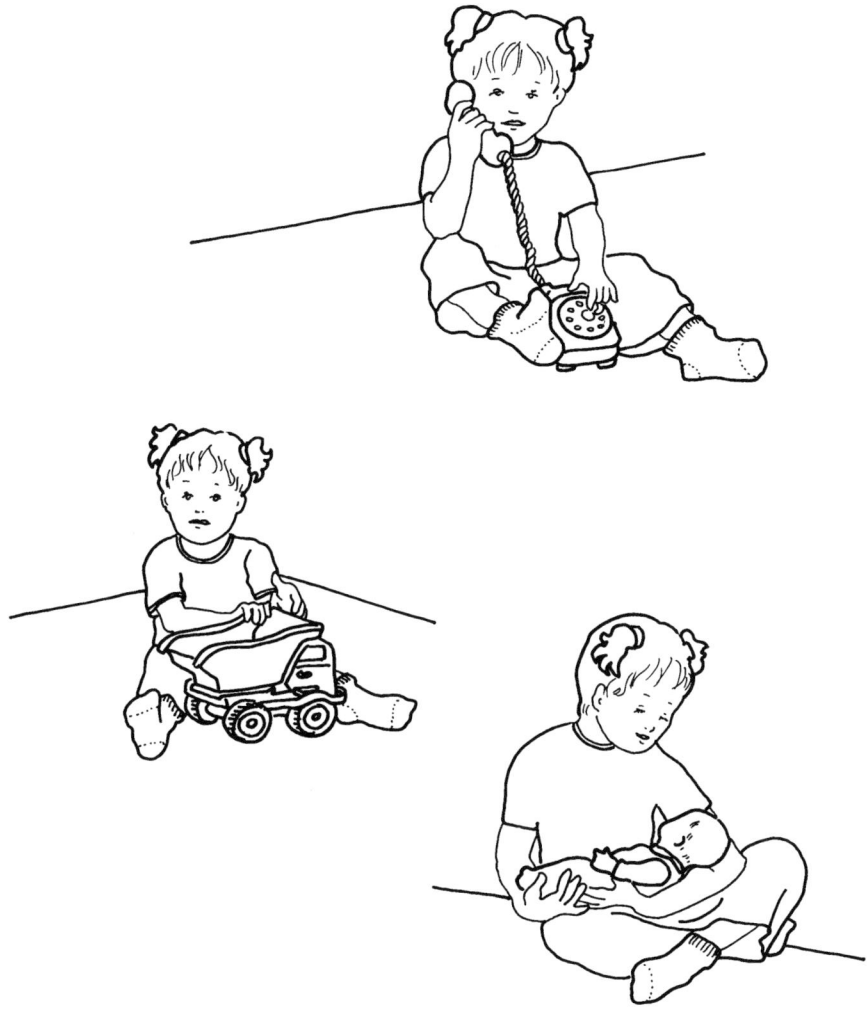

**Learning basic concepts**

The capacity for representative thought also helps the child develop basic concepts based on the perceptual characteristics of objects.[7,13,18] Draw the child's attention to these concepts by talking to him in contextualized situations in daily life. Call his attention to the size of objects, such as a big ball and a small one; it is important to choose household objects or toys that are identical save for the difference in their size (Figure 3.21, Activity 59). Vary this activity to include daily life situations, e.g. ask him whether he wants a big or small piece of cake and so on. Concepts of spatial location will help give him greater independence in familiar settings; in day-to-day situations, ask him to reach for objects that are under or on top of furtniture (Figure 3.22, Activity 60) or ask him to retrieve objects that had been placed in a container (Figure 3.23, Activity 61). You can gradually create other situations in which the child can experience different spatial location concepts such as front, back, side and others that are associated with the child's and family's context. Other activities can also help the child understand concepts such as similar and different; for example, present him with 3 familiar objects, two identical and one different and ask him to point out the one that is unlike the others. At first, the differences between the objects can be very obvious, such as their color, size or shape because he may have difficulties paying attention to small details. Later on, he can be presented with objects with more subtle differences, which demand a greater capacity for abstact thinking (Figure 3.24, Activity 62).

**Figure 3.21    Activity 59**
Small and big

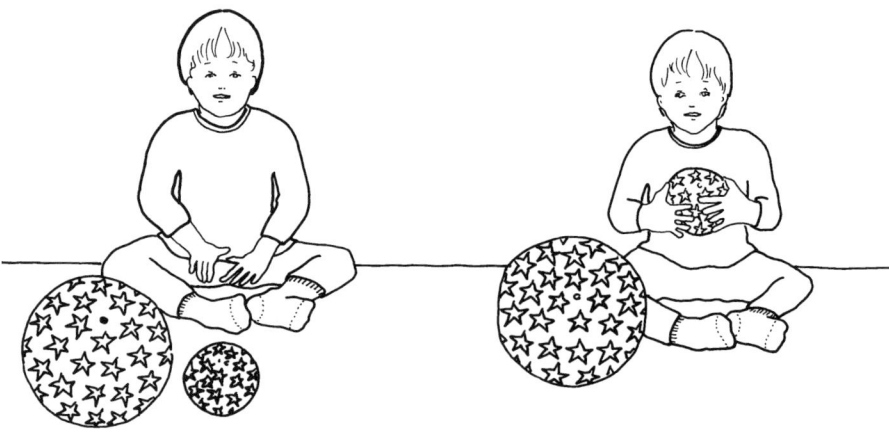

**Figure 3.22    Activity 60**
On top or on the bottom

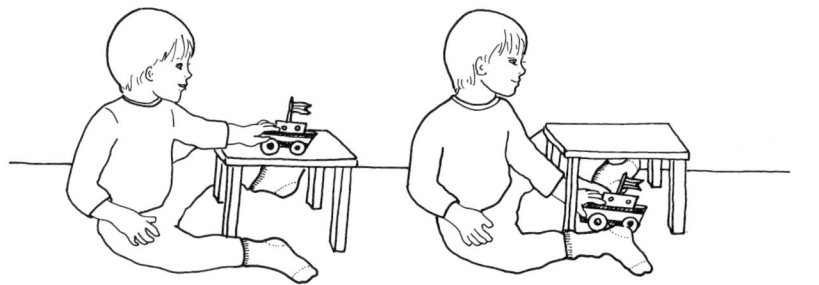

Puzzle boards are toys that can also promote the child's percetual development and his representative thinking (Figure 3.25, Activity 63). Furthermore, during conversations with the child, you may include the concept of shapes, for example, and call his attention to round objects such as the tires on a car, a CD, and others. Gradually the child will create these associations on his own. These are but a few of the day-to-day situations that you can explore to help the child develop basic concepts of size, similarity, spatial location and shapes.

**Figure 3.23   Activity 61**
Place and remove

**Figure 3.24 Activity 62**
Same and different

**Figure 3.25   Activity 63**
Shape board

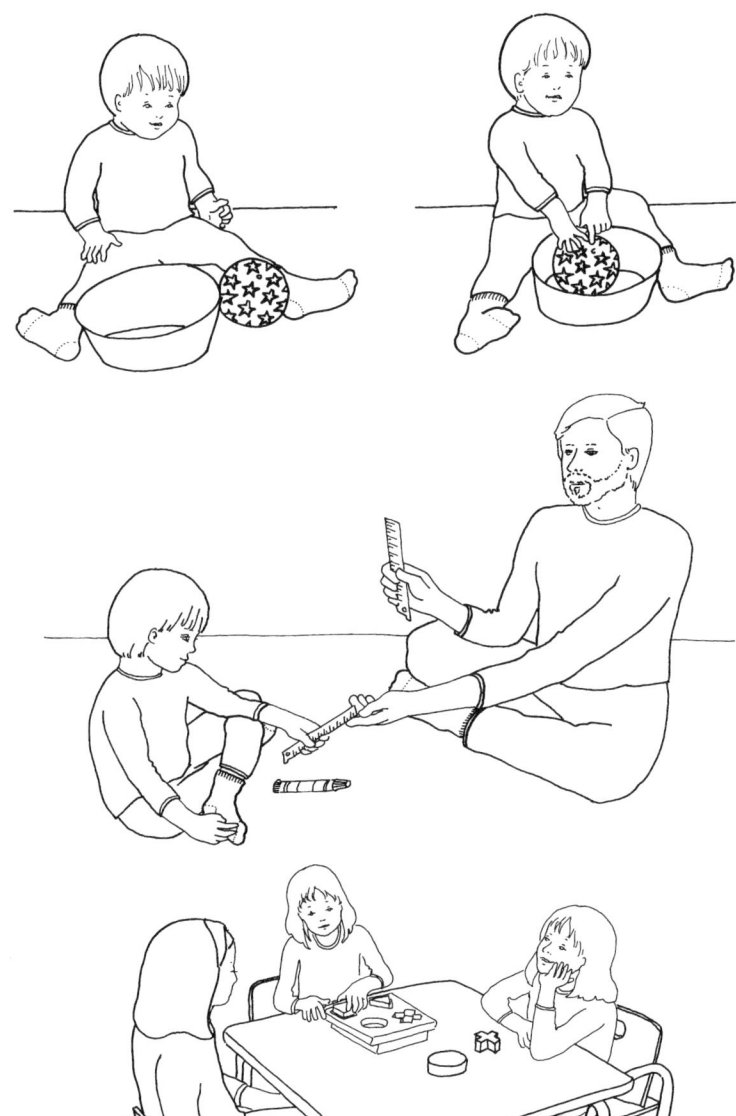

**Identifying body parts in a picture**

During this same stage of development, the child begins to understand simple symbolic processes, such as drawings and pictures. This acquisition can be stimulated, initially, by showing the child photographs of familiar people or drawings of simple objects or animals. You can also show him a picture of someone and ask him to help identify the parts of that person's body (Figure 3.26, Activity 64).

**Figure 3.26   Activity 64**
Identifying body parts in a picture

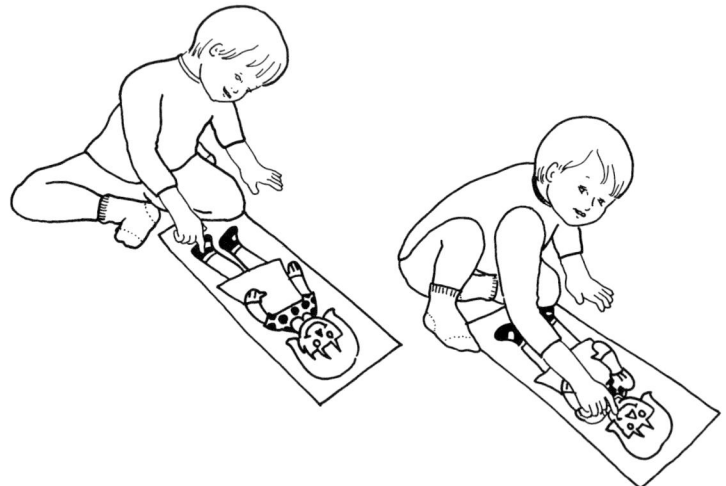

Numbers are abstractions. It is difficult to know exactly when a child begins to understand what a number is.[22] Before he is even aware of it, the child lives in a world pervaded by numbers: he has one mother, one body, several limbs, toys, family members, and so on. Daily life contains situations that naturally reinforce the notion of numbers and allow the child to formulate an analogical representation of quantity that precedes language.[23] As his language skills develop, the child starts to name numbers.

**Understanding quantity**

Children have many opportunities for counting during their daily routine. At first, show the child objects while working the concepts of one, two and many; then, the concepts of one, two, three and so on, successively. Later, add counting the child's fingers and toes out loud, buttons on a shirt, or the cookies placed in the jar. You can also gradually incorporate numeric concepts into conversations with the child. Asking him to reach for one or two or three toys is another way of helping him practice notions of quantity (Figure 3.27, Activity 65). Use children's songs to help him memorize number sequences.

**Figure 3.27    Activity 65**
Understanding quantity

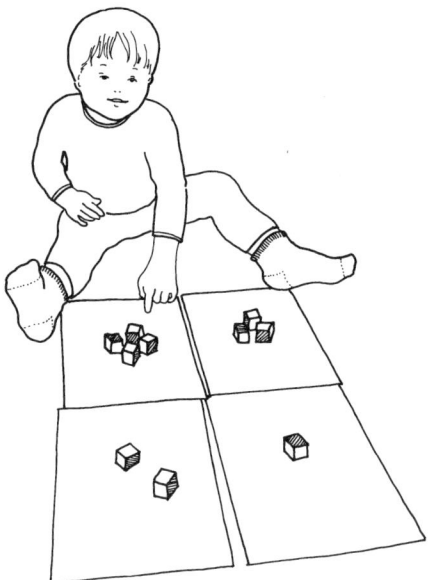

## Concept Development

The way that social activities are structured helps strengthen the child's cognitive organization.[4] The child partakes of different daily scripts in the context of the family's domestic life, in routines that include taking a bath, eating, and sleeping. Scripts are designs or plans that specify who participates in an event, what their social roles will be, which objects they will use and how the sequence should play out.[7] The child gradually becomes more adept at certain activities and takes on a larger role in that process. Scripts are guidelines for actions, mental representations that children and adults use to predict and plan the probable sequence of events in familiar circumstances. They can be generalized, providing a means for organizing concepts that apply to many types of events. An organized activity can take on many forms; for example, the child can group objects, people, events, or ideas into a structured whole: toys, members of the family, eating utensils, small objects, and so on. The child is, in all of these situations, building concepts and organizing his thoughts and ideas.[24–25]

The child's ability to learn, understand and express meaningful language and maintain adaptive behavior is dependent on clues found in familiar surroundings.[4] Daily life naturally affords the child various opportunities that foster his cognitive organization.

## Daily scripts

From an early age, the child begins to participate in, and understand, the interrelationship of daily events. He starts to formulate associations based on scripts that comprise his home life; for example, a very small child learns that when he is put to bed and the lights are turned off that it is time to go to sleep. The child's attention should be drawn to the different sequences of events that take place throughout the various activities inherent to daily domestic routines, and he will benefit from discussions about the details that comprise them (Figure 3.28, Activity 66).

**Figure 3.28   Activity 66**
Daily scripts

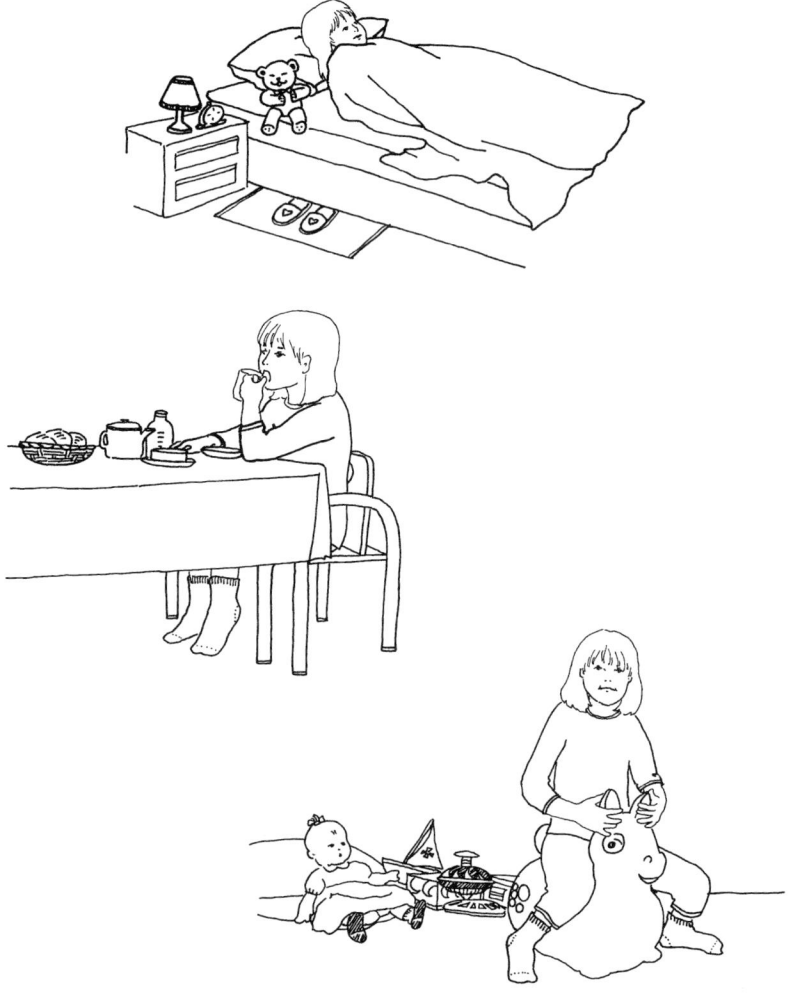

## Orientation

Encourage the child to pay attention to sounds inside and outside the home, name each one, ask him if he can hear them, and then help him associate them with the events that are taking place. Help him associate smells and aromas with the person or object that emanates them. Gradually, he will start to anticipate daily situations based on the clues provided by specific activities, and this will help him organize and orient himself in his day-to-day life (Figure 3.29, Activity 67).

**Figure 3.29   Activity 67**
Orientation

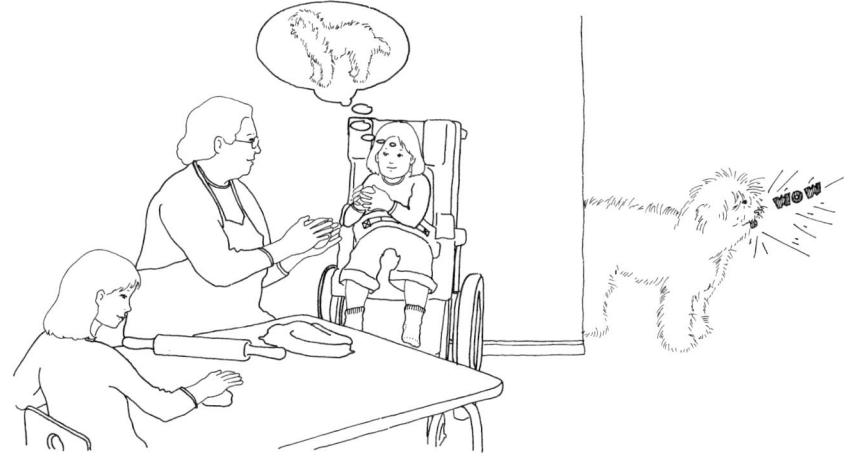

## Matching pairs

Identify situations that stimulate the child's interest in the basic properties of groups of objects. At first, the groups can be comprised only of objects that are identical and not those that share one common characteristic or function. When helping the child get dressed, for example, ask him to get the other shoe (after he already has one on), or request that he get a spoon identical to the one already on the table, or help him pair objects with which he is familiar (Figure 3.30, Activity 68).

**Figure 3.30   Activity 68**
Matching pairs

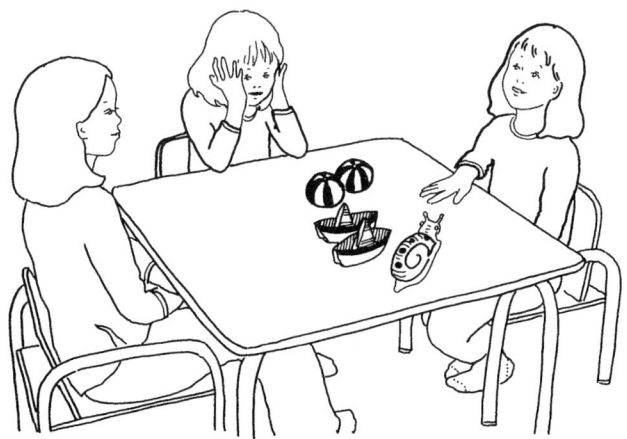

**What something does**

As the child's understanding of these concepts progresses, encourage him to use and improve his ability to identify these properties. It is important to talk to the child during day-to-day activities, helping him name and organize different objects that he uses for different tasks. For example, ask the child to help you set the table before a meal and separate the silverware, plates and cups. He will gradually form associations between the objects and their function. Show appreciation for this newly acquired knowledge and play at separating various items of his personal use such as toothpaste and toothbrush, plate and spoon, pencil and eraser, and then group them accordingly, all the while talking to him and helping him establish associations and organize groups (Figure 3.31, Activity 69).

**Figure 3.31    Activity 69**
What something does

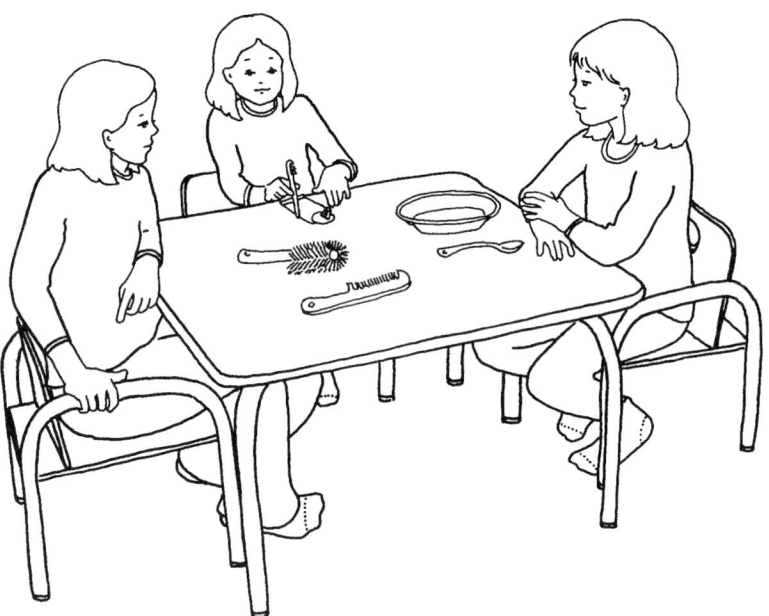

Concept formation is a creative process that helps solve problems.[26] As children acquire complex knowledge about objects and develop a greater capacity for language, they will be able to make more abstract conceptual representations.[27]

**Sorting by one physical characteristic**

When the child is engaged in an activity that involves classifying a group of objects such as wooden blocks of various colors, shapes, and sizes, help him choose one given trait and form a group of those items alone. Initially, he may use different associative principles during the task; for example, he may begin by sorting all the round blocks and then include a round yellow one in the group, after which he will continue grouping according to the color yellow (Figure 3.32, Activity 70). Organize daily life situations in a way that will provide opportunities for the child to establish associations, such as sorting his clothes from those of his brother, separating large spoons from small ones, forming small collections of boxes, lids, figures, or whatever else he fancies.

**Figure 3.32   Activity 70**
Sorting by one physical characteristic

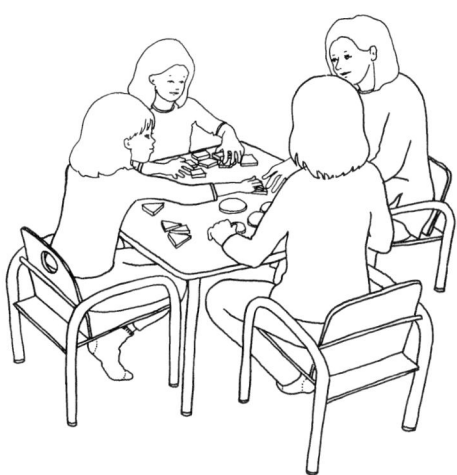

**Grouping by two physical characteristics**

As you begin to perceive the child's developmental progress, make playtime a little more complex by asking, for example, that he engage in activities that involve sorting groups of objects according to two physical characteristics, such as separating his socks from his sister's or gathering all the large, blue toys into a box (Figure 3.33, Activity 71).

**Figure 3.33   Activity 71**
Grouping by two physical characteristics

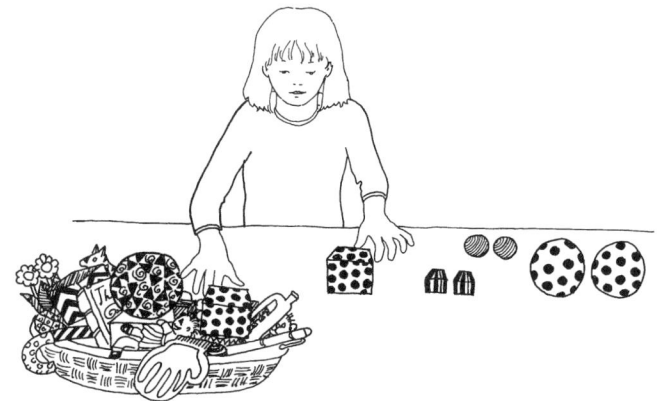

## Sorting and calculating

The child formally learns logical mathematical reasoning in school. Nevertheless, the knowledge that the child acquires during the first few years of life will reinforce his academic learning.[28] You can help the child count and associate the name of the number with the quantity, as well as the spatial order of the counting (Figure 3.34, Activity 72).

**Figure 3.34   Activity 72**
Sorting and calculating

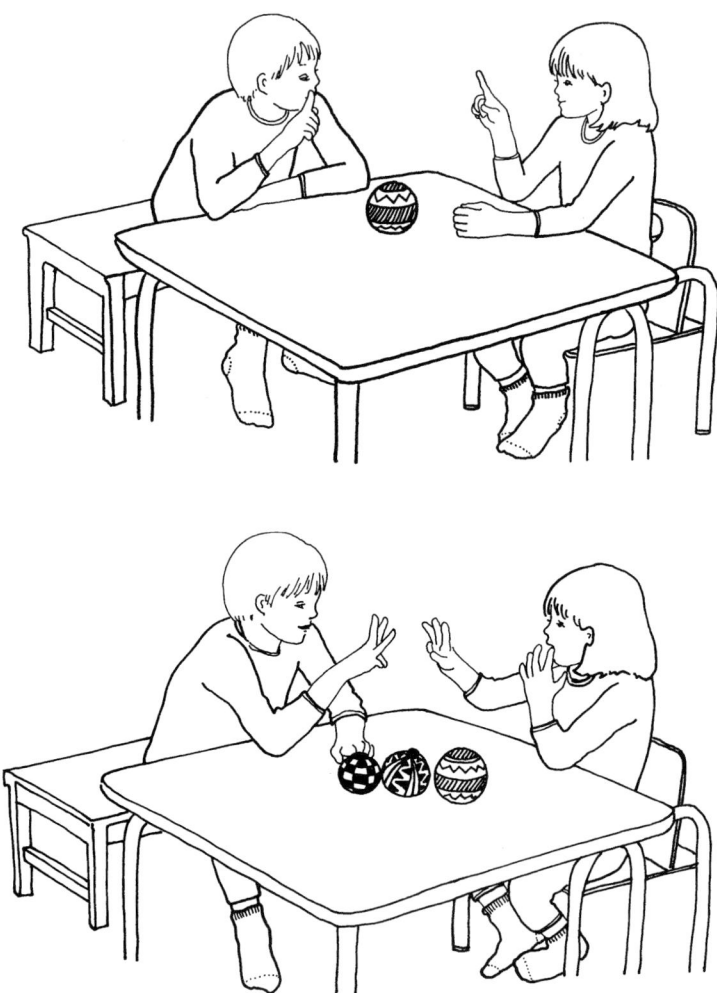

**Seriation**

You may also encourage the child to organize toys by size, such as the smallest to the biggest, and to place one inside the other or to form groups of a given item. You can ask him to point out the group that has fewer objects or play with him at separating things (Figure 3.35, Activity 73).

**Figure 3.35    Activity 73**
Seriation

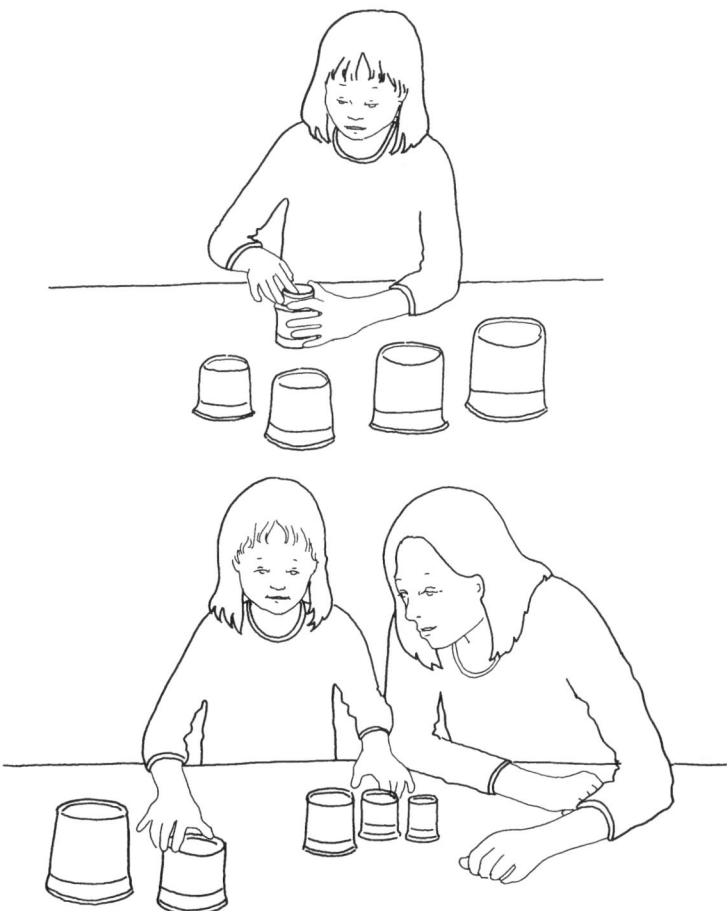

*Playing Games*

Group games entail interacting with others, which presupposes a reciprocal action between the participants. By interacting socially, the child anticipates the other's action and develops complex, self-regulatory behaviors; his emotions are both regulated by, and regulators of, the situation.[29]

Culture helps determine the types of games a child will play throughout childhood. Children's games are characterized by the incorporation and transformation of values passed on from generation to generation. Children with brain injury can benefit greatly from interactive games with siblings or friends. It is important for the child to experience situations that foster the development of behaviors that require emotional control.

**Group play**

Throughout development, children modify both their participation in and organization of interactive games. The child's first experiences with interactive games can begin with simple activities such as playing ball with siblings (Figure 3.36, Activity 74).

**Figure 3.36   Activity 74**
Group play

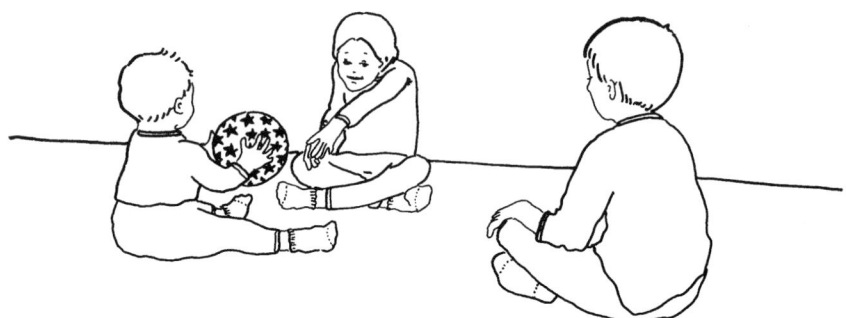

Games that involve children with various levels of knowledge open up the gateways to learning.[30] Furthermore, group games promote attention development. During an interactive game, the child needs to pay attention to what he is doing, what the others are doing, and how the game is proceeding.

**Role playing**

During games of make-believe, the child confronts, reorganizes and integrates the cognitive complexities of the adult world into his range of cognitive schemata.[3] Gradually, symbolic play becomes more complex; children start to represent and engage in various roles, routines and social scripts. The child naturally acquires an interest in these games during his developmental process. You can motivate him in his daily representations by giving him household items, articles of clothing, hats, accessories, and the like (Figure 3.37, Activity 75).

**Figure 3.37   Activity 75**
Role playing

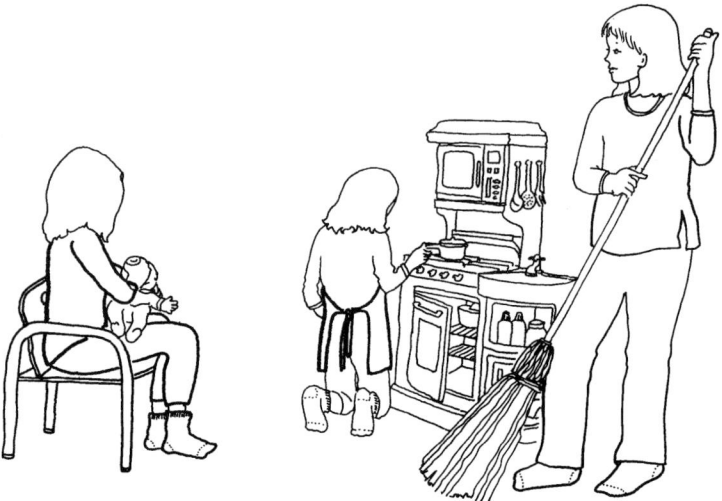

**Playing with figurines**

Children also engage in symbolic play when they are alone, frequently using miniatures such as farm sets, kitchen utensils, toy gas stations, and doll-houses (Figure 3.38, Activity 76). Children with fine manual coordination deficits can benefit from having magnets affixed to certain objects, making them easier to handle. A child uses games of make-believe to experiment with activities he is not yet allowed to do by himself, such as carrying a tray with cups or holding and changing a baby.[7]

**Figure 3.38   Activity 76**
Playing with figurines

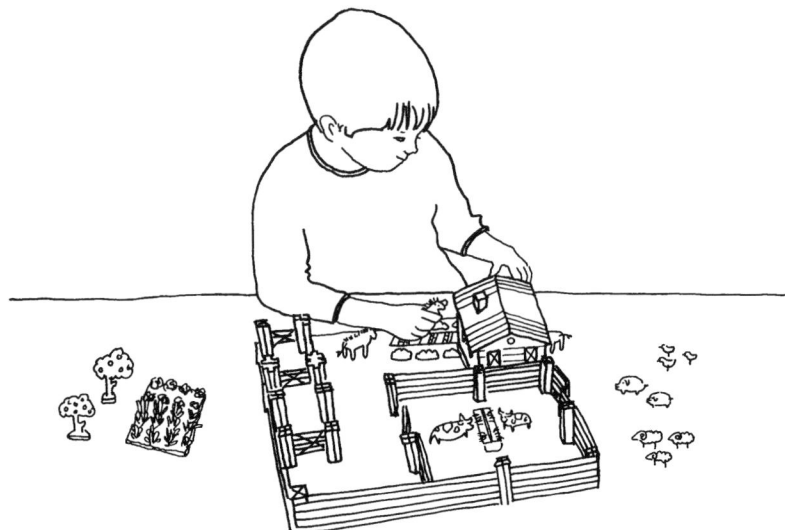

## Adult–Child Interaction and Cognitive Development

Several studies have shown an association between the adult style of inter-acting and the child's development of various cognitive skills, including memory, planning, organization of thoughts, and organization of lan-guage.[31–36] Ylvisaker and colleagues[37–38] captured this style with the terms col-laboration and elaboration, and have applied the themes to cognitive intervention for children with disability (see Table 3.1). A collaborative style is one in which the adult refrains from quizzing the child and from being overly directive, but rather cooperates with the child in producing interest-ing and connected thoughts as they converse. An elaborative style is one in which the adult introduces more and more connected ideas so that the child's understanding grows even as they enjoy the conversation. Much of the research has been based on adult–child co-constructed narratives about life experiences that they have shared, but the topic of conversation can be anything interesting and the context can be shared book reading, dinner con-versation, or any other opportunity for relaxed interaction.

---

**Table 3.1**
**Interactive collaboration and elaboration competencies associated with cognitive development in children**

**Collaboration competencies**

*Collaborative intent*
The conversation partner:
• Shares information (versus quizzing)
• Uses collaborative talk (e.g., "Let's think about this")
• Communicates understanding of the child's contribution
• Invites the child to evaluate own contribution
• Confirms the child's contributions
• Shows enthusiasm for the child's contributions
• Makes effort to establish equal leadership roles

*Cognitive support*
The conversation partner:
• Gives information when needed (within statements or questions)
• Makes available memory and organization supports (e.g., calendar, photos, graphic planning systems, memory book, gestures)
• Gives cues in a conversational manner
• Responds to errors by giving correct information in a nonthreatening, nonpunitive manner

*Emotional support*
The conversation partner
• Communicates respects for the child's concerns, perspectives and abilities
• Explicitly acknowledges difficulty of the task (e.g., "It's hard to put all these things in order, isn't it?")

*Questions: positive style*
The conversation partner
• Asks genuine questions (i.e., not a quiz) in a nondemanding manner
• Asks questions in a supportive manner (e.g., questions include needed cues: "Do you need to get the paint first?")

*Collaborative turn-taking*
The conversation partner
• Takes appropriate conversational turns
• Helps the child express thoughts when struggle occurs (e.g., word finding difficulties)

**Elaboration competencies**

*Elaboration of topics*
The conversation partner
• Introduces/initiates topics of interest with potential for elaboration
• Maintains the topic for many turns
• Contributes many pieces of information to the topic
• Invites elaboration (e.g., "I wonder what happened ...''; "What do you think would happen if ...").

*Elaborative organization*
The conversation partner
• Conversationally organizes information as clearly as possible:
  • sequential order of events (e.g., "First we ..., then we ...")
  • physical causality (e.g., "The radio's not working because it got wet.")
  • psychological causality (e.g., "Maybe you don't want to do it because you're scared.")
  • similarity and difference (e.g., "Yes, they're the same because ...")
  • analogy and association (e.g., "That reminds me of ... because ...")
• Explicitly reviews the organization of information
• Makes connections when topics change
• Makes connections among day-to-day conversational themes

*Elaborative explanation*
The conversation partner
• Conversationally adds an explanation for events (e.g., "Maybe the fact that you were sick at the time had something to do with it.")
• Invites explanations for events (e.g., "Why do you suppose ...?")
• Invites discussion of problems and solutions (e.g., "I wonder whether we can think of a better way to handle this if it comes up again.")
• Invites the child to address problems and solutions
• Reflects on the child's physical and psychological status (e.g., "You must have felt miserable about that.")
• Invites the child to reflect on his physical and psychological states

This positive style of adult–child interaction is associated with the developmental theories of Lev Vygotsky[26] and has been described with two popular metaphors: *apprenticeship*,[39] suggesting that children serve an apprenticeship in thinking as they interact with adults, and *scaffolding*,[40] suggesting that adults support the child by providing the information and connections that the child is not yet able to provide as they jointly construct increasingly complex thoughts in their interaction. Remembering, planning, organizing, problem solving, valuing, and other cognitive processes thus begin as social interaction and gradually become internalized or appropriated by the child with repeated exposure to the more mature level of thinking. In this sense, the verbal-cognitive mediation of adults or more mature children shapes the developing thought processes and cognitive self-regulation of less mature children.

In this way, everyday conversation can be a powerful tool in cognitive rehabilitation. Much of the research is based on preschool cognitive development. However, since Plato wrote his Socratic dialogues, it has been recognized that conversation is a useful context for teaching higher levels of thought. Thus these themes apply to rehabilitation of children and adolescents of all ages beyond infancy.

Consistent with this Vygotskyan theme, Landry and colleagues have more recently documented a significant relation between parents' interactive style and growth in the child's executive self-regulatory functions, specifically problem-solving skills.[41–42] Parental scaffolding (including hints, prompts, and other verbal supports) at age 3 predicted scores on executive function measures at age 6. Because many adults take over the executive, self-regulatory aspects of functioning for children with disability, they should be alerted to the importance of engaging their children in executive function scripted routines, providing whatever support may be necessary.

Ylvisaker and Feeney[43] proposed a rehabilitation framework within which the executive, self-regulatory aspects of behavior become a component of everyday adult–child interaction. Table 3.2 includes examples of executive function scripts that should be delivered in a supportive, conversational manner, using language that the child understands and to which the child reacts positively.

Similar scripts can be devised for problem-solving routines, strategy exploration routines, and the like. The goal is to associate the scripts with the everyday occurrences for which that self-regulatory thought process would be helpful. With repetition and gradual reduction of supports, these scripts can then be internalized by the child as relatively automatic self-regulatory thought processes, triggered by relevant environmental events.

**Table 3.2**
**Examples of executive function/self-regulatory interactive scripts**

**Goal–Plan–Do–Review script**

- This is the goal (what you want to accomplish, make happen)
- We need a plan; how about . . .?
- Do it
- Review it: How did it work out? What worked for you? What didn't work?

**Hard/easy script**

- This seems to be kind of hard (or easy) for you
- I think it's hard (easy) because . . .
- Because it's hard, you should probably . . .
- There's always something that works

**Big deal/little deal script**

- I think this is a big deal (or not a big deal)
- It's a big (or little) deal because . . .
- Because it's a big (little) deal, you . . .
- There's always something that works.

# School

School is an environment for adult–child interaction and for children to interact with their peers. There are various issues related to the education of this group of students and it is essential that the educational program be flexible enough to accommodate these needs; the program must be organized around the strategies that tend to change over time.[5] It is important to place the child in nursery school or preschool as early as possible. The activities engaged in during the first few years of life are naturally reinforced and given continuity through formal schooling. Furthermore, it is in school that children will encounter different opportunities for gradually developing and exercising their independence, deepening their social relationships and integration while in a protective setting that is organized to foster their development.

# School-aged children and adolescents with traumatic brain injury

After hospitalization, parents and children are confronted with immediate difficulties in day-to-day life and uncertainties about the future. When the child or adolescent returns to school, their educational and emotional needs will be different from what they were prior to the TBI.[43] It is a delicate moment. Many children and adolescents are aware of the changes that took place in their lives; close friends, classmates and teachers tend to compare what they are like post-injury with their behavior and performance before the injury. This is a natural process that many times signals a special concern for and interest in the child or adolescent; however, classmates and teachers will also need assistance in dealing with the post-TBI reality. Despite the tendency to make comparisons between the child's performance before and after, these should be avoided, especially in front of him, for they may affect his self-esteem. Instead, everyone around him should try to think about the progress that he has made since the injury and consider how they, together, can help him resume his developmental process.

The following section will describe some of the main difficulties that the school-aged child and adolescent may experience after TBI, as well as activities that can be performed in a contextualized manner, in spontaneous and informal settings.

## Consciousness and Orientation

Orientation, in other words, consciousness of the "I" in relation to one's environment or setting, requires consistency and integration of attention, perception, and memory.[44] The immediate effects of a sudden trauma to the brain can cause loss of consciousness, which can last from a few minutes to several months.

As children and adolescents begin to regain consciousness, they become increasingly responsive to external stimuli. During this phase, considerable movement is common and they may become agitated, at times even irritable or aggressive. They may be able to respond to simple commands and can concentrate for short periods of time, but will have difficulties sustaining their focus. These children and adolescents may also be disoriented with regards to personal, spatial and temporal information.

Some aspects of this disorientation may result from impaired memory of events prior to the injury (loss of retrograde memory) and/or difficulties with memory and retention of new post-injury information (loss of antero-grade memory). At the same time, the child or adolescent may be unaware of the deficits acquired after the TBI (anosognosia); in other words, he may not be able to perceive his difficulties.

**Personal orientation**

In the early stages of post-TBI recovery, the family can help orient the child or adolescent by explaining where he is, telling him stories about his childhood, and providing a few personal facts about who he is. If the child is still in the hospital, the room should be decorated with photos and other familiar objects from home (Figure 3.39, Activity 77).

**Figure 3.39   Activity 77**
Personal orientation

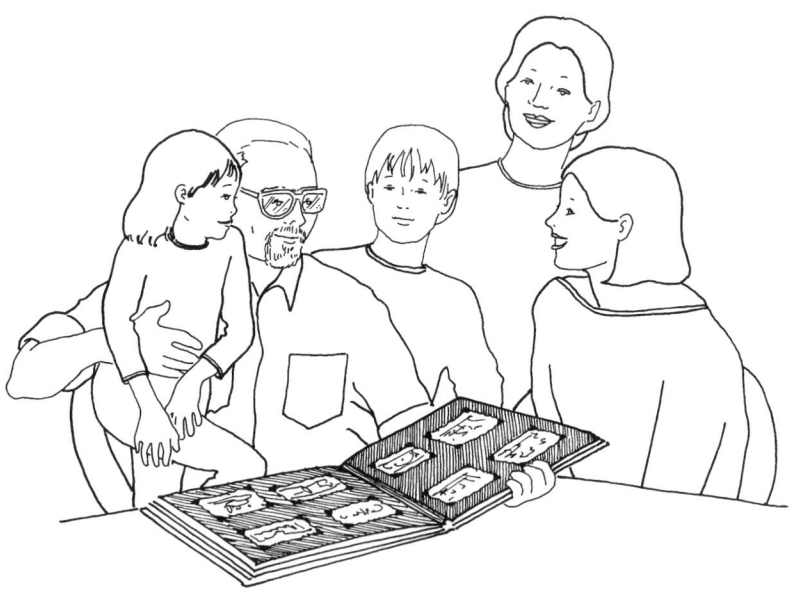

**Temporal orientation**

Having a calendar on hand with information about the day of the week, month, and year can help the child or adolescent recover his temporal orientation. This calendar should be placed where he can easily see it, and should be large enough and brightly colored to capture his attention and interest (Figure 3.40, Activity 78).

**Figure 3.40   Activity 78**
Temporal orientation

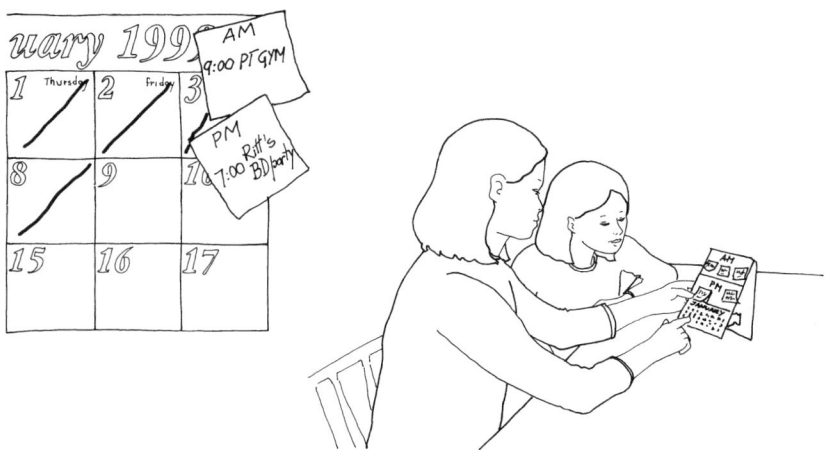

**Daily routines**

Agendas can also serve as a place to note down the child's activities and events for the day, week, or month. You can help or mediate the creation of the chart, whose contents should be written in with the child's or adolescent's participation, whenever possible. The schedule of activities should not be excessive. Try to include recreational activities and moments for relaxation, which are important for recovery (Figure 3.41, Activity 79).

**Figure 3.41   Activity 79**
Daily routines

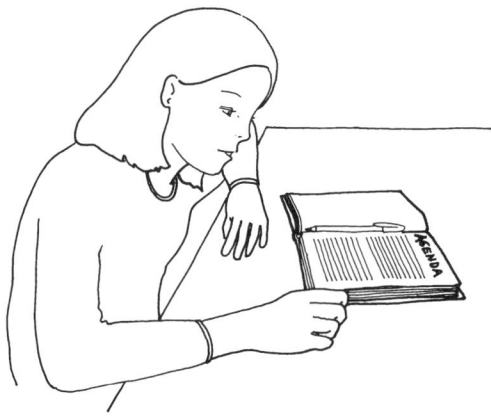

## *Attention*

Attention is a basic function, one of the prerequisites for effective learning and adequate functioning of all the domains, such as memory, language, and perception.[44] Intact attention is necessary for the execution of tracking activities (e.g., problem solving and following a sequence of ideas) and concentration.

After the TBI, the child's and adolescent's attention may be impaired on various levels and they may have such deficits as delayed response to specific visual, auditory or tactile stimuli (focal attention) and difficulties concentrating and sustaining a constant response during an activity, which results in fragmented, confused perception of a situation (sustained attention). Furthermore, they may not yet be able to focus and stay focused on a situation without being distracted by what is taking place around them, in other words, focusing on what is relevant while isolating other interferences (selective attention). These factors can compromise the learning process.[45]

In addition to focusing, sustaining and selecting, it is important to know how to efficiently alternate and divide attention among the different stimuli in the surroundings. A child or adolescent with TBI may also have difficulties in these two dimensions: he may not be able to alternate his focus from one task to another, which will interfere in his ability to efficiently switch and change activities (alternating attention). Finally, he may lose his capacity to perform and pay attention to two or more things at once (divided attention); for example, in the classroom, the child may have trouble reading what is written on the blackboard and copying it down in a notebook.

Attention problems interfere with different aspects of the child's and adolescent's life, and the potential for new learning may be impaired.[45] There are a variety of ways to help them cope with attention deficits.

---

**Focusing attention**

In daily life, it is very important to reduce or eliminate the distractions and stimuli that compete with the child's objective; this will help him remain focused long enough to complete the activity. Homework should be done in a quiet place, as devoid as possible of distracting stimuli such as television, radio, nearby toys, or too many people (Figure 3.42, Activity 80).

**Figure 3.42   Activity 80**
Focusing attention

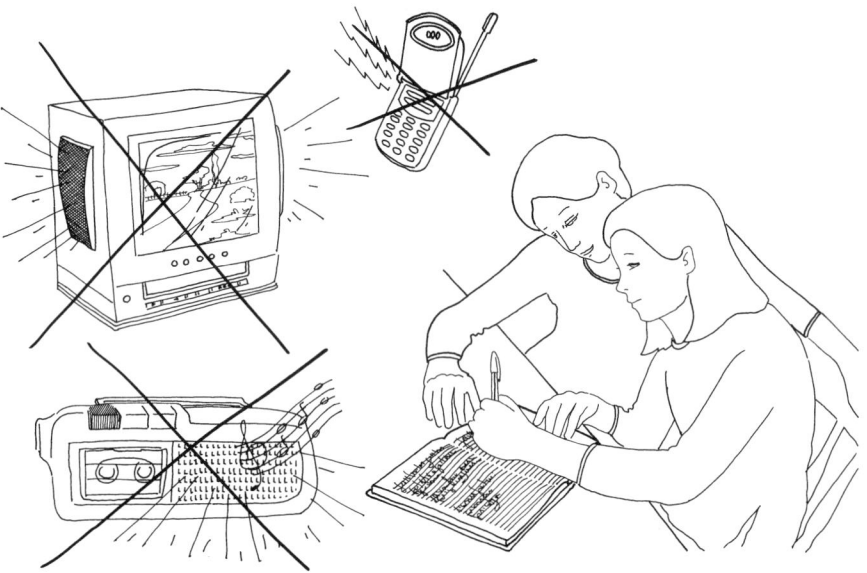

The team of school professionals may have difficulties dealing with the child's attention problems in the classroom. It is not always easy to apply strategies that worked well at home to the school setting. Sometimes a smaller school with fewer students per classroom and well-structured routines is best for the post-TBI child or adolescent, and, whenever possible, this option should be considered. An open, ongoing dialogue with the school team helps facilitate joint problem solving.

After the brain injury, it is common for the child and adolescent to tire more easily, and to perform activities at a slower pace. The intensity with which information is offered should be regulated, allowing for rest periods during and between activities. After the child or adolescent has completed an activity, be it academic or recreational, ask him to review what he has just done or is doing, and give him the chance and the supervision, when necessary, to make eventual corrections.

## Heminegligence

After brain injury, an adolescent may be unable to direct his attention to one side of his body, causing him to perceive only the objects, individuals and stimuli situated on the other side (heminegligence). This disorder is often reflected in activities of daily life and school tasks. For example, if the neglected side is on the left, he may not touch the food on the left side of his plate or, during a reading exercise, he may not read the words or phrases written on the left side of the page.

### Body and spatial perception

Development of contextualized activities is the most efficient path to discovering alternative means of compensating or overcoming these difficulties, which will be most evident in day-to-day activities. These strategies are generally simple and basically involve presenting stimuli on the neglected side. For example, at home, when approaching the child, do so from the neglected side as often as possible; this will help him explore his setting as a whole. In the bedroom, furniture such as nightstands or lamps, personal items, bedtime books, stereo, television, and others, can be placed on the neglected side. However, make these changes in the child's environment gradually and be attentive to his response to each change. If, for example, the child or adolescent stops watching television because it is positioned on his neglected side, the set should be moved to the midline where he will be better able to see it; then, it should be slowly moved by degrees, each day, towards the neglected side, but only if he continues to pay attention to the television as it moves to the other side. During reading and writing tasks, inserting a catchy stimulus in the margins of the neglected side, such as a red label, can stimulate the child or adolescent to use and perceive the entire page (Figure 3.43, Activity 81).

**Figure 3.43    Activity 81**
Body and spatial
perception

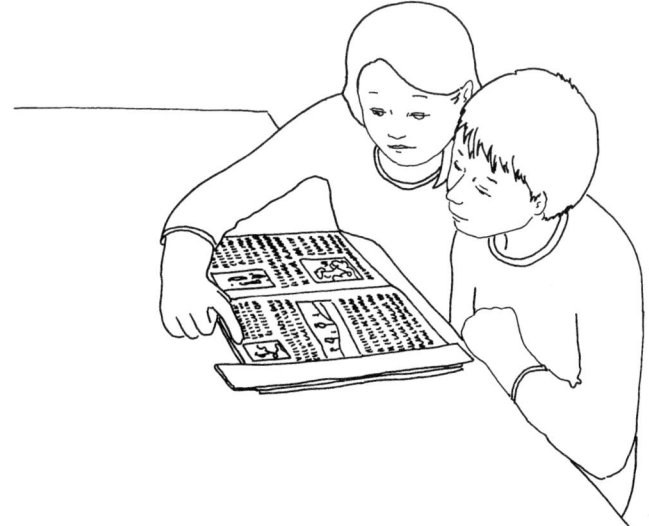

The child and adolescent can be encouraged to explore both sides of their bodies in a more symmetrical way during self-care activities such as bathing or showering, dressing or personal hygiene, e.g., while combing their hair.

## Memory

Memory is a function that allows the brain to store information and later retrieve it. There are various types of memory: *declarative* or *explicit memory* is the conscious access of stored information, the memory of facts and events such as the names of people and cities, and historical data; *non-declarative* or *implicit memory* is unconscious access resulting from automatization, such as the ability to drive, walk, ride a bike and tie a shoelace.[44]

As there are different types of memory, there are also different stages in memory processing: one refers to the capacity to store small amounts of information for a limited time (*short-term memory*) and the other is the ability to store large quantities of information for an indefinite period of time (*long-term memory*).

Memory impairment is one of the most common disorders after TBI. The child or adolescent may have problems learning new things, as well as difficulties retaining and, consequently, retrieving information,[46] even though it is not yet known for certain at what stage this failure occurs. This impairment is one of the main reasons that students with TBI often fail when they return to school and when they attempt to perform some activities of daily life.

There are a variety of ways to help children and adolescents cope with memory deficits in the home, school and social settings. Strategies include alternative means of remembering and retaining new information (compensating the deficits) and others involve modifying and adapting the environment.[47] For example, at home, place the child's belongings, such as school materials, books, and personal items, always in the same place, which will make it easier for him to find them.

When interacting with the child, try to simplify and reduce the amount of information that you give him to help him retain this new data. Often while conversing with their child, the family will have to repeat themselves more than once and/or provide clues such as saying the first letter or part of a word to help his recall. The child and adolescent should be assisted in establishing their own pathways to remembering what is necessary, instead of promptly being given the complete answer.

## Visual and auditory retention

Some strategies may be useful to the teachers to help the student organize his behavior and not forget what he has to do, as well as to promote new learning at school and in daily life. It is helpful to reinforce verbally communicated information with drawings that facilitate his visualization of what is being said (Figure 3.44, Activity 82). When the information is similar to something he has already learned, the connection between the two should be pointed out and explained.

**Figure 3.44    Activity 82**
Visual and auditory retention

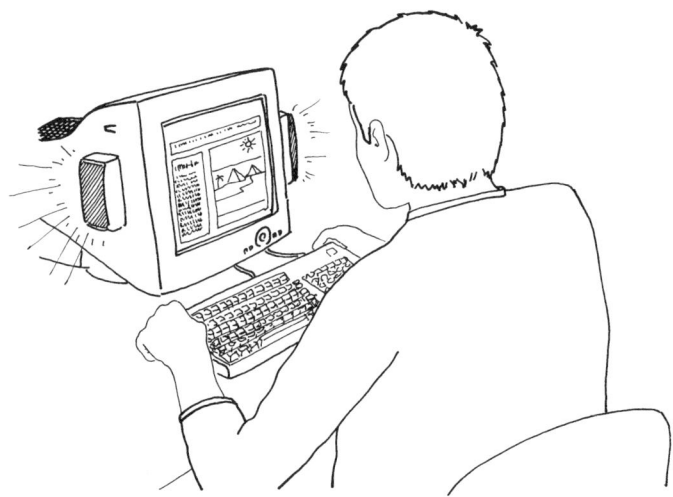

## Devices for memory

External resources that foster memorization of the activities to be performed can be very useful. Notebooks, schedules, agendas, and electronic devices such as calculators and digital watches with functions like alarms or fields for written messages can help the student who occasionally forgets to check his schedule (Figure 3.45, Activity 83).

**Figure 3.45    Activity 83**
Devices for memory

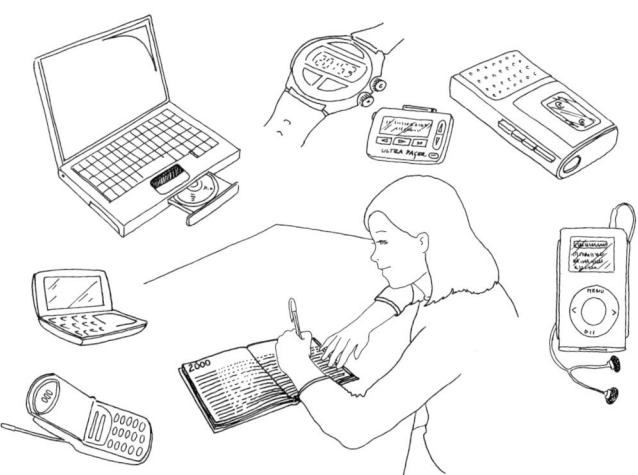

**Auditory retention**

If the child or adolescent is experiencing great difficulties retaining information that is verbally taught during class, using a tape recorder to tape the class so that he can listen to the information again at home can increase his chances of remembering the material (Figure 3.46, Activity 84).

**Figure 3.46 Activity 84**
Auditory retention

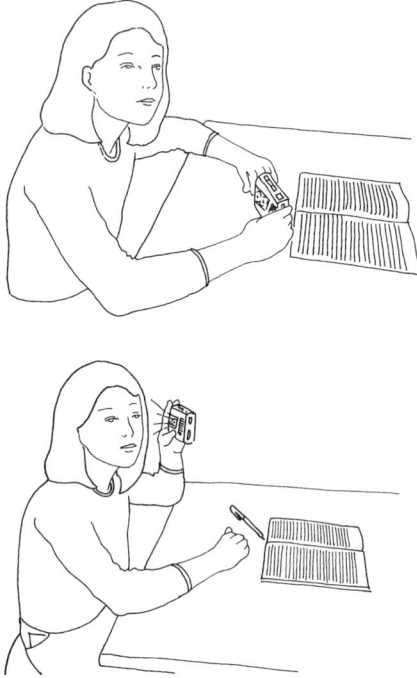

Memory deficits can be long term after TBI. Choosing which strategy to use is a very individualized issue and depends on the difficulties, potential and context of each child's or adolescent's life. It is important for the parents, rehabilitation team and teachers to discuss the child's difficulties and, together, consider what would be the best rehabilitation program for him, specific to his level of recovery and development.

## Executive Functions

The executive functions are skills and abilities that enable a person to successfully engage in and perform activities in an independent, intentional, and self-serving manner. They include components such as:

- volition
- planning
- purposive action
- effective performance

Traumatic brain injury can cause impairment of these executive functions.[4;45]

Impairment of the executive functions can also damage the child's or adolescent's ability to perform tasks that involve specific preserved skills. After a TBI, children and adolescents generally have difficulties organizing their lives and dealing with learning situations. For example, they are often unable to begin a task without first receiving considerable encouragement to do so. While doing their homework, they may read a problem but be unable to start solving it, not because they did not understand what they read, but for lack of a planning strategy that indicates a starting point. In other cases, the child or adolescent may present impulsive or perseverative behaviors, which can keep them from successfully performing a task. During a game, for example, they may have difficulties following the rules, even when the instructions are repeated. They may also have difficulties starting a conversation or adhering to logical reasoning, with their ideas in correct order and sequence.

**Following instructions**

At home and in school, parents and teachers can help the child compensate for his organizational and planning difficulties by helping him structure his daily tasks. Graphic organizers such as photos, figures, pictures, and symbols can help children through organizationally demanding tasks. It is important to verbalize the plan of action step-by-step and ask him to do the same before, during and after the task. When requesting a given action, your speech can help orient the child's or adolescent's attention and facilitate the completion of what is solicited.[48] Use situations in the child's daily routine to ask him to do simple, sequential tasks with which he is already familiar, such as opening a container, taking out a snack, and then putting the container away (Figure 3.47, Activity 85).

**Figure 3.47    Activity 85**
Following instructions

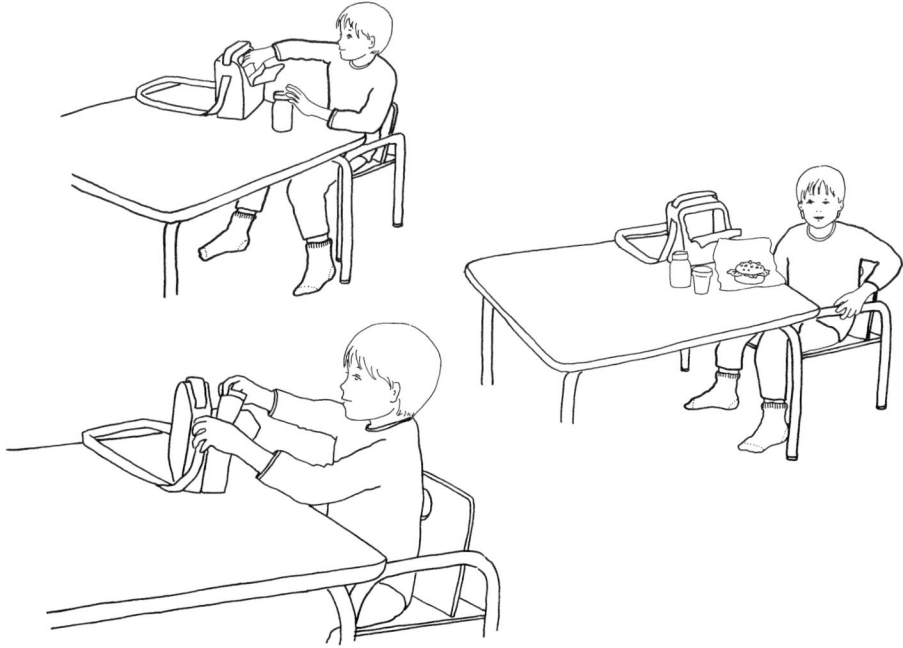

**Logical sequence**

Activities that simulate and reinforce the learning of practical situations and that involve a chain of sequential actions are also beneficial (Figure 3.48, Activity 86). Start with simple, well-structured activities, and provide the child with as much information and clues as possible. As the child and adolescent acquire greater initiative, planning, and organizational skills, clues will no longer be necessary and the tasks can gradually become more complex.

**Figure 3.48    Activity 86**
Logical sequence

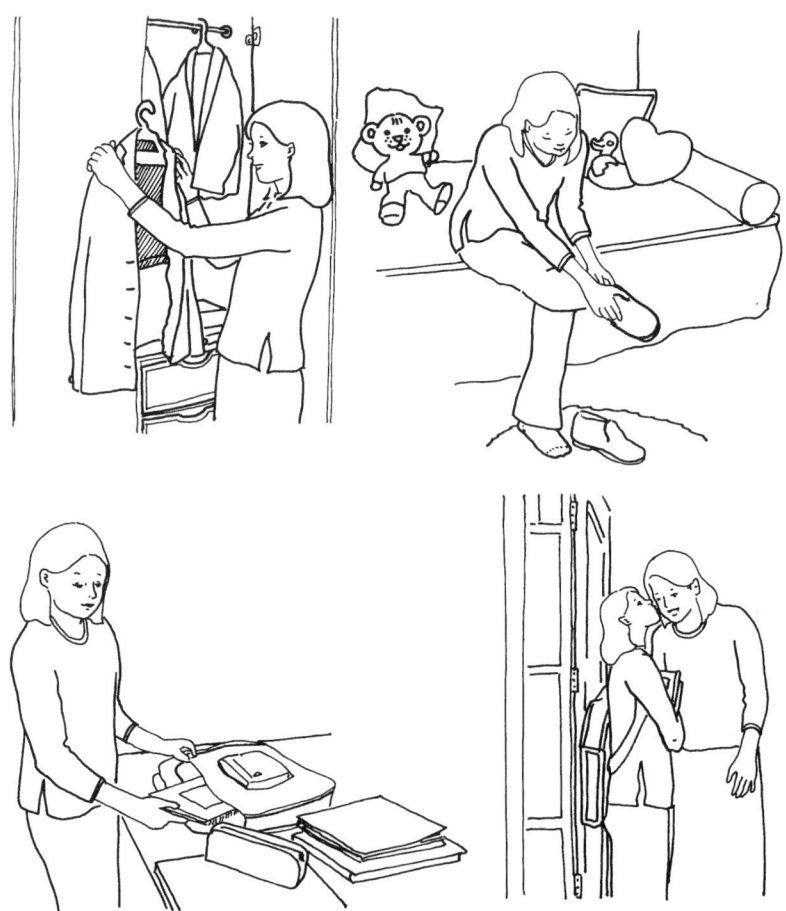

## Calculation

After a brain injury, children and adolescents may have several different types of calculation disorders; they may have difficulties dealing with numbers in their day-to-day life or their capacity to learn arithmetic concepts may be damaged.

## Calculation in daily life

Calculation skills are used in various daily life situations. An effective way to encourage the child and adolescent to train their calculation skills is to incorporate activities into their daily life routine. Using money to do calculation stimulates math skills and also helps them find solutions for day-to-day problems (Figure 3.49, Activity 87). To help, you can promote situations that are based on the child's or adolescent's interests, life context and individual potential. Attentiveness to his responses is important for he may experience specific difficulties and need different levels and types of assistance.

**Figure 3.49    Activity 87**
Calculation in daily life

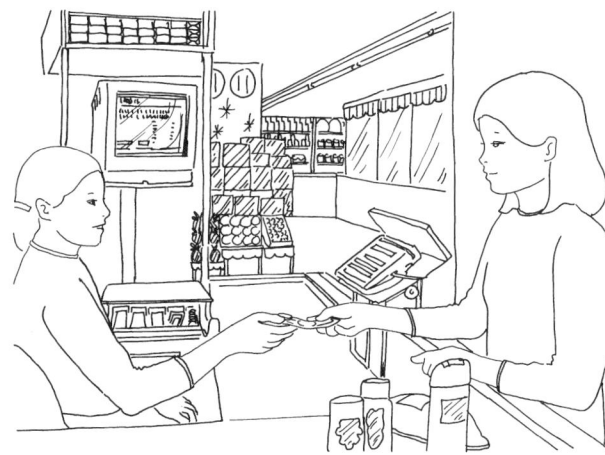

## Calculation strategies

Children and adolescents may have difficulties calculating because of damage to their *working memory* functions. This occurs when they are unable to store and manage information in a short period of time, a skill that is very important, for example, in doing mental-oral calculation or solving a more complex math equation. Mental-oral calculation is used extensively in daily life activities; in these situations, having support materials on hand such as pencil and paper, and writing down each step of the math problem may help the child and adolescent perform the calculation. Sometimes the child or adolescent may benefit from using a calculator (Figure 3.50, Activity 88).

**Figure 3.50    Activity 88**
Calculation strategies

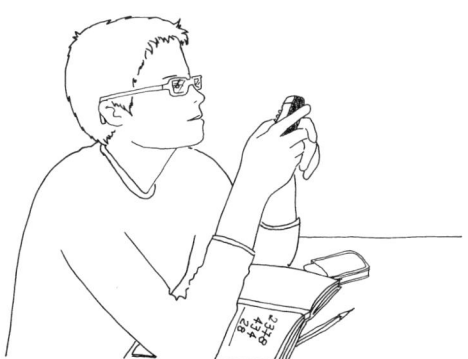

Another factor associated with post-TBI calculation disorders is difficulties *reading and writing numbers*. For example, the child is able to complete a simple two-plus-two calculation, but when giving the answer he says four and writes down five. Similar difficulties can also occur in dictations or reading of numbers; for example, the child reads the numeral thirteen (13) and writes it down as number three (3). This condition can also include difficulties understanding arithmetical signs, leading to mistakes in completing math problems. You can provide clues and help him understand the differences, but always be attentive to signs that he may be having too much difficulty. Remember to reassure him so that he does not feel like a failure, which can affect his self-esteem.

## Motor Apraxias

After TBI, children and adolescents may have problems performing voluntary movements, even if they do not have any difficulties controlling their movements or any sensory deficits (motor apraxias).[49] This can occur in various situations. For example, the child or adolescent may not be able to imitate a movement, but may be able to do it within a given context, i.e. he may be incapable of imitating the movements of locking a door, but when asked, he is able to open the actual door, even if with a certain degree of difficulty (ideomotor apraxia); or he may have difficulties using household items due to his inability to perform a complex sequence of coordinated movements, despite having an intact capacity for imitating (ideative apraxia); or he may have lost the ability to draw or copy a geometric figure or organize blocks in a certain way (constructive apraxia).[44]

It is important to try to show the child or adolescent the sequence of motor acts necessary for completing a task, and to try to contextualize the activity in such a way that he is able to use environmental clues to assist his motor behavior. For example, it is one thing to ask the child to do a hypothetical gesture, such as the motion of brushing his teeth; it is another to contextualize the motor act by, for example, having him brush his teeth in the bathroom, alongside his siblings or other family members, before bedtime.

Using models or fragments of motor sequences broken down into different components as a reference may also help. For example, you can perform with the child the activity that he is having difficulties with: stand beside him, make slow studied gestures, and give him enough time to keep up. Gradually, as his skill improves, reduce the amount of external references and, if possible, help him develop an awareness of reference points that can help him organize his behavior.

This chapter presented examples of activities for cognitive development and for minimizing the effects of neuropsychological disorders. More importantly, however, is the manner in which the child and the adult interact, the process of co-construction. Daily sharing of experiences can permit adults, whether members of the family or of the rehabilitation team, to construct increasingly complex cognitive processes in their interactions with the child. The cognitive development of the child with brain injury is ideally pursued within the context of supported routines of everyday action and interaction at home and in school.

# References

1.    Liptak GS, Accardo PJ. Health and social outcomes of children with cerebral palsy. J Pediatr 2004; 145(Suppl 2):S36–S41.

2.    Braga LW, Campos da Paz AJ. Neuropsychological pediatric rehabilitation. In: Christensen AL, Uzzell B, editors. International handbook of neuropsychological rehabilitation. New York: Kluwer Academic/Plenum, 2000: 283–295.

3.    Encyclopedia of Psychology. Washington, DC: American Psychological Association; Oxford: Oxford University Press, 2000.

4.    Ylvisaker M, Feeney T. Executive functions, self-regulation, and learned optimism in paediatric rehabilitation: a review and implications for intervention. Pediatr Rehabil 2002; 5(2):51–70.

5.    Braga LW. Cognição e paralisia cerebral: Piaget e Vygotsky em questão. Salvador: Sarah Letras, 1995.

6.    Talbot LR, Joanette Y. Postcomatose unawareness in a brain-injured population. J Neurosci Nurs 1998; 30(2):129–134.

7.    Cole M, Cole SR. O desenvolvimento da criança e do adolescente. 4th ed. Porto Alegre, Brazil: Artmed, 2004.

8.    Poggi G, Calori G, Mancarella G et al. Visual disorders after traumatic brain injury in developmental age. Brain Inj 2000; 14(9):833–845.

9.    Jacobson L, Ygge J, Flodmark O, Ek U. Visual and perceptual characteristics, ocular motility and strabismus in children with periventricular leukomalacia. Strabismus 2002; 10(2):179–183.

10.   Vasta R, Haith MM, Miller SA. Child psychology: the modern science. 2nd ed. New York: John Wiley & Sons, 1995.

11.   Zeman A. Consciousness. Brain 2001; 124(Pt 7):1263–1289.

12.   Piaget J, Inhelder B. A psicologia da criança. 19th ed. São Paulo: Difel, 2003.

13.   Piaget J. Seis estudos de psicologia. 24th ed. Porto Alegre, Brazil: Forence Universitária, 2003.

14.   Ylvisaker ME. Traumatic brain injury rehabilitation: children and adolescents. 2nd ed. Woburn, MA: Butterworth-Heinemann, 1998.

15.   Bauer PJ, Wiebe SA, Waters JM, Bangston SK. Reexposure breeds recall: effects of experience on 9-month-olds' ordered recall. J Exp Child Psychol 2001; 80(2):174–200.

16.   Chugani HT, Phelps ME. Maturational changes in cerebral function in infants determined by 18FDG positron emission tomography. Science 1986; 231(4740):840–843.

17. Piaget J. O nascimento da inteligência na criança. Rio de Janeiro: LTC, 1987.

18. Piaget J. A formação do símbolo na criança imitação, jogo e sonho, imagem e representação. 3rd ed. Rio de Janeiro: LTC, 1990.

19. Ylvisaker M, Hanks R, Johnson-Greene D. Perspectives on rehabilitation of individuals with cognitive impairment after brain injury: rationale for reconsideration of theoretical paradigms. J Head Trauma Rehabil 2002; 17(3):191–209.

20. Iavorskii AB, Sologubov EG, Nemkova SA. Kinesthetic characteristics of vertical stability in patients with infantile cerebral palsy. Zh Nevrol Psikhiatr Im S S Korsakova 2004; 104(2):21–26.

21. Piaget J. A linguagem e o pensamento da criança. 7th ed. São Paulo: Martins Fontes, 1999.

22. Lacert C. Les troubles du calcul chez l'IMC. In: Hout AV, Meljac C, editors. Troubles du calcul et dyscalculies chez l'enfant. Paris: Masson, 2001: 213–223.

23. Gaillard F, Braga LW. Calcul et langage dans le développement et troubles de l'apprentissage. In: Hout AV, Meljac C, editors. Troubles du calcul et dyscalculies chez l'enfant. Paris: Masson, 2001: 179–200.

24. Wilson RA, Keil FC. The MIT encyclopedia of the cognitive sciences. Cambridge, MA: MIT Press, 1999.

25. Courage ML, Howe ML. From infant to child: the dynamics of cognitive change in the second year of life. Psychol Bull 2002; 128(2):250–277.

26. Vygotsky LS. Thought and language. Cambridge, MA: MIT Press, 1962.

27. Vygotsky LS, Luria AR, Leontiev AN. Linguagem, desenvolvimento e aprendizagem. 6th ed. São Paulo: Icone, 2001.

28. Geary DC. From infancy to adulthood: the development of numerical abilities. Eur Child Adolesc Psychiatry 2000; 9(Suppl 2): II11–II16.

29. Cole PM, Martin SE, Dennis TA. Emotion regulation as a scientific construct: methodological challenges and directions for child development research. Child Dev 2004; 75(2):317–333.

30. Vygotsky LS. A formacao social da mente: o desenvolvimento dos processos psicologicos superiores. 8th ed. São Paulo: Marins Fontes, 2000.

31. Fivush R, Reese E. The social construction of autobiographical memory. In: Conway MA, Rubin DC, Spinnler H, Wagenaar WA, editors. Theoretical perspectives on autobiographical memory. Dordrecht: Kluwer Academic, 1992: 115–132.

32. Fivush R. Event memory in early childhood. In: Cowan N, editor. Development of memory in childhood. Hove, East Sussex: Psychology Press, 1997: 193–261

33. Haden CA, Haine RA, Fivush R. Developing narrative structure in parent-child reminiscing across the preschool years. Dev Psychol 1997; 33(2):295–307.

34. Haden CA. Joint encoding and joint reminising: implications for young children's understanding and remembering of personal experiences. In: Fivush R, Haden CA, editors. Autobiographical memory and the construction of a narrative self. Mahwah, NJ: Lawrence Erlbaum, 2003: 49–69.

35. Nelson K. Language in cognitive development: the emergence of the mediated mind. New York: Cambridge University Press, 1996.

36. Reese E, Haden CA, Fivush R. Mother–child conversations about the past: relationships of style and memory over time. Cognit Dev 1993; 8:403–430.

37. Ylvisaker M, Sellars C, Edelman L. Rehabilitation after traumatic brain injury in preschoolers. In: Ylvisaker M, editor. Traumatic brain injury rehabilitation: children and adolescents. Boston, MA: Butterworth-Heinemann, 1998: 303–329.

38. Ylvisaker M, Feeney T. Supported behaviour and supported cognition: an integrated, positive approach to serving students with disabilities. Educ Psychol in Scotland 2001; 6(1):17–30.

39. Rogoff B. Apprenticeship in thinking: cognitive development in social context. New York: Oxford University Press, 1990.

40. Wood D, Bruner JS, Ross G. The role of tutoring in problem solving. J Child Psychol Psychiatry 1976; 17(2):89–100.

41. Landry SH, Smith KE, Swank PR, Assel MA, Vellet S. Does early responsive parenting have a special importance for children's development or is consistency across early childhood necessary? Dev Psychol 2001; 37(3):387–403.

42. Landry SH, Miller-Loncar CL, Smith KE, Swank PR. The role of early parenting in children's development of executive processes. Dev Neuropsychol 2002; 21(1):15–41.

43. Hawley CA. Behaviour and school performance after brain injury. Brain Inj 2004; 18(7):645–659.

44. Lezak M, Howieson DB, Loring DW. Neuropsychological Assessment. 4th ed. New York: Oxford University Press, 2004.

45. Sohlberg MM, Mateer CA. Introduction to cognitive rehabilitation: theory and practice. New York: Guilford Press, 1989.

46. Yeates KO, Ris MD, Taylor HG. Pediatric neuropsychology: research, theory, and practice. New York: Guilford Press, 2000.

47. Limond J, Leeke R. Practitioner review: cognitive rehabilitation for children with acquired brain injury. J Child Psychol Psychiatry 2005; 46(4):339–352.

48. Luria AR. Curso de Psicologia Geral. Rio de Janeiro: Civilização Brasileira, 1991.

49. Caldas AC. A herança de Franz Joseph Gall: O cérebro a serviço do comportamento humano. Lisbon: McGraw-Hill, 2000.

# 4 *Speech, Language, and Communication*

*Ingrid L Gil and Flávia Y Shikida*

This chapter will discuss typical elements of speech, language and communication, and the problems encountered by the child with cerebral palsy (CP) or traumatic brain injury (TBI). It will also present illustrated activities to foster language development as well as strategies for overcoming or compensating for the difficulties presented by post-TBI school-aged children and adolescents who had previously learned to read and write.

Language is a system of symbols whose expression and comprehension involve motor, sensory, linguistic and neuropsychological skills that require attention and memory, abstraction and generalization, analytic and synthetic abilities. It also involves knowledge of language sounds (phonology), word construction and sentence structure (morphosyntax), word meanings and concepts (semantic aspect), and the intention and means to communicate (pragmatic aspect).

Brain injury can cause problems in speech production and/or language development that range from mild to severe. These impairments can be divided into two dimensions: motor difficulties in speech, and language disorders.[1]

Dysarthria is the motor-related speech impairment most often found in children and adolescents with CP and TBI.[2] This disorder in coordinating and executing speech interferes with the production of sounds, articulatory precision, and control of speech rhythm. In some cases, this deficit is almost imperceptible, while in others it can render speech unintelligible, resulting in mild to severe limitations in social interactions.[3]

Language disorders in CP often involve phonological, semantic, morphosyntactic and pragmatic aspects. The phonological capacity of children with spasticity may be better than that of children with choreoathetosis, but in choreathetosis the impairment is more related to expressive than phonetic discrimination difficulties. Morphosyntactic disorders in language result in decreased discourse due to the physical strain of communicating, leading to the use of more restricted vocabulary and grammatical simplifications.

Finally, on a pragmatic level, children with CP do not usually have as many opportunities to practice language in different contexts and situations because of the difficulties inherent to their communicative interactions.[1]

The disorders in children with TBI differ from those in adults,[4] and vary according to the severity and location of the lesion, the presence of a focal or diffuse brain injury, the age when the injury occurred and their prior language development.[5] Post-TBI children and adolescents may also bypass typical pathways in search of ways to compensate for or overcome their language difficulties.

Trauma that occurs before the age of 2 may cause a significant reorganization of function as well as developmental impairments, such as difficulties with lexical acquisitions.[6] The child may be slow in attaining phonological, semantic and morphosyntactic functions, and may also present a decrease in pragmatic aspects associated with interactive communication opportunities.

When the injury occurs after a linguistic framework has been established, specific deficits may result, such as aphasias. These disorders vary depending on the nature of the insult to the brain. Although uncommon, TBI may produce significant aphasic disturbances in children. However, subtle deficits are seen in comprehension and expression of words, lexical and discourse levels, as well as in pragmatic skills,[7] which interfere in language reorganization, recovery and development.[8] These language processing disorders frequently affect academic, communicative and social skills.[9]

Language results from the integration of a network of areas in the brain.[10] The consolidation of a language framework, i.e., the formation of these brain systems, occurs during childhood and adolescence and can be improved throughout life.[11] Communication is a broad concept not limited to speech and language, and is a fundamental aspect of the development of the child with brain injury.

## Program of Activities

In general, the approach to children with brain injury should aim at improving their capacity for expression and making it more efficient, promoting communication comprehension, enriching their linguistic environment, and fostering a more active participation in social interactions. It should encompass the children's communicative needs in various contexts, since it is through interaction that they will express themselves and comprehend the world.

The activities described in this chapter were designed to foster the development of speech, language and communication in all children. These activities have been contextualized into familial or school settings and organized into dialogue, gestures, reading and writing, and alternatives forms of communication.

Children are surrounded by a world that talks, gesticulates, and communicates with them in verbal and nonverbal ways. The family plays an important role in the development of language and communication by giving meaning and context to the child's vocalizations and gestures, words and sentences.

## Motherese

Family members have a special way of talking to a small child, called "motherese", which pervades the daily parent–child interactions. This way of speaking includes modulating the rhythm and tone of voice to resemble melody, emphasizing facial expressions, repeating words, and often involves the use of nicknames, nursery rhymes and folksongs. The discourse is adapted to the child's day-to-day vocabulary and language capacity (Figure 4.1, Activity 89).

**Figure 4.1    Activity 89**
Motherese

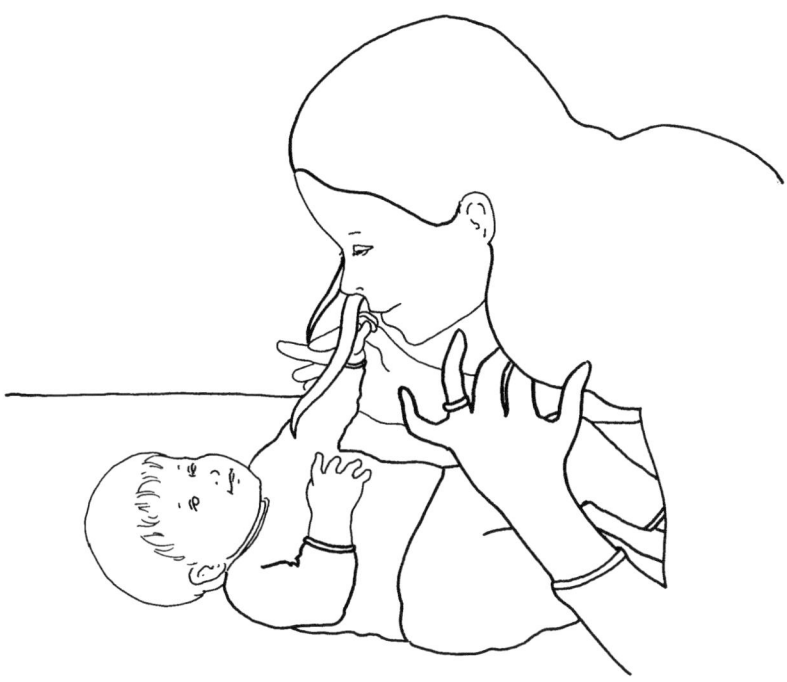

## Eye contact

Individuals usually sustain eye contact when speaking to one another. You can position yourself in front of the infant baby to get his visual and auditory attention. This will give him the chance to explore your facial expressions while you observe his communicative intentions and actions (Figure 4.2, Activity 90). In cases of sensory or cognitive deficits, touching and drawing close to the child's face can help you get his attention and establish eye contact.

**Figure 4.2    Activity 90**
Eye contact

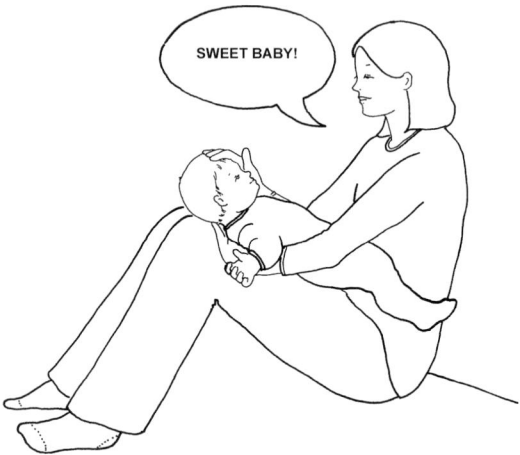

## Vocal play

During the first few months of life, children make nonsensical noises and rehearse tongue movements involved in the act of talking, although they do not yet attribute any linguistic meaning to these sounds. Talk to the child using melodic vocal sounds, encouraging him to vocalize and respond to your vocalizations. The child then begins to perceive that by emitting sounds he elicits responses from those around him, which will help initiate his experience with dialogue (Figure 4.3, Activity 91).

**Figure 4.3    Activity 91**
Vocal play

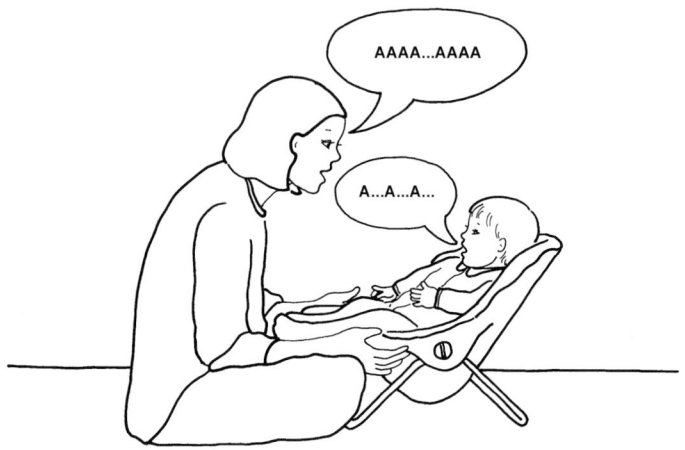

## Babbling

With vocal practice, small children start to better control the sounds they make, which can lead to the formulation of "noises" that resemble, for example, dadadada, babababa. Babbling is the child's attempts at reproducing what he hears. You can repeat the sounds he makes or say words that contextualize his sounds, such as "dadadada (means) ... Daddy" (Figure 4.4, Activity 92). Social interaction helps shape the child's babbling.

**Figure 4.4    Activity 92**
Babbling

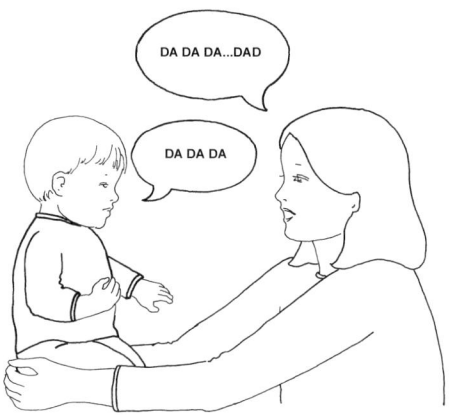

## Eye-gaze

When you notice that a child is gazing at an object, you will normally ask what he wants and then retrieve it for him. Children thus learn that directing their eyes towards a specific target makes that object come to them; through this discovery, they will start interacting with their surroundings with your help. Try to be attentive to day-to-day situations involving the child. Another way to encourage him to manifest choices through eye-gazing is by placing various types of a given object (e.g., toys or snacks) in front of him, asking which one he prefers, and then waiting for him to respond with the movement of his eyes (Figure 4.5, Activity 93). The eye-gaze is also a common form of communication for children with CP and severe motor impairments throughout development. Children and adolescents recovering from TBI usually initiate their communication efforts through indicative gestures such as these.

**Figure 4.5    Activity 93**
Eye gaze

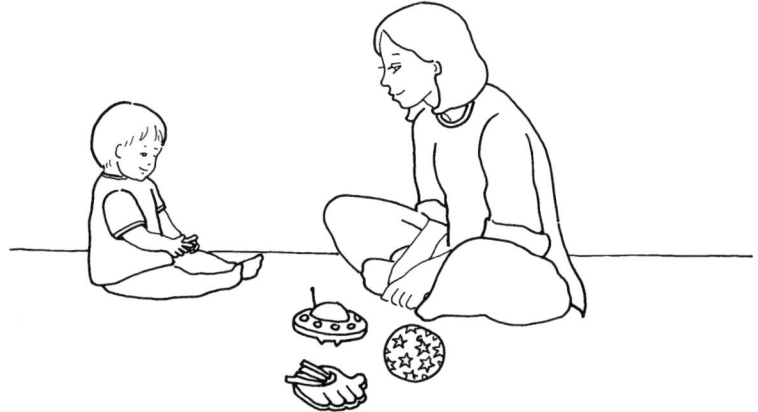

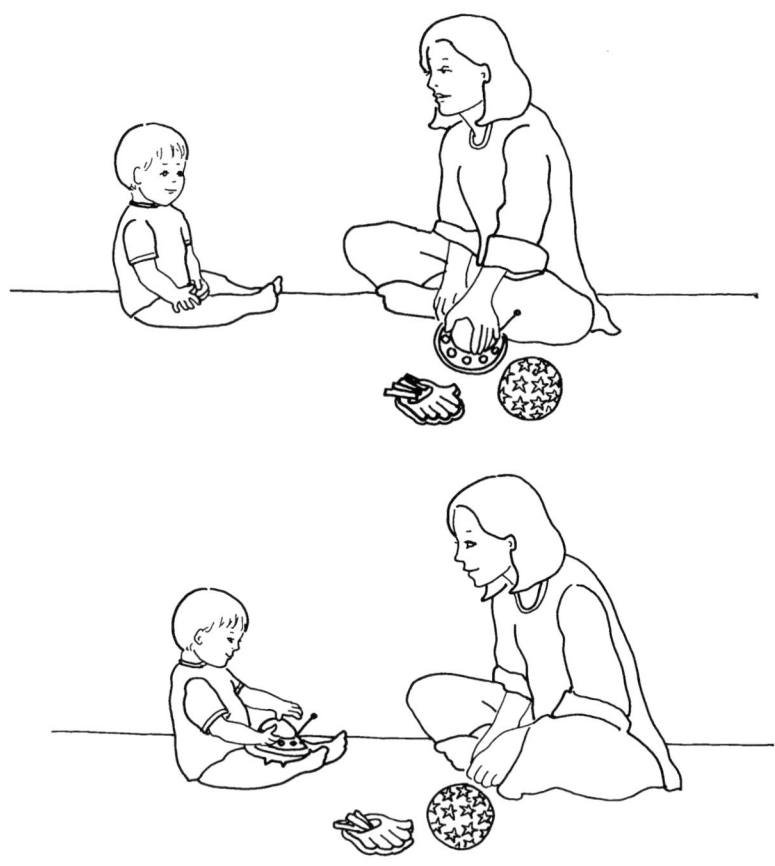

## Joint attention

Joint attention is a synchronicity of focus between the child and the individual who is speaking to him. You can establish eye contact with the child and direct his interest towards a person or toy, thereby guiding his attention so that you are both focused on the same thing (Figure 4.6, Activity 94). Joint attention is an evolution of the eye contact that pervades communicative interactions and promotes learning processes.[12] Children with CP may need more time to direct their attention to an appointed focus due to motor impairments.

**Figure 4.6   Activity 94**
Joint attention

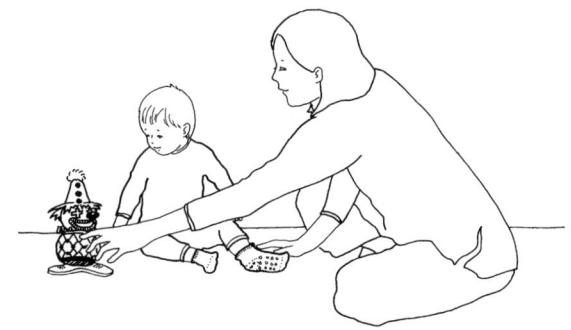

## Pointing

When a child attempts to reach for objects, he will extend his arm in the direction of an object; individuals around him notice his movement, point to it and then ask if he wants it. This teaches a child what pointing accomplishes: it calls attention to the object he desires. You can place toys out of the child's reach and ask that he point to the object he wants (Figure 4.7, Activity 95). It is important to observe the individual behavior of the child with brain injury and value the pointing movement that he is capable of performing.

**Figure 4.7    Activity 95**
Pointing

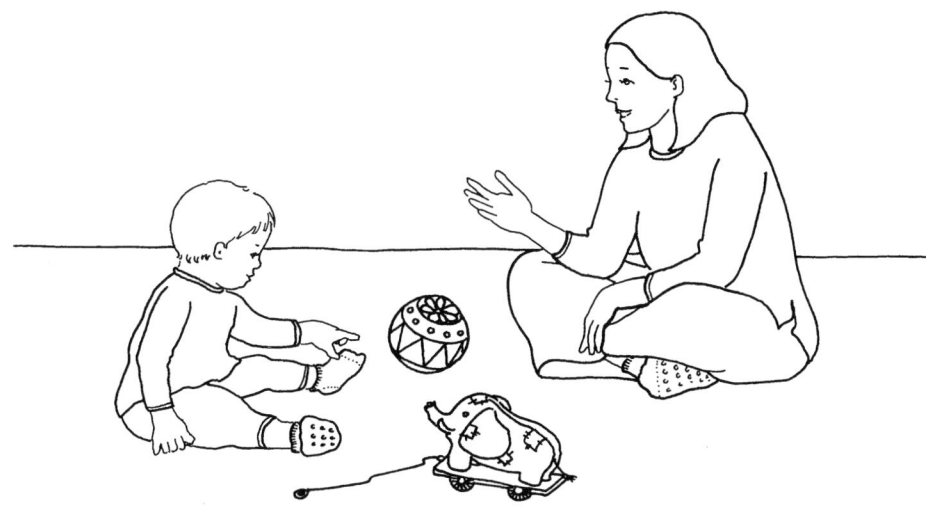

## Understanding gestures

Learning to speak and make social gestures involves first imitating cultural sounds and movements. Encourage the child to reproduce these motor or gestural motions by offering examples and helping him imitate and perform these movements. Understanding a gesture entails appropriation of the social meaning of a motor act that expresses ideas or feelings. The first gestures that the child sees are usually related to daily routines and are included in play, feeding time and bedtime, for example (Figure 4.8, Activity 96).

**Figure 4.8    Activity 96**
Understanding gestures

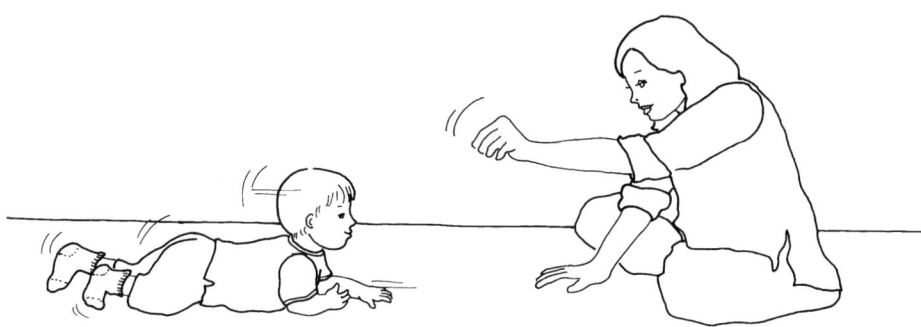

**Word comprehension**

Children associate sounds with familiar people and objects, for example the word "mommy" with the maternal figure. Naming the individuals who interact with the child and the objects that are offered to him during play and other daily life situations fosters these associations. You can ask the child "Where is daddy?" or say "Here is the ball!" (Figure 4.9, Activity 97).

**Figure 4.9   Activity 97**
Word comprehension

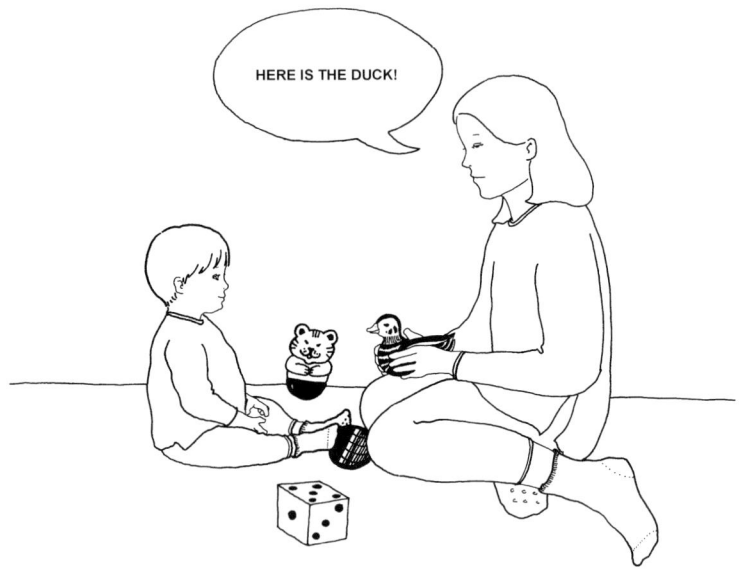

**Following simple instructions**

Listening comprehension is fostered by the practice of associating gestures with instructions. While playing with the child, position yourself in his line of vision and ask, for example, "Can you give me the ball?" (Figure 4.10, Activity 98). Children and adolescents with TBI who have information processing deficits may take longer to respond to your commands. Care should be taken not to interrupt the adolescent's attempts with further directives or questions. In cases of aphasia, the use of visual clues or gestures facilitates the comprehension of the instruction.[13]

**Figure 4.10   Activity 98**
Following simple
instructions

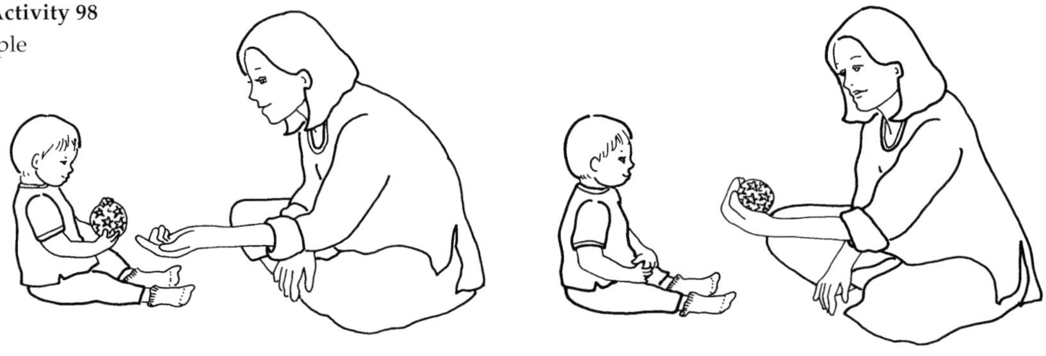

**First words**

Before learning to actually say words, the child becomes acquainted with various aspects of the verbalization of language related to speech intonation: melody, rhythm and tone. Initially, his speech may be in the form of "jargon". As he practices his vocal production, his ability to sequentially articulate different syllables and use distinct intonations such as those for questions, exclamations, affirmations or negations grows. Children enter the universe of words when they begin to make sounds to denote specific things. The first words take place within an immediate context. Initially, the child's vocalizations resemble social sounds that name objects, such as "oll" for "doll". When a child vocalizes a sound in reference to a given object, you should engage him in dialogue, emphasize melodious and rhythmic aspects of language in your speech, confirm his communicative intention and provide the complete name of the object, e.g., "Doll? Yes, it's a doll!" (Figure 4.11, Activity 99).

**Figure 4.11   Activity 99**
First words

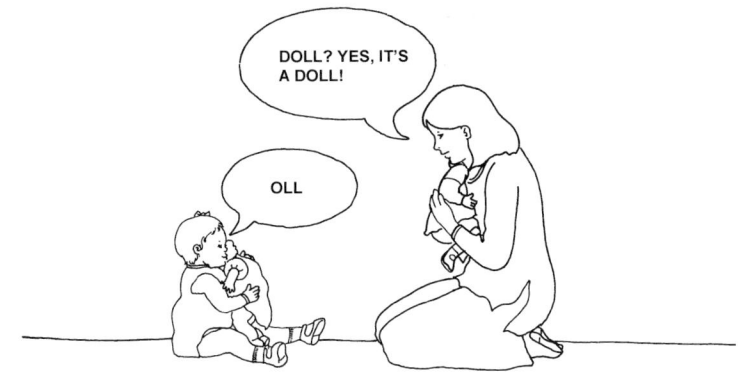

**Onomatopoeias**

It is not uncommon for children to use onomatopoeias in naming things. Onomatopoeias are terms whose pronunciations resemble the sounds of that which they refer to, such as "wow-wow" or "knock-knock". You can include onomatopoeias in games of pretending by imitating, for example, the sound of a car (Figure 4.12, Activity 100). Onomatopoeias foster vocal practice of phonetic language sounds and entail the representative use of words.

**Figure 4.12   Activity 100**
Onomatopoeias

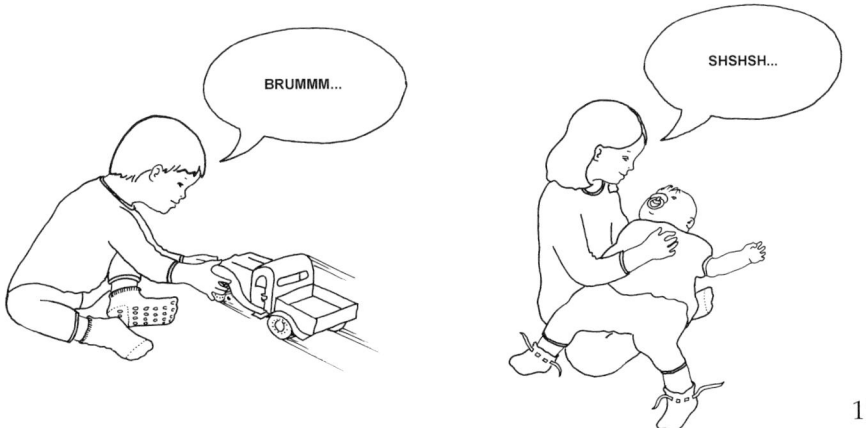

**One-word sentence**

Children may apply the same word to different situations due to still limited vocabularies. Furthermore, an idea may be equivalent to a whole phrase when coupled with gestures. The child may use the word "me", for example, when expressing "I want the truck" or "Give me cookies". His intentions are given meaning or made clear through interpretations that you make, based on clues in the immediate context. During communicative interactions, you can complement the child's one-word sentences by saying short, but complete, sentences (Figure 4.13, Activity 101). Post-TBI children and adolescents may initially use one-word sentences in spoken language. Adolescents with aphasia may use them as a predominant means of communication, to the extent that they tend to develop telegraphic and grammatically simple speech because of problems with verbalization.[14]

**Figure 4.13   Activity 101**
One-word sentence

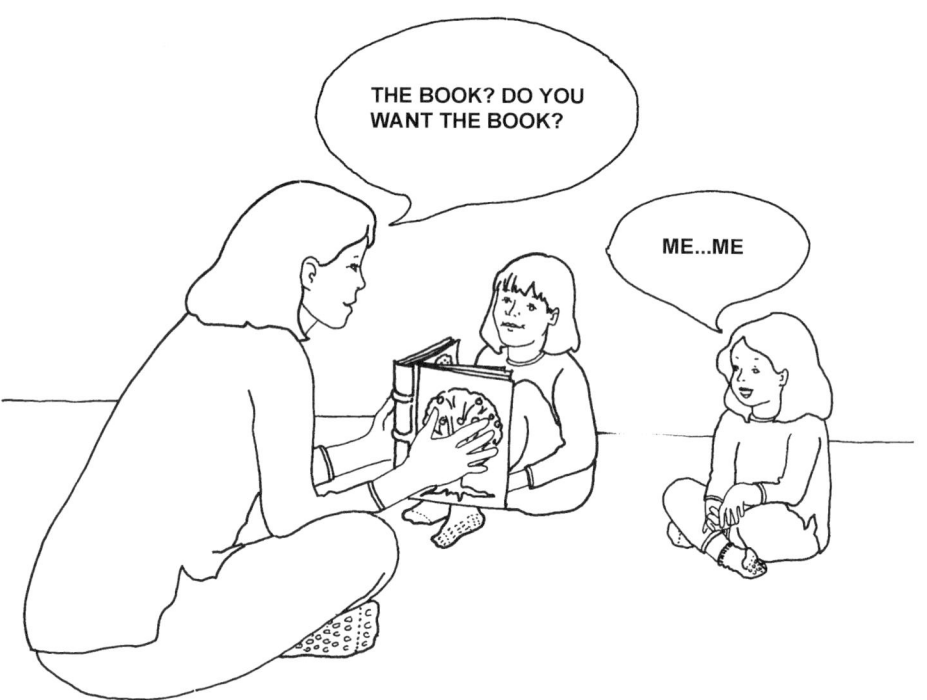

112

## Naming

Naming contributes to the expansion of the child's vocabulary. You can take household items and show them to the child, say the name of each object and highlight its meaning, purpose or function.[15] These naming games can be worked into daily domestic routines, e.g., naming articles of clothing during grooming or kitchen utensils during cooking (Figure 4.14, Activity 102). If the child with TBI has problems naming objects (anomia), or commits errors in selecting words by approximation of the word concepts (semantic paraphasias), or repeats the same oral or gestural response that is unrelated to the context (stereotypies), you can facilitate the task by giving him clues.

**Figure 4.14   Activity 102**
Naming

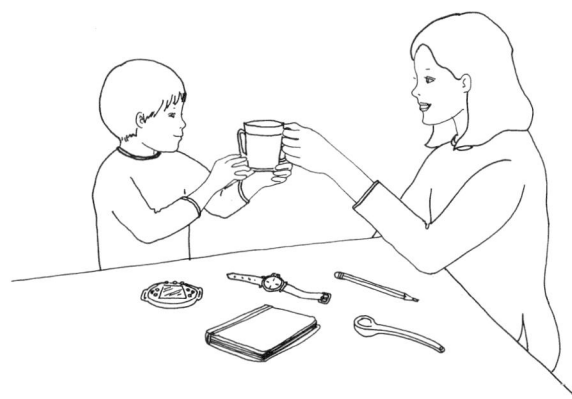

## Mouthing words

Using the wrong phoneme is common until a child becomes adept at vocalizing all phonetic language sounds. You can position yourself in front of the child and, in a playful manner, enunciate words correctly and slowly, and then encourage him to imitate the phonoarticulatory, or mouthing, movements involved in verbalizing those words. A mirror can be used to perform this activity, permitting him to see his own facial movements (Figure 4.15, Activity 103).

**Figure 4.15   Activity 103**
Mouthing words

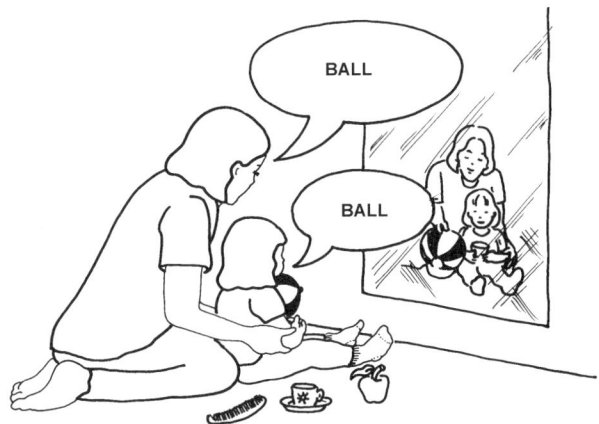

**Mouthing mimics**

The imitation of mouth and facial movements aids the oromotor coordination of speech. You can engage the child in throwing kisses, blowing out a candle on a cake or making bubbles out of water and soap (Figure 4.16, Activity 104). Children with CP or TBI may have trouble performing or coordinating these movements, but practicing these motor actions can help improve the intelligibility of their speech.[16]

**Figure 4.16    Activity 104**
Mouthing mimics

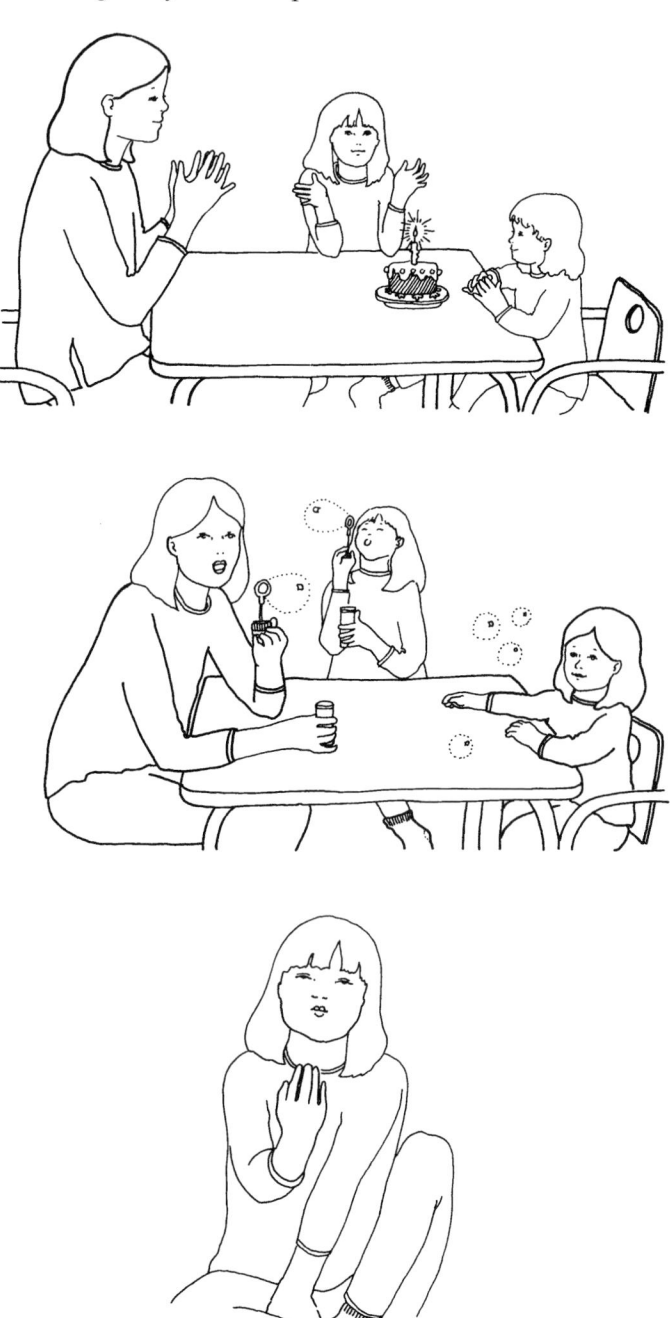

**Listening to stories**

Recounting and discussing a story with a child promotes comprehension and ordering of facts into a logical sequence. It is important to highlight noteworthy elements such as the main character in the story, the events involved and their succession. Children appreciate and benefit from visual and verbal clues, such as images, onomatopoeias, facial expressions and varied intonations. Questions should be included during the story to stress facts, encourage the child to infer what happens next, and convey the notion of beginning, middle and end (Figure 4.17, Activity 105). Stories should be selected according to the reality of the child or adolescent, and kept relatively short so as to facilitate attention, comprehension of facts and how they play out, especially with children or adolescents who have attention deficit disorders or post-TBI aphasia.

**Figure 4.17    Activity 105**
Listening to stories

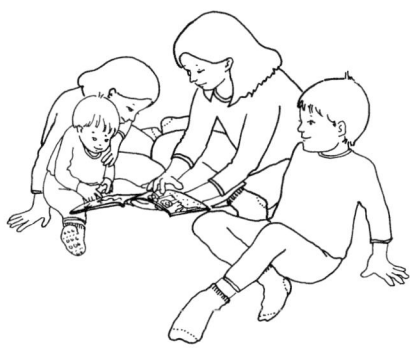

**Using gestures**

The child's first gestures usually represent day-to-day ideas or actions, such as grooming or eating. You can use gestures specific to a given context (for example, at bedtime, the motion representative of sleeping), verbalize their meaning and encourage the child to imitate them (Figure 4.18, Activity 106). Children with brain injury and motor impairments may experience problems in performing gestural movements and may develop their own unique gestures. The communicative intention and the gesture's context should be given more value than the actual precision of the movement. Gestural communication is common in adolescents with CP or TBI and severe speech or language impairment even if they know how to read and write, and it is also present in the use of Augmentative and Alternative Communication (AAC) because it facilitates the comprehension and dialogical dynamic of social interactions.[17]

**Figure 4.18    Activity 106**
Using gestures

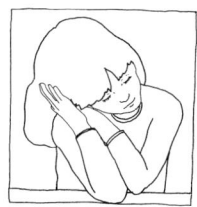 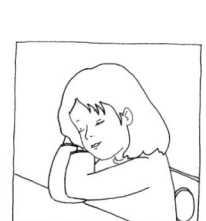 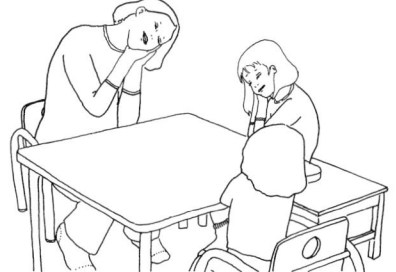

## Forming sentences

A child should be stimulated to form sentences and develop contextualized speech. Open-ended questions that encourage the child to respond with phrases, such as asking "What are we going to do?" during a game, can be beneficial. If the child replies with one-word answers or simple sentences (noun and verb), help him by contributing elements of the reply. However, care must be taken not to offer the whole sentence, but rather components that encourage the child to complete it (Figure 4.19, Activity 107).

**Figure 4.19   Activity 107**
Forming sentences

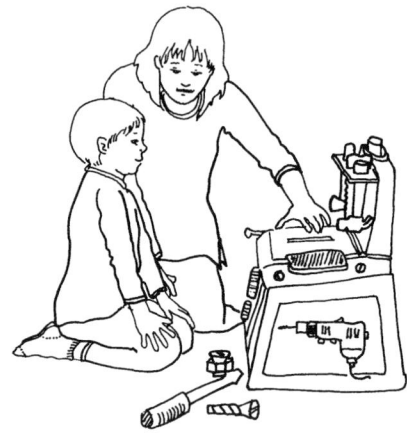

## Taking turns

Play-talking with children teaches them that dialogue is organized by turns and that each speaker respects the other's turn to speak. You can pose questions or make comments, and then wait for the child's answers in an alternating exchange that allows each a chance to talk. The child's response may manifest in various distinct forms such as facial expressions, babbling, gestures, words or phrases (Figure 4.20, Activity 108). A child's awareness of his active participation in a verbal exchange, your attention to his communication signals, and your response to his attempts at self-expression are fundamental to constituting dialogue.

**Figure 4.20   Activity 108**
Taking turns

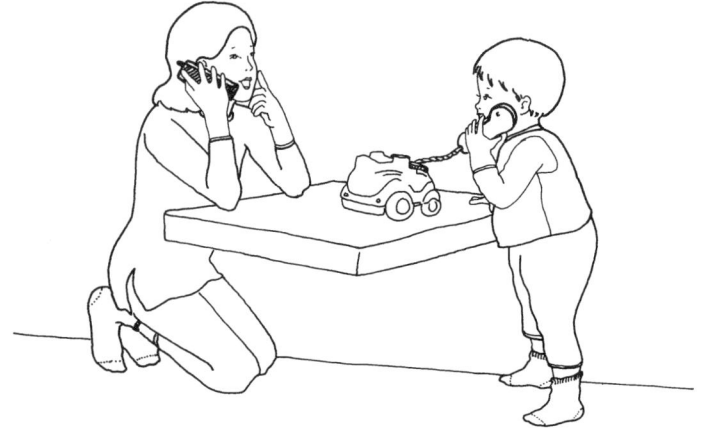

**Figure identification**

Exploring images with the child during storytelling fosters his listening comprehension skills and his ability to remember the storyline. You can refer to the illustrations in a book, draw images on a piece of paper, or use gestures and facial expressions related to the tale (Figure 4.21, Activity 109). The ability to recognize and explore images is of great value to children with brain injury who have severe speech impairment because the use of graphic symbols helps expand their vocabulary and facilitates the use of AAC systems.

**Figure 4.21   Activity 109**
Figure identification

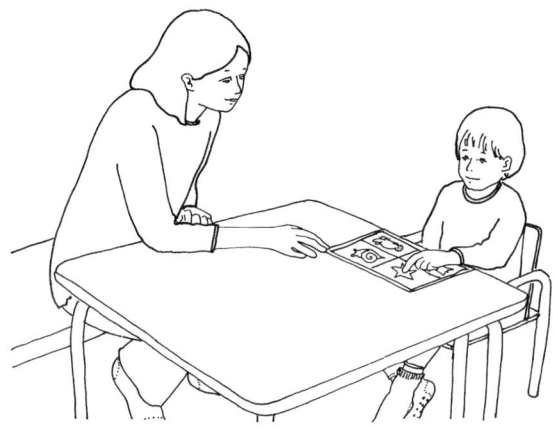

**Folksongs**

Folksongs vary from culture to culture and constitute oral narratives. Singing with children is also a way of telling stories. In addition to verbalizations and sequential events, songs usually involve gestures or mouthing mimics, integrating motor, perceptual, linguistic, and neuropsychological systems. You can explore the song's story and gestures, stressing narrative elements, the sequence of events and their relationship to the gestures involved (Figure 4.22, Activity 110).

**Figure 4.22   Activity 110**
Folksongs

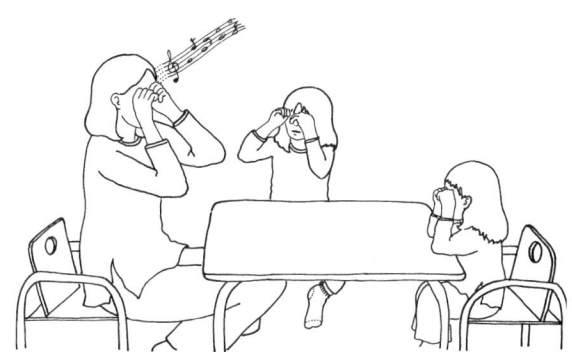
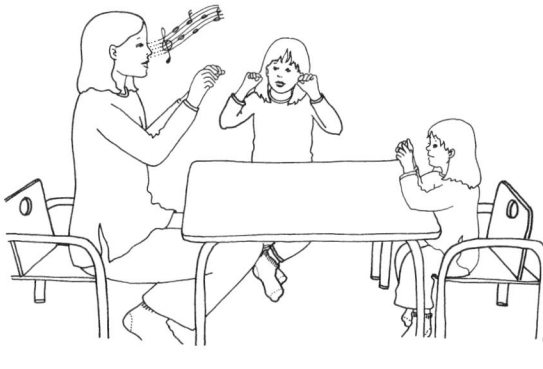

## Music play

Musical instruments, toys or objects that produce different sounds, enhance the child's experience with sounds and help establish auditory identification. You may select flutes, whistles, tambourines or bells, for example, and play them and sing along to familiar songs or compose new melodies with the child (Figure 4.23, Activity 111).

**Figure 4.23    Activity 111**
Music play

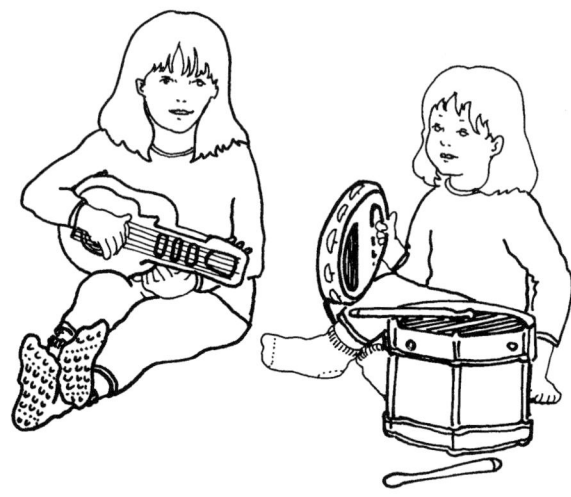

## Sound play

Playing with the phonetic sounds of words helps children organize and become familiar with language structure. Selecting objects whose names have similar phonemes, such as "ball" and "doll" or "pick" and "put", and practicing their phonemic similarities and differences with the child is a way to exercise these skills. You can also show the child an item, say its name, and then ask that he say another word that begins or ends with the same phoneme (Figure 4.24, Activity 112).

**Figure 4.24    Activity 112**
Sound play

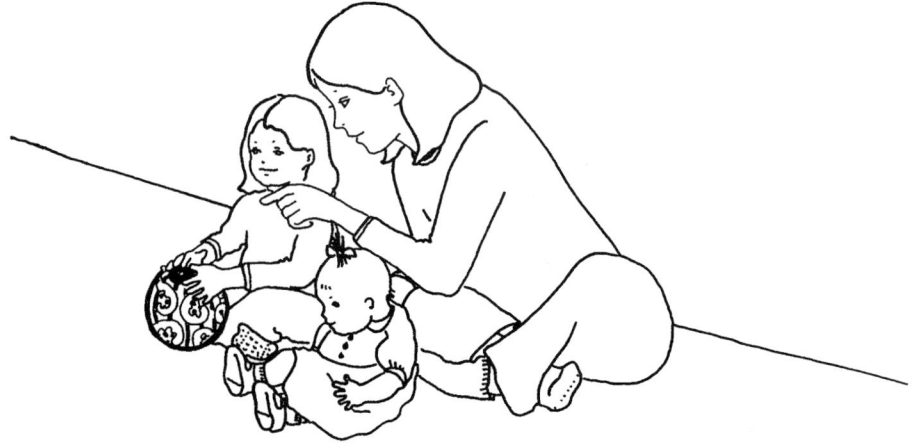

**Forming groups**

Words contain ideas or concepts that the child elaborates with use.[18] Children may associate a series of words if they refer to the same situation, or if they belong to the same category, such as animals. You can select objects that are related because they pertain to animals, clothing, or toys, or because they are involved in the same task, such as making a cake: bowl, spoon, flour and milk. The selected items should be mixed and given to the child to name and separate into matching groups (Figure 4.25, Activity 113). By so doing, the child learns to form groups and organize semantic fields.[15;18]

**Figure 4.25    Activity 113**
Forming groups

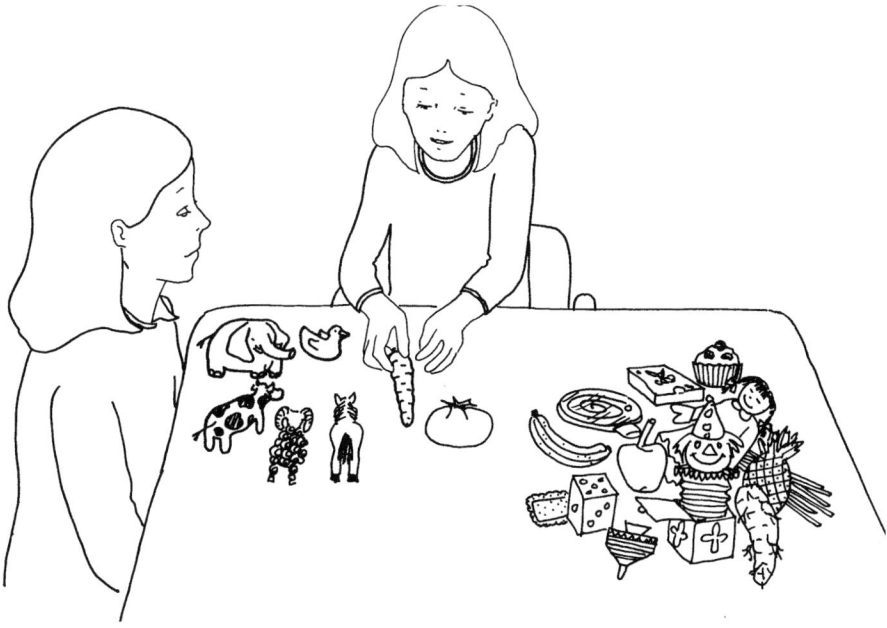

## Guessing

The development of language and thought can be fostered by simple guessing games that involve thinking with, or about, language. You can place several familiar objects on a shelf, select one without telling the child which one it is and give him one clue at a time until he guesses what the item is. The clues can be phonetic, semantic, or they can be about the object's properties or qualities. The child and adolescent should also be encouraged to invent and lead guessing games, with defined subjects such as people, types of fruit or actions, and be allowed time to formulate questions, to which you respond with yes/no (Figure 4.26, Activity 114). This activity practices more refined language use because it calls for linguistic, communicative, cognitive and neuropsychological abilities, such as memory processes, mental flexibility, analysis, synthesis, and inference.

**Figure 4.26   Activity 114**
Guessing

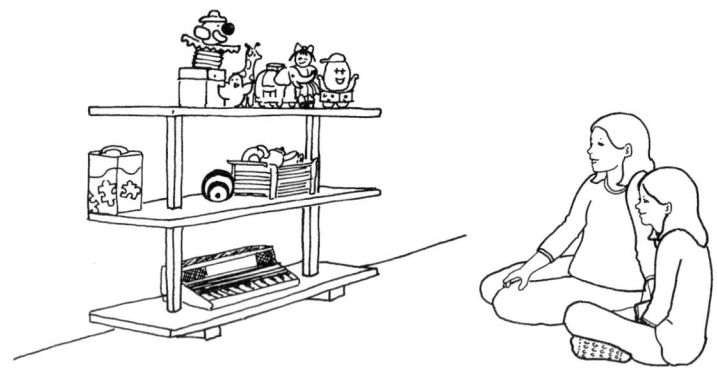

## Logical story sequence

Playing at arranging the facts of a story in successive order can help foster the child's ability to develop sequential ideas. Some children's games include illustrated narratives that mark the beginning, middle and end of the story. You can arrange these drawings in a non-sequential order and ask the child to describe the scenes before putting them in their right sequence. Once the images are organized again, encourage the child to tell the story (Figure 4.27, Activity 115). Day-to-day situations, such as the sequence of daily routines or events from the child's experience, can also be used in this activity.

**Figure 4.27   Activity 115**
Logical story sequence

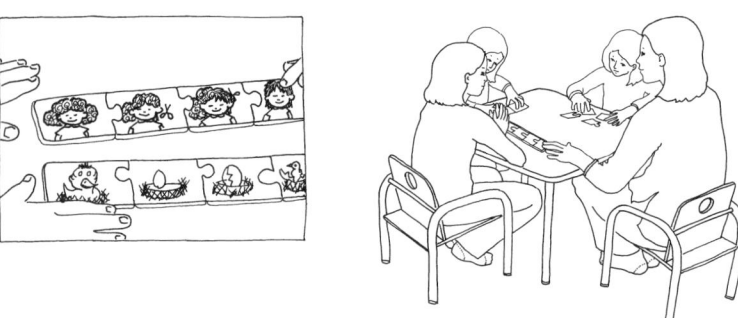

**Storytelling**

In order to tell a story, a child needs to organize a logical sequence and maintain narrative coherency about subject, space and time, as well as cognitive organization and working memory.[19] You can ask the child to recount or invent a story using books, personal experiences or puppets. If the child has difficulties organizing the facts, help him by asking questions (Figure 4.28, Activity 116).

**Figure 4.28    Activity 116**
Storytelling

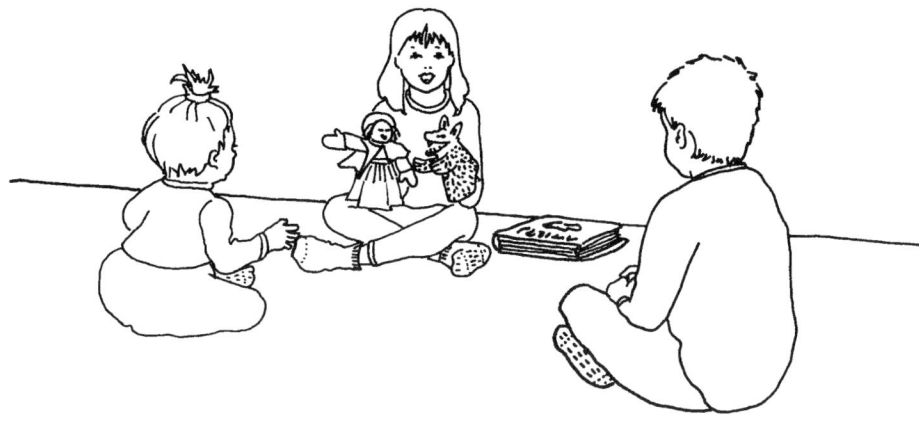

**Improving the dialogue**

It is important to be attentive to the richness of the child's linguistic environment in order to facilitate his observation and formulation of language, and promote more refined use. You can help by contextualizing the child's discourse, presenting new words, telling stories, and encouraging him to engage in or initiate a dialogue (Figure 4.29, Activity 117).

**Figure 4.29    Activity 117**
Improving the dialogue

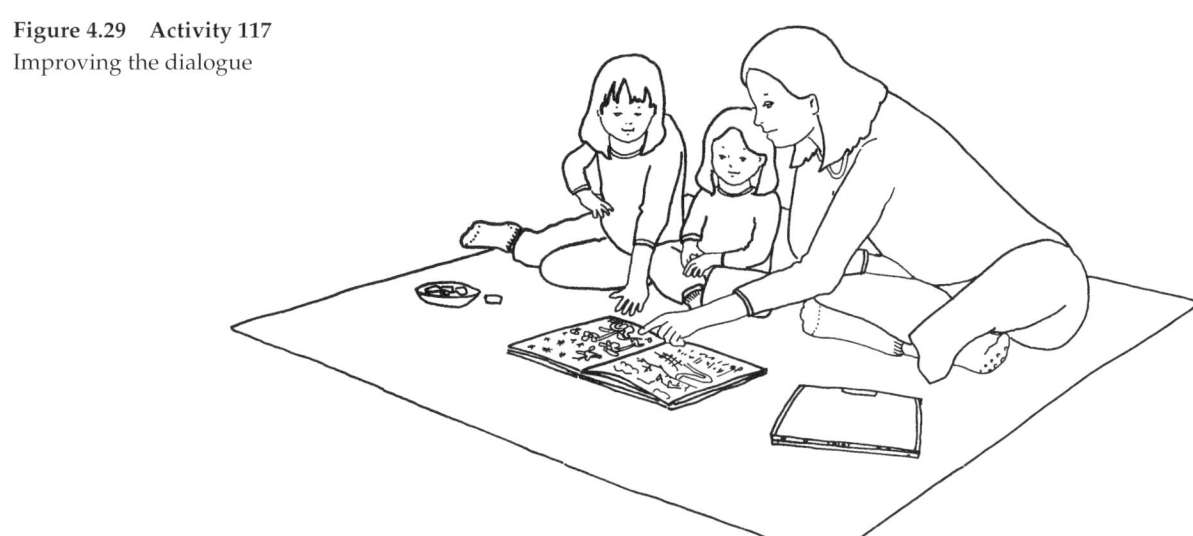

## *Reading and Writing*

By listening to and telling stories, scribbling, drawing, identifying brands of toys or names of stores, and watching people read and write, children enter the world of written language, a world represented by letters and numbers. An understanding of the complex organization of written language derives from a slow, gradual process within which children pass through various stages of experimentation. When formally learning to read and write, they learn to identify characters that represent letters, and also learn some of the forms (graphemes) that represent distinct sounds (phonemes). Reading and writing teaches the child new rules, such as spatial positioning. They also follow specific guidelines that vary from culture to culture. In western languages, sentences are written horizontally from the left to the right side of the page, which is different from the way they are written in some cultures. Over time, other rules are introduced, such as punctuation, promoting the expansion of communication skills.

Reading and writing are activities usually learned in school. You can help improve the performance of the child with brain injury who is experiencing difficulties with these skills by using simple activities.

### Games with letters and sounds

To help the child develop awareness of each sound and its representation (phonological awareness) in a playful manner, you can display objects or illustrated objects that begin with specific letters and sounds, and play with the child at trying to group them according to the first letter or sound (Figure 4.30, Activity 118). Other games include saying names that begin with a given letter or sound, circling or cutting out images from magazines that start with the same letter as the child's name.

**Figure 4.30   Activity 118**
Games with letters and sounds

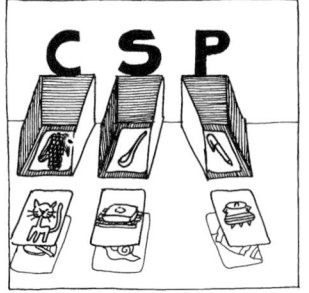

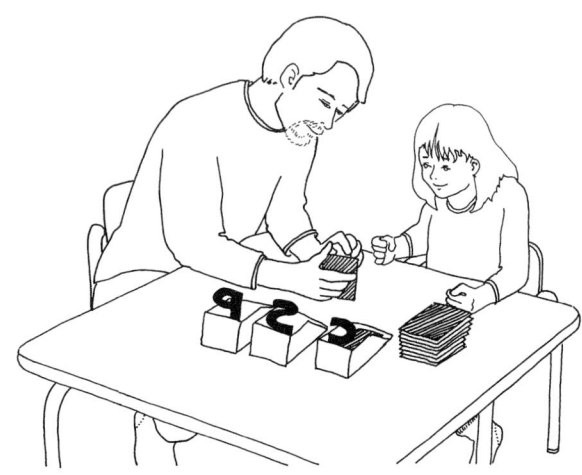

**Reading and writing words**

You can help the child by giving him objects and labels that have the objects' names on them for him to decode and associate. Include the child in activities such as making grocery lists or creating a schedule or writing in a journal (Figure 4.31, Activity 119). Children with CP and unintelligible speech or those with motor deficits that affect the ability to write need to use adapted material or alternative resources for communication, depending on the nature and level of impairment.

**Figure 4.31 Activity 119**
Reading and writing words

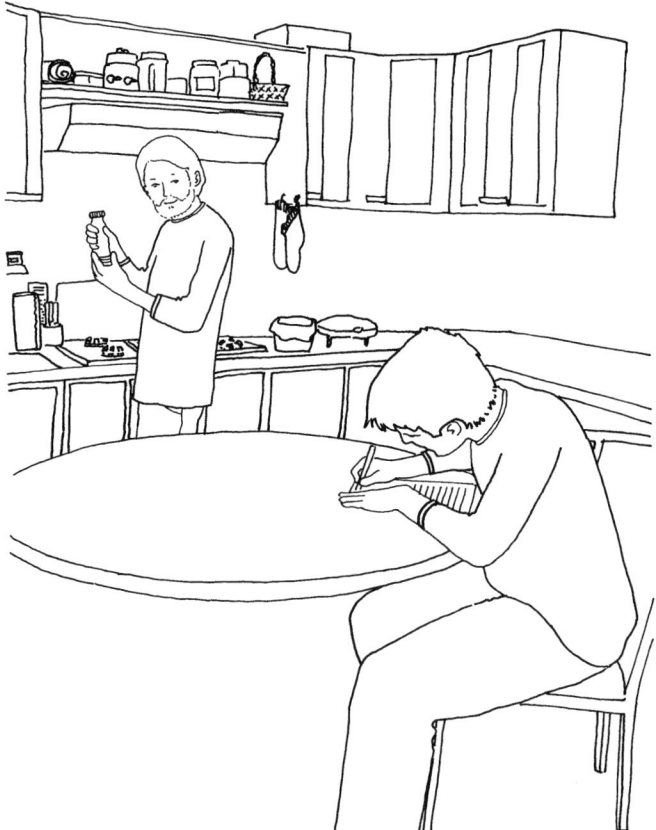

Children and adolescents with CP can have persistent problems with spelling, such as switched, substituted and/or missing letters, that may be related to limited phonological experience or speech disorders. Post-TBI children and adolescents may have phonological dyslexia, i.e., the inability to recognize familiar words, mostly nouns, and great difficulties reading words or phrases. There are ways to help these children or adolescents read and write words, such as by isolating letters or providing phonological clues.

## Short notes

You can help by asking the child or adolescent to read and write short notes, showing him how to jot down messages, and other activities that are part of his daily life (Figure 4.32, Activity 120).

**Figure 4.32    Activity 120**
Short notes

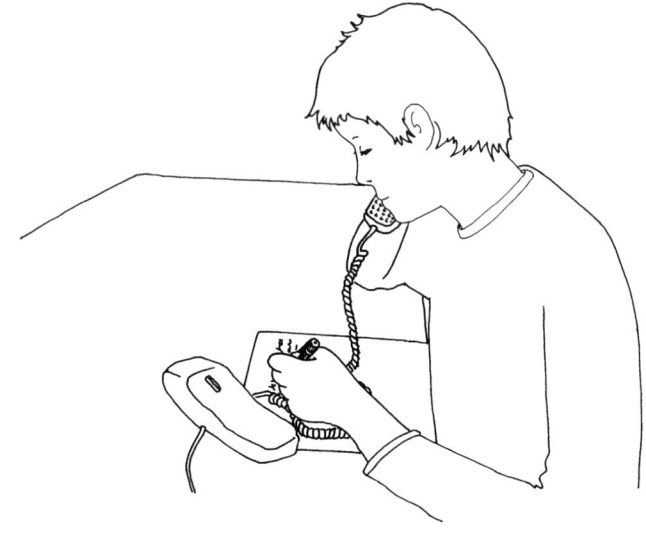

## Reading and writing stories

Reading and writing are present in various daily life activities in the family, school and social settings. The incentive to read magazines, books or newspapers, depending on the child's or adolescent's interests, helps him develop efficient reading skills. It is important to enrich the linguistic environment, emphasizing details, logical sequences in stories, and associating facts that take place in day-to-day routines. Incentives for writing stories can come from recounting what is heard, keeping a diary, sending and receiving emails or letters from friends (Figure 4.33, Activity 121).

**Figure 4.33    Activity 121**
Reading and writing
stories

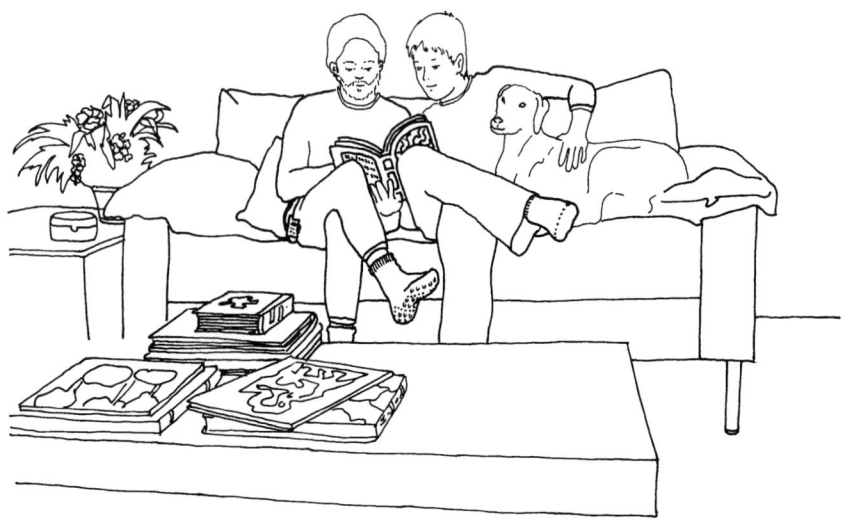

## *Alternative Forms of Communication*

Children and adolescents with severe motor impairments and minimally intelligible speech rely heavily on nonverbal forms of communication to express themselves. Furthermore, children or adolescents are not always able to give the answers usually expected of them, or to do so in the allotted time, leading to a decline of speech comprehension and fluency.[20] To foster the development of communication and language, alternative forms of exchange that expand the child's means of self-expression, and adjustments of the temporal dynamic of dialogue are required; this involves instructing the individuals who communicate with the child,[21] as well as enriching the linguistic environment to promote the development of the child's language and thought processes.

**Head nods**

Communicative yes/no signals permit the speech-impaired child to answer questions related to specific contexts. Children should be taught socially conventional signals such as head nods, gestures, "okay" motions, or vocalizations like "eh" for yes and "o" for no; these signals are also easier to understand outside the family context. You can start with simple requests, selected from daily routines, such as offering a snack or a toy and asking, "Do you want this truck?" (Figure 4.34, Activity 122). When motor impairment limits the development of social gestures, you and the child can stipulate specific signals such as looking up or down, lifting or lowering the arms or legs. These signals can be understood in other contexts so long as their meanings are shared with others who are not familiar with the signals.

**Figure 4.34   Activity 122**
Head nods

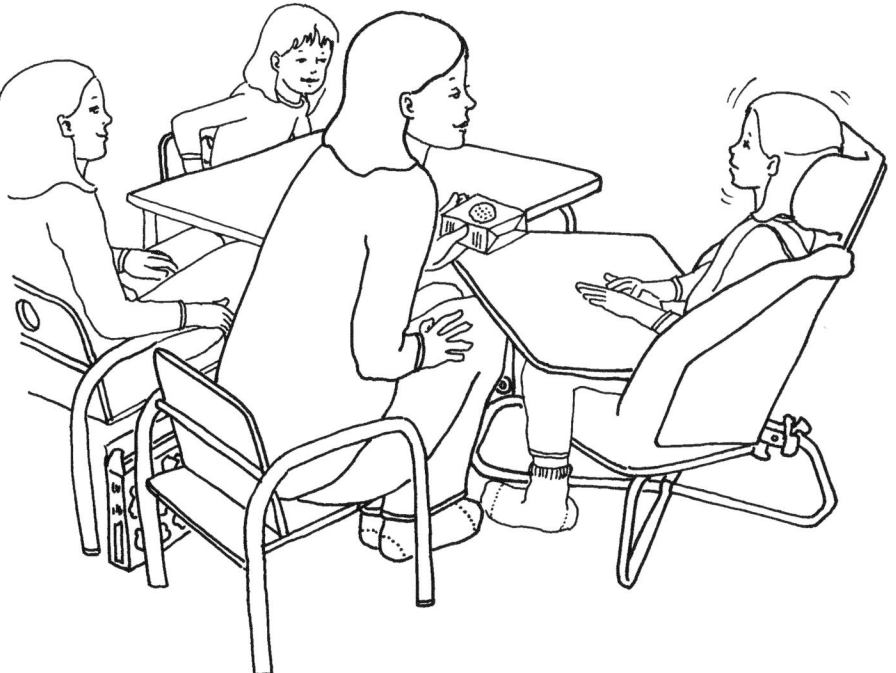

**Switches**

Switches, such as buttons that activate toys and appliances, should be adapted to the child's movement abilities. They can also be used to activate AAC systems. A playful way to teach and motivate the child to use switches is to show him electronic toys and demonstrate how the switch works by explaining the effect that it has on a toy and by using oral commands until the child is able to activate it on his own (Figure 4.35, Activity 123). Sound switches can be an alternative means of expressing yes/no and may be used for calling someone nearby when motor impairments restrict gesturing in children and adolescents with CP or in the initial stages of post-TBI recovery.[22]

**Figure 4.35   Activity 123**
Switches

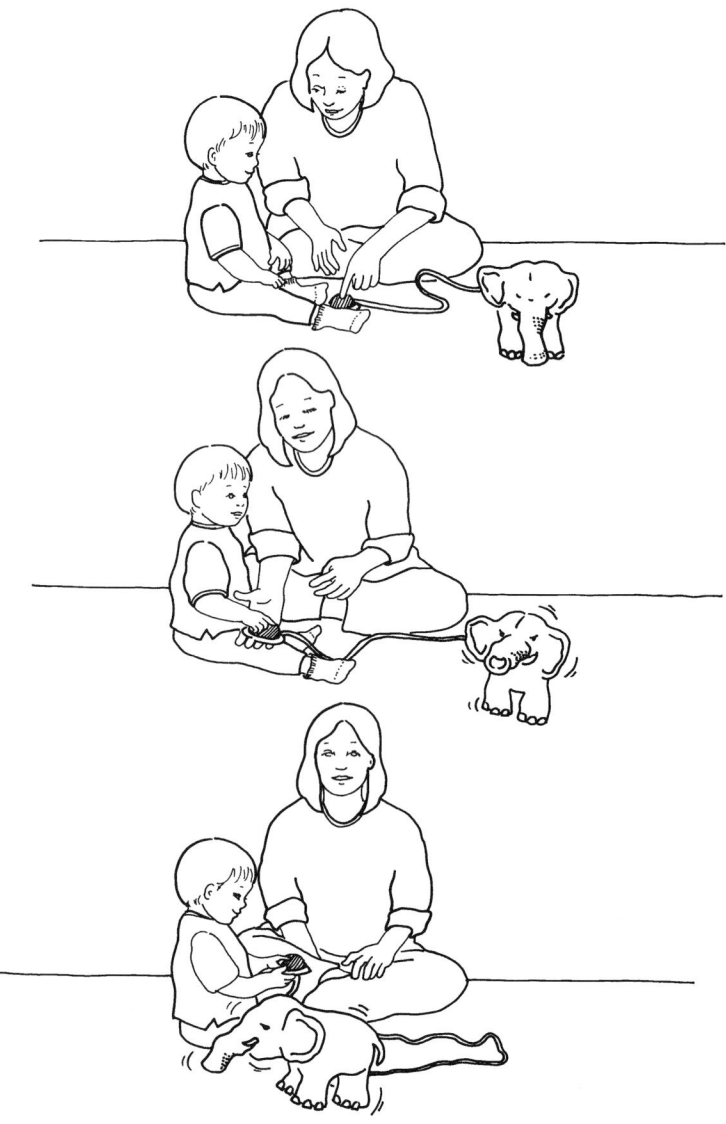

**Scanning**

With restricted possibilities for self-expression, a child's communication relies on how the adult uses language, which can include offering answer choices, interpreting the child's communicative intentions, and enriching the linguistic environment with details and facts about the subject or language. Scanning involves offering choices, one at a time. For example, place three toys in front of the child and ask, "Which one of these do you want? Phone? Car? Doll?" A pause should be made after each choice, allowing the child time to communicate; the dialogue's temporal dynamic should also be adjusted to the amount of time a child needs to respond (Figure 4.36, Activity 124). Little by little the choices can be increased and figures can be included. There are various forms of scanning: one at a time, line/column, or by groups. Scanning is one of the organizational principles of AAC systems and should be adjusted to the motor, perceptual, linguistic and neuropsychological abilities and communication needs of each child.

**Figure 4.36   Activity 124**
Scanning

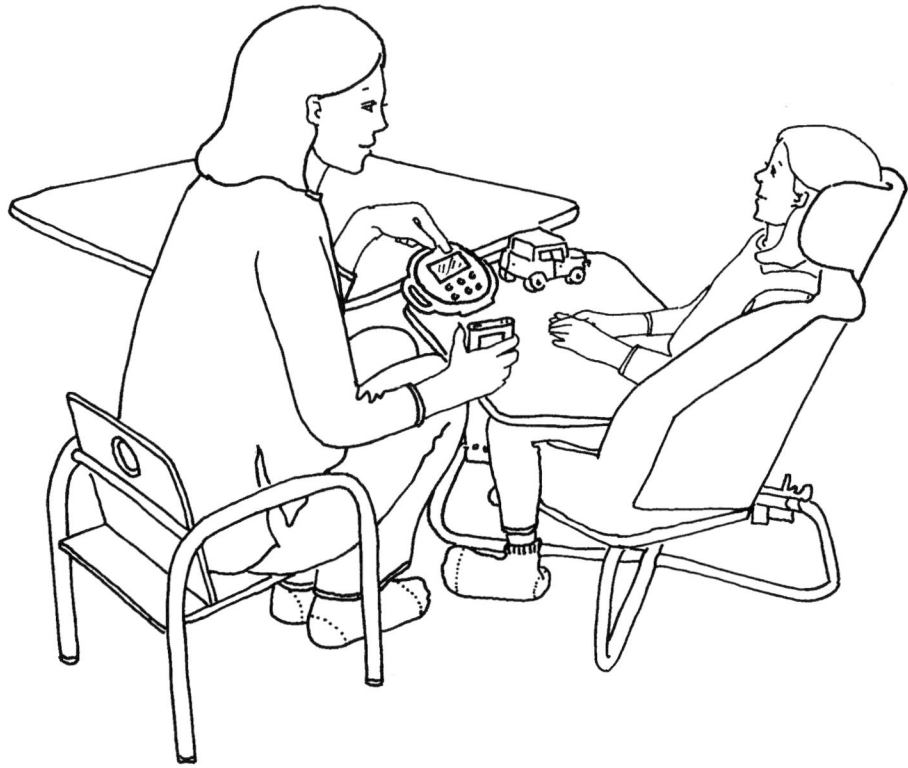

**Communication boards**

The construction and use of communication symbol boards enhances the vocabulary of children with unintelligible speech and improves their possibilities for self-expression. The child's level of mental representation will determine his choice of symbols; these can be photographs, drawings, graphic symbols, letters, words and/or sentences. The rehabilitation team and family should explore the child's communication needs and contexts, choose the symbols,[23-24] and create the boards according to the child's abilities, mode of selection, and scanning. It is recommended that the first board be based on the family's daily routines, such as choice of food, toys or leisure activities. In addition to formulating the questions and scanning the boards for the child to answer, you should encourage him to initiate interaction (Figure 4.37, Activity 125). The boards can be made for various communication needs and organized in such a way as to permit formulation of words, sentences and short texts. It is important to try to meet the child's communication needs within family, school and social contexts. Communication boards can be used by post-TBI children before they recover speech or if they have aphasia. In cases of post-TBI aphasia, the boards permit communication and may facilitate verbalization. The visual support provided by the communication boards also fosters understanding of language in children with learning difficulties.

**Figure 4.37 Activity 125**
Communication boards

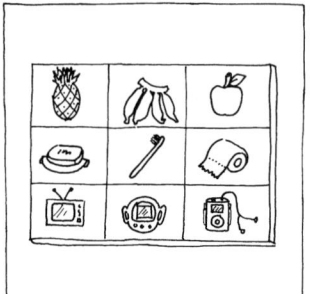

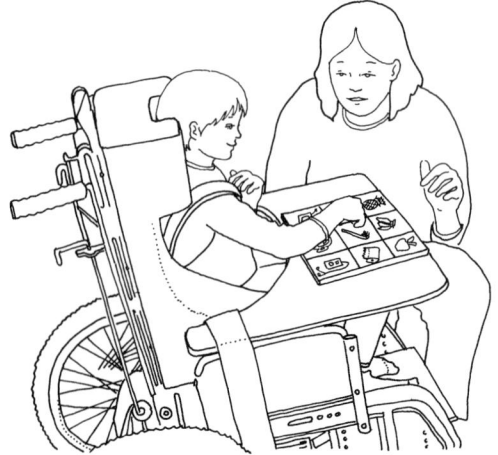

**Talkers**

Talkers are electronic devices that permit the elaboration or recording and reproduction of various communicative intentions. These tools vocalize prearranged messages and/or messages constructed by the child during dialogue using a text editor. The symbols used (images, letters or sentences) may be visual and correspond to specific sounds. The parents play a fundamental role in the arrangement, use and improvement of these tools because they are usually the facilitators closest to the children and more apt to understand their communication needs. Furthermore, the parents are usually the first to communicate with the child who uses AAC systems in daily life. This close interaction facilitates the inclusion of talkers in the child's day-to-day routines, games, outings, as well as the mediation and encouragement of the child in his attempts at beginning and conducting a dialogue, such as how to make a purchase or ask others for information (Figure 4.38, Activity 126).

**Figure 4.38    Activity 126**
Talkers

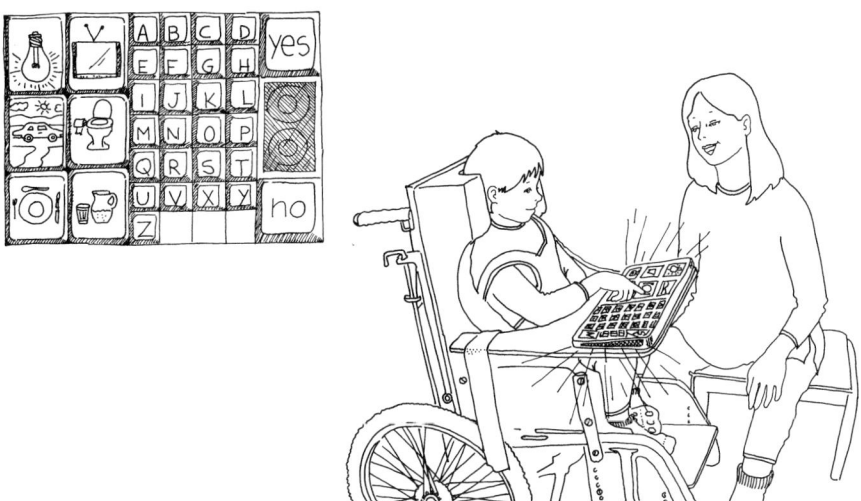

AAC systems are tools that can broaden the opportunities for expression and foster the development of language and thought in children with severe motor impairments and minimally intelligible speech. The systems should be adjusted periodically throughout development, and made to adapt to the communication needs and contexts of the child. Implementing the use of an AAC system is a gradual process that requires adaptation to changes in the child's daily context, as well as practice and persistence on the part of the child and family. Initially, the system may appear to be ineffective because the child will likely need time to express a communicative intention, and you may have to adapt your conversational style to the child's new forms of self-expression. It is important to remember the benefits that communication will bring to the child's socialization and academic processes. Although AAC systems facilitate more autonomy and independence in social interactions, they do not substitute speech nor do they guarantee real time in dialogue, thus demanding that speakers adapt to and respect the child's temporal dynamic.

# Speech and Language Disorders in TBI

Post-TBI children and adolescents may have specific disorders in speech and/or language that affect their independence in activities of daily life, as well as their performance in school. It is important to be familiar with the child's or adolescent's current communicative and linguistic abilities so that you can adapt your conversations to include strategies that facilitate their expressive efforts, oral and writing comprehension.

## Dysarthria

Dysarthria refers to problems coordinating and executing speech due to brain injury. Speech disorders can be observed in the child's or adolescent's breathing, which marks the beginning of the speaking process, in the manner in which sound is made (phonation), and in impaired speech-related articulation.[25]

The child or adolescent with TBI who is in the process of spontaneous speech recovery may have a weaker voice due to decreased respiratory support, which is essential to speaking, and lack of coordination between breathing and phonation.[2] Subsequently, voice and speech quality may be impaired, and can manifest as hypernasality and incorrect articulation of words. During rehabilitation, children's vocal intensity tends to adapt naturally once breathing has been adjusted and they have recovered their speech functions.

Some children or adolescents with TBI present dysarthria due to motor deficits. When there is a predominance of spasticity, the act of speaking may demand too much effort and the speech may sound distorted. With athetosis, the intensity of the voice can constantly vary (high–low), with frequent pauses or stops during speech. In children with ataxia, the main characteristics are tremulous voice and difficulties performing fine motor tasks with precision, which results in slow and monotonous speech.[25]

Dysarthria and communication can be rehabilitated at the same time. When you notice that the child or adolescent has difficulties saying a word, help him by providing correct feedback e.g., if he says "wa" to mean water, answer with the whole word and contextualize it by inserting it in a question, "Water? Do you want water?" This is a natural way for children or adolescents to experience and perceive the different ways words are articulated while having their errors corrected and increasing their chances to improve the articulation of their speech.

It is essential that speech rehabilitation in children and adolescents be conducted in a playful, contextualized manner. Oromotor exercises can be included in day-to-day activities, for example, stimulating the tongue muscles during oral hygiene. A soft-bristled toothbrush can be used to brush the tongue with gentle strokes over, inside to outside and around the edges of the tongue, sensorially stimulating the tongue. Associating exercises such as these with activities of daily life makes it easier to perform them consistently and more frequently without the child or adolescent being aware that they are engaging in rehabilitation exercises.

It is important to bear in mind that rehabilitation of dysarthria should focus on the functional aspect of communication. In cases of dysarthria that significantly impair the intelligibility of speech, alternative forms of communication may be used. When the dysarthria is mild to moderate, speech stimulation should aim at increasing intelligibility and adjusting the conversational dynamic to the best of the child's or adolescent's capabilities.

## Speech Apraxia

Another speech disorder observed in children and adolescents with TBI consists of difficulties programming and executing the orofacial movements essential to speaking, i.e., apraxia of speech.[26] Children with this disorder commit articulation errors and have impaired rhythm and prosody. Generally, the errors are not systematic, for example, the child may say "umbrella" incorrectly, omitting the first syllable "um", but might, at other times, leave out a different phoneme or syllable or may even say the whole word correctly.

There are several signs that characterize apraxia of speech, such as the struggle to find the appropriate movement for saying a given word, i.e., children may perform various oral motions in search of the one that will permit them to properly articulate that word. This struggle usually triggers constant interruptions in speech and may compromise its intelligibility, or cause a slowing down of what is being said. Difficulties sequentializing speech sounds is another characteristic of this disorder. When trying to say the word "elephant" the child may switch the order of the phonemes and utter "ephalent".

The ability to count numbers (automatic speech) in children or adolescents with these speech problems is usually less impaired than their capacity for spontaneous speech. They may also commit more mistakes when asked to repeat or read nonsense words. Apraxia of speech can compromise the development of reading and writing, as it may interfere with the child's ability to choose the sound and represent it in writing (phonological awareness).

The rehabilitation of speech apraxia involves activities that demand attention and promote the capacity to say words correctly. The child or adolescent should be encouraged to read texts that contain new words or sentence structures, for these will demand that they use phonological pathways of speech, such as decoding words letter by letter while trying to reproduce the sound. Activities that repeat movements, phonemes, words or songs can also be beneficial. Tape recorders can be useful tools that provide a source of feedback for the child or adolescent for they allow him to hear his own voice.

# Language Specific Disorders

## Aphasias Acquired during Childhood

Aphasias acquired during childhood are communication disorders that result from partial or total loss of language expression and/or comprehension due to brain injury. These are characterized by the inability to understand what is being heard or read and/or difficulties expressing oneself through speech or writing after a linguistic framework has already been established.[27] These comprehension and expression disorders interfere in the functionality of day-to-day communication because they affect the child's or adolescent's linguistic skills, but they are not related to sensorial aspects such as visual or auditory acuity or to motor functions associated with speech.[7]

Language deficits in children whose neurological impairments precede their first linguistic acquisitions are considered dysphasias.[28] In these cases, the child may be slow in attaining phonological, semantic and morphosyntactic functions, and may also have a decrease in pragmatic aspects associated with interactive communication opportunities.

With regards to oral expression dysfunctions in the initial stages of recovery, the child or adolescent may exhibit major difficulties verbalizing any sound or might present reduced spontaneous speech, occasionally saying only isolated words (initial mutism).[29] This speech deficit can also be observed in how gestures are performed, severely compromising the child's independence. At that moment, the parents and treatment team should be alert to any signs of communicative attempts on the part of the child or adolescent, including indicative gestures such as eye-gazing or pointing, and should also encourage the utterance of sounds. Based on these signals, you can try to interpret the child's intention by asking questions and by encouraging him to verbally express the meaning of what he wants. The use of familiar songs can also help the child verbalize.

Automatic speech and almost involuntary verbalizations, such as asking the other "what is your/my name?", are also sometimes observed. Creating situations that encourage oral responses in varied contexts, such as always greeting the child or adolescent, singing familiar songs or counting during physical activities help facilitate the recovery of oral expression.

Difficulties with naming significantly affect communication and language use. This function demands the recall of the names of objects, in other words, searching for, remembering and saying the object's name. The child or adolescent may use compensatory mechanisms, such as saying a word from the same word category when he is unable to recall the name of a certain object, e.g., "table" instead of "chair" (semantic paraphasia). Another mechanism involves saying a word that entails similar pronunciation sounds, such as "people" instead of "purple" (phonemic paraphasia).[25] These mechanisms help the listener better understand what the child or adolescent is trying to communicate because they offer clues about the action or object in question. Likewise, you can use semantic and phonetic clues that can help the child recall names, for example, by providing information about the word's semantic category, its characteristics and function, followed by phonetic clues such as mimicking the oral movement that produces the first sound of the word so he can try to complete it.

Because of their difficulties with expression, children and adolescents with TBI tend to have limited vocabulary and construct phrases and sentences with simple syntax, and omit connective elements (telegraphic speech). You can encourage the child to complete sentences by introducing connective language elements in conversation and stimulating him to continue the narrative[7].

Deficits in comprehension may be observed in childhood aphasia to a greater or lesser degree. This disorder is commonly perceived when, upon being asked to perform a given action, the child or adolescent may perform it inadequately or only partially. Many times, comprehension impairments are more pronounced when children or adolescents start or return to school, when greater mastery, or refined use, of language becomes necessary.

During the initial stages of post-TBI recovery, children and adolescents with severe comprehension deficits might not be aware of their own dysfunction and may give inadequate responses or use meaningless words to communicate, i.e., jargon. Furthermore, they may not perceive that their discourse is incomprehensible, as in the case of anosognosia. Another dysfunction that interferes with comprehension is agnosia, i.e., the inability to recognize familiar objects through sensory perception (visual, auditory or tactile). The child or adolescent might not, for example, visually recognize a key but upon touching and handling it, may be able to identify it and say its name or purpose. The same occurs with hearing and touch.[30] Auditory agnosia is related to the naming of objects, e.g., the child hears the word "shirt" but does not associate it with a piece of clothing that he wears, an incapacity that may be interpreted as a hearing impairment. Adjustments in conversational style are beneficial, such as short phrases with simplified vocabulary, contextualized in daily life, and reinforced with gestures. Communicative activities aimed at improving listening comprehension and facilitating expression should be contextualized within situations of daily life, and may include other settings with which children or adolescents are familiar such as a visit to the library, a trip to the movies, sports or musical activities.

When associated with acquired childhood aphasia, the difficulties in written language disorders are similar to those observed in listening comprehension and oral expression, and can affect functions that range from understanding isolated written words to partial or total impairment of text interpretation. Problems with written language in children and adolescents with TBI can also occur and may not be associated with aphasia, such as focal deficits that affect written comprehension, e.g., reading (acquired alexia or dyslexia) or written expression (acquired agraphia).[31]

With regards to written comprehension, children or adolescents may not be able to read an entire text because of deficits in visual analysis that impair their comprehension. Because of deficits in phonological access, e.g., difficulties recalling the association between phonemes (sounds) and graphemes (letters), they may be able to read words only letter by letter, or by syllable, which affects the synthesis of the word or sentence and, consequently, comprehension of the text (dyslexia). Children may be able to read or write words they are familiar with, but are not as successful with unfamiliar words.

Impairments of written expression can be the result of visuo-constructive or praxic disorders that affect the act of writing. When writing dysfunctions are associated with aphasia, the child or adolescent may have writing difficulties that are similar to those in oral expression. Problems with naming interfere with the writing of words and with more automatic responses, such as the writing of one's own name; furthermore, switching of words in the same category (semantic paragraphia) or spelling errors due to switches or substitutions of letters (phonetic paragraphia) may also be observed.

Encouraging the automatic writing of familiar names or words is one of the first exercises usually assigned to post-TBI children and adolescents for rehabilitating their writing functions. This activity can be performed in a contextualized manner and associated with other skills such as writing comprehension, for example, the filling in of personal information in ID questionnaires. Copying requires the integration of motor, perceptual and neuropsychological abilities and, as previously mentioned, activities should be contextualized in day-to-day life, such as transferring information to a new address book, or should be associated with other activities, such as naming or identifying words. Writing activities can be performed with the assistance of printed letter cards, isolated letters, or even a computer. If children or adolescents present impaired phonological access (difficulties evoking the letters of a word), writing can be facilitated by providing them with the letters that comprise a given word, but in a disordered fashion, so that they can put the word together themselves. Another tactic is to provide the letters of the words and add two or three extra ones that they must leave out when writing the word. These activities allow the child's or adolescent's world of letters to gradually expand. For written naming, crossword puzzles can be used, as well as the jotting down of messages and short texts.

Children and adolescents with brain injury may have speech and/or language disorders, in varying degrees of severity, that interfere with the intelligibility and quality of expression and comprehension, compromise communication and, consequently, impair academic performance and social interactions.[32] Being conscious of the child's or adolescent's difficulties, facilitating their language comprehension and expression, and looking for ways to adapt conversations to meet their capacities can help establish a more harmonious and productive dialogue.

# References

1. Puyuelo-Sanclemente M. Psychology, audition and language in different disorders of childhood: communication and neuropsychological aspects. Rev Neurol 2001; 32(10):975–980.

2. Rosenthall R. Rehabilitation of the adult and child with traumatic brain injury. 3rd ed. Philadelphia, PA: FA Davis, 1999.

3. Cogher L, Savage E, Smith MF. Cerebral palsy: the child and young person. London: Chapman and Hall, 1992.

4. Bates E, Reilly J, Wulfeck B et al. Differential effects of unilateral lesions on language production in children and adults. Brain Lang 2001; 79(2):223–265.

5. Ewing-Cobbs L, Barnes M. Linguistic outcomes following traumatic brain injury in children. Semin Pediatr Neurol 2002; 9(3):209–217.

6. Van Hout A. An outline of acquired aphasia in children. Saggi: Child Dev & Disabil 2000; 26(1):13–21.

7. Didus E, Anderson VA, Catroppa C. The development of pragmatic communication skills in head injured children. Pediatr Rehabil 1999; 3(4):177–186.

8. Ewing-Cobbs L, Barnes MA, Fletcher JM. Early brain injury in children: development and reorganization of cognitive function. Dev Neuropsychol 2003; 24(2–3):669–704.

9. Catroppa C, Anderson V. Recovery and predictors of language skills two years following pediatric traumatic brain injury. Brain Lang 2004; 88(1):68–78.

10. Luria AR. Pensamento e linguagem: as ultimas conferencias de Luria. Porto Alegre, Brazil: Artes Medicas, 1987.

11. Leontiev AN. O desenvolvimento do psiquismo. Lisbon: Livros Horizonte, 1978.

12. Slaughter V, McConnell D. Emergence of joint attention: relationships between gaze following, social referencing, imitation, and naming in infancy. J Genet Psychol 2003; 164(1):54–71.

13. Records NL. A measure of the contribution of a gesture to the perception of speech in listeners with aphasia. J Speech Hear Res 1994; 37(5):1086–1099.

14. Morse S, Haritou F, Ong K, Anderson V, Catroppa C, Rosenfeld J. Early effects of traumatic brain injury on young children's language performance: a preliminary linguistic analysis. Pediatr Rehabil 1999; 3(4):139–148.

15. Gelman SA, Coley JD, Rosengren KS, Hartman E, Pappas A. Beyond labeling: the role of maternal input in the acquisition of richly structured categories. Monogr Soc Res Child Dev 1998; 63(1):1–148.

16. Cahill LM, Murdoch BE, Theodoros DG. Articulatory function following traumatic brain injury in childhood: a perceptual and instrumental analysis. Brain Inj 2005; 19(1):55–79.

17. Clarke M, Kirton A. Patterns of interaction between children with physical disabilities using augmentative and alternative communication systems and their peers. Child Lang Teach & Ther 2003; 19(2):135–148.

18. Vygotsky LS. Pensamento e linguagem. São Paulo: Martins Fontes, 1991.

19. Ylvisaker M, Szekeres SF, Haarbauer-Krupa J. Cognitive rehabilitation: organization, memory, and language. In: Ylvisaker M, editor. Traumatic brain injury rehabilitation: children and adolescents. Boston: Butterworth-Heinemann, 1998: 181–220.

20. Pennington L, McConachie H. Interaction between children with cerebral palsy and their mothers: the effects of speech intelligibility. Int J Lang Commun Disord 2001; 36(3):371–393.

21. Pennington L, Goldbart J, Marshall J. Speech and language therapy to improve the communication skills of children with cerebral palsy. Cochrane Database Syst Rev 2004; (2):CD003466.

22. Chester CC, Henry K, Tarquinio T. Assistive technologies for children and adolescents with traumatic brain injury. In: Ylvisaker M, editor. Traumatic brain injury rehabilitation: children and adolescents. Boston: Butterworth-Heinemann, 1998: 107–120.

23. Fallon KA, Light JC, Paige TK. Enhancing vocabulary selection for preschoolers who require augmentative and alternative communication (AAC). Am J Speech Lang Pathol 2001; 10(1):81–94.

24. Fallon KA, Light J, Achenbach A. The semantic organization patterns of young children: implications for augmentative and alternative communication. AAC Augment Altern Commun 2003; 19(2):74–85.

25. Code L, McDonald S, Togher L. Communication disorders following traumatic brain injury. Hove, East Sussex: Psychology Press, 1999.

26. Murdoch BE. Dysarthria: a physiological approach to assessment and treatment. Cheltenham: Stanley Thornes, 1998.

27. Murdoch BE. Desenvolvimento da fala e disturbios da linguagem: uma abordagem neuroanatomica e neurofisiologica. Rio de Janeiro: Revinter, 1997.

28. Castano J. Clinical forms of infantile dysphasias. Rev Neurol 2002; 34 (Suppl 1):S107–S109.

29. Dayer A, Roulet E, Maeder P, Deonna T. Post-traumatic mutism in children: clinical characteristics, pattern of recovery and clinicopathological correlations. Eur J Paediatr Neurol 1998; 2(3):109–116.

30. Lezak M, Howieson DB, Loring DW. Neuropsychological assessment. New York: Oxford University Press, 2004.

31.    Cherney LR. Aphasia, alexia, and oral reading. Top Stroke Rehabil 2004; 11(1):22–36.

32.    Yeates KO, Swift E, Taylor HG et al. Short- and long-term social outcomes following pediatric traumatic brain injury. J Int Neuropsychol Soc 2004; 10(3):412–426.

# 5

# Visuo-motor Coordination

*Luciana Rossi, Katia S Pinto and Eliane G Catanho*

Brain injury causes restructuring not only of the neuronal networks, but also of the manner in which daily life activities are performed. Children may be able to discover alternative pathways to attaining their goals. The more natural, spontaneous forms of movement are frequently those at which the child is most dexterous.

The main objectives of manual coordination are functional independence and the ability to accomplish a task. Some children with brain injury may take longer to perform a manual activity and may be clumsy or uncoordinated when doing so, but they will nonetheless achieve efficient results. These children tend to choose the more effective strategy for performing the activities that require less time, planning or concentration.[1]

The notion that speed equals efficiency has been widespread, but the fact that one child is faster than another does not necessarily mean the final product will be qualitatively better. For example, students with brain injury may be slower at writing, which can put them at a disadvantage in relation to their classmates because they write fewer words per minute. However, the qualitative results of their writing, what they are able to express, the manner in which they are able to organize their ideas, and their level of creativity are factors that are not automatically associated with how fast they are able to write.

Nevertheless, a student may take so long to perform a given task that it becomes tiring, and he can end up losing his motivation and interest in what he is doing. Going back to the example of school: when the child has a brain injury, his writing pace may be significantly impaired for various reasons, and this can cause him to always be the last one to finish. All of these repercussions can also have a negative influence on his learning abilities as well as his self-esteem.[2] Some children may require special adaptations and assistance from bioengineering technology.[3]

The goal of adaptations is to improve skill and dexterity. If the student takes too long to copy items from the blackboard, and if he is incapable of going any faster, a fact that may be upsetting him, then certain strategies, such as special adaptations may be called for. These can include writing on a computer or making photocopies of a classmate's notes, or even using a tape recorder. This is just one example of adjusting the situation to meet the child's needs.

# Program of Activities

When planning an activities program for the child or adolescent with brain injury, it is beneficial to first discuss the meaning of the development, improvement or recovery of manual skills. Helping a recovering child or adolescent develop different forms of grasping, and explore movement precision and speed are components that can optimize his motor acts. However, it is important to understand that performance varies from one individual to another.

To develop a program for recovering manual function, the rehabilitation team and the family should discuss the child's interests in games and daily manual activities, in other words, what he likes to do and what strategies he has already developed on his own. Select the objects for manipulation based on the child's current interests and, if possible, allow him to help choose them. Present stimuli gradually and observe the child's reactions, gestures, attempts and ways of solving problems.

Every child has an appropriate position for his hands that allows him to free them up, keep them together and visualize what he is doing.[4] Some smaller children will manipulate objects better if they are sitting on someone's lap, or when seated with support, or even when lying on their side. The best positioning should be chosen for each child individually. In the absence or deficit of trunk balance, a corner-chair or table adapted to the child's size can be used, or even a board-table adapted to the wheelchair.

The following program of activities is organized based on the functions of reaching and grasping, bimanual skill, vertical coordination, fine movements, planning exercises, and games. Although this program is structured to introduce gradually increasing levels of complexity, children with brain injury may bypass certain sections without having had to complete the previous one, depending on their potential. For adolescents with traumatic brain injury (TBI), the need for some of the activities in this first section may be transitory.

## *Reaching and Grasping*

The hands play an important role in children's daily life. They are important for playing, exploring and attaining independence. Throughout the first year of life, children undergo a significant change in behavior; they mature from reflexive reactions to intentional actions, learn different forms of exploring a toy, and gradually acquire a greater capacity for acting on objects and coordinating different movements to reach an object.[5–7] To reach for an object, children must be able to move their hands from one point to another.[8]

### Tactile exploration with the hands

The child's first sensory and tactile experiences will help him discover his hands, establish body awareness, and develop reaching and grasping movements. Children with cerebral palsy (CP) can benefit from activities such as singing and performing rhythmic motions, or passing one hand over the other, which will allow them to feel and relax their hands (Figure 5.1, Activity 127).

**Figure 5.1    Activity 127**
Tactile exploration with
the hands

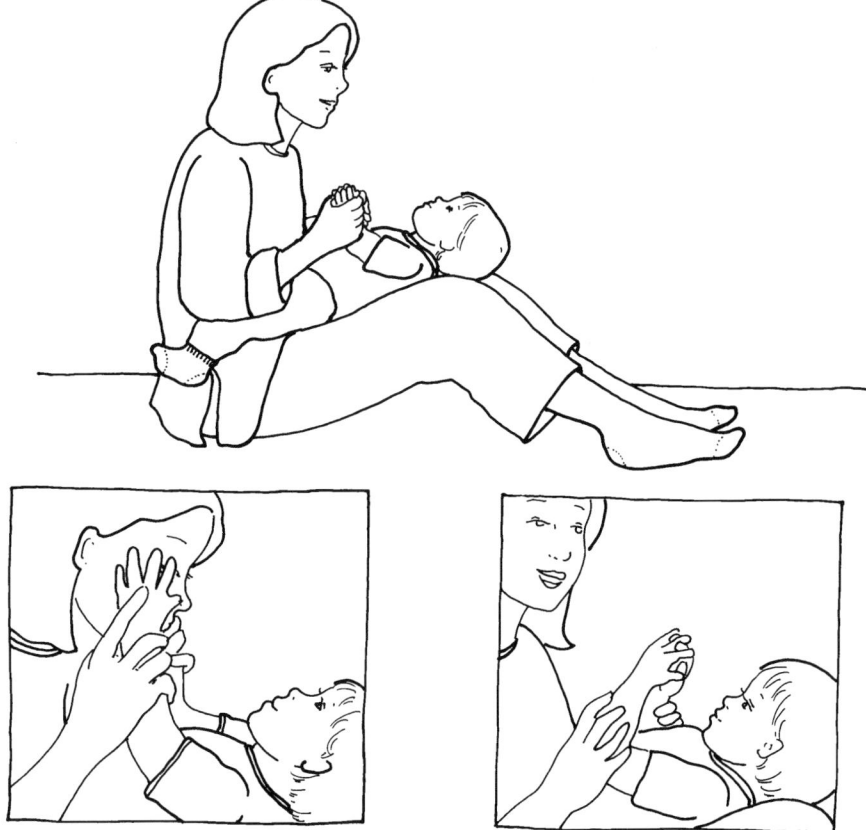

141

**Visual fixation and reaching movements**

The child uses tactile and visual information to become skillful at using visual input to adjust his hands to the size and shape of the object before grasping.[9-10] You can place within the child's reach a variety of objects that help foster visual perception and stimulate attempts, for example, grasping at a toy so that he can examine it. By using spontaneous, unintentional movements, he begins to touch or shake the toys placed within his visual field. As he repeats these attempts, he starts to perceive that his actions impact on his surroundings (Figure 5.2, Activity 128).

**Figure 5.2    Activity 128**
Visual fixation and
reaching movements

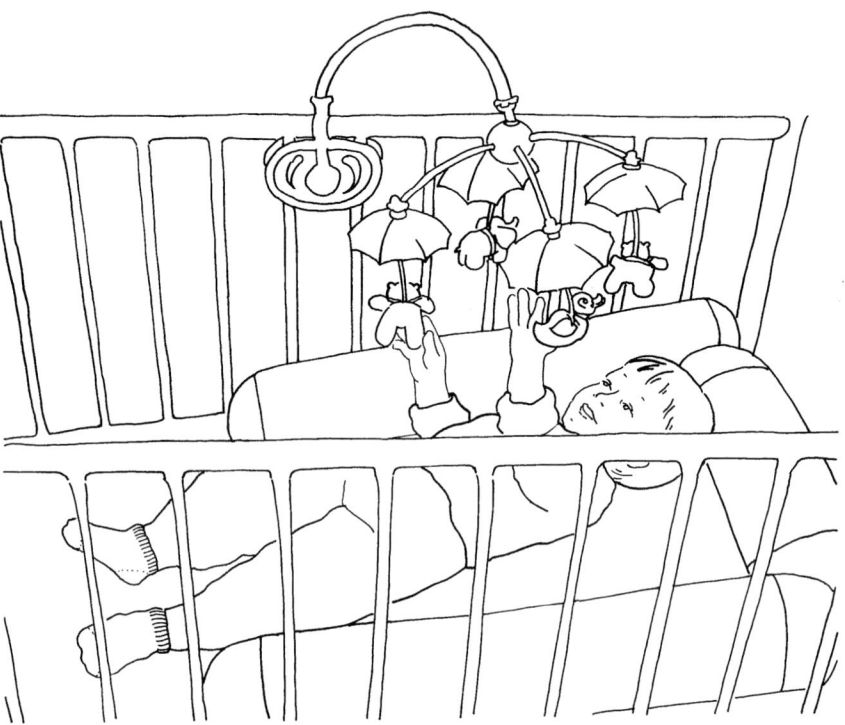

It is important to choose or adapt the type of toys that will most pique and sustain the child's attention and change them frequently. Light/dark contrasts such as checkers or intense colors can help maintain the attention of children with visual disorders.[11]

**Playing on his side**

Lying on their side helps children sustain their head in the midline and bring their hands together for reaching and exploring toys. Use a pillow to support the child's back, helping him maintain this position, and place easy-to-handle toys within his reach (Figure 5.3, Activity 129).

**Figure 5.3    Activity 129**
Playing on his side

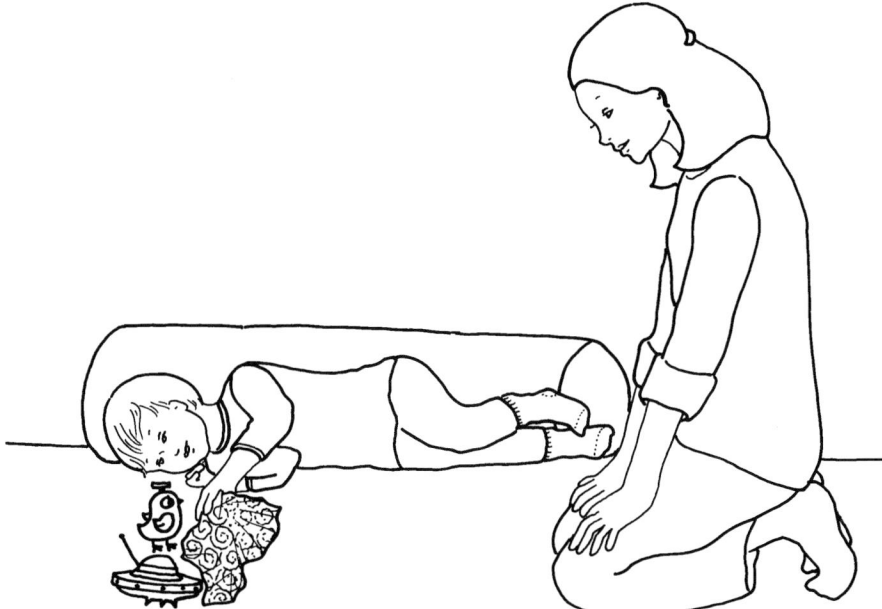

Some children with CP may develop uncommon forms of reaching for and exploring an object or toy. Observe these alternative pathways developed naturally by the child and, if possible, respect and encourage them, for they may help him to attain a goal in his own way.

Visual disorders secondary to brain injury are common. These are often multiple and complex, and can interfere in the process of development.[12] Observe the child's responses and reactions to visual stimuli. It is often necessary to bring an object close to the child's face so that he can see it better; at other times, he will have a better response to objects that are distant or placed to the left or right of his field of vision. By being aware of these possibilities, you can adjust the presentation of the visual stimuli to promote the child's perception and manipulation of objects. Another way to stimulate the first reaching movements in the child who is beginning to develop this function is to place objects very close to his hands so that he can begin practicing reaching and grasping movements.

## Holding and Releasing Objects with Both Hands

The evolution of bimanual skill implies the ability to move the hands in different directions and use their actions to complement each other. The use of the hands must be coordinated and, at the same time, disassociated. Control of the movements for grasping objects precedes the ability to release them.[8]

**Grasping with both hands**

The child acquires the ability to grasp an object with both hands by simultaneously using, at first, the region of the palm and base of the thumb. Positioning the child in a seated or reclining position facilitates visualization of the object and helps free up his hands for bimanual activity. You can give him large, light-weight objects such as a ball, or flexible items with different textures, because they facilitate grasping, bimanual function and sensory integration (Figure 5.4, Activity 130).

**Figure 5.4  Activity 130**
Grasping with both hands

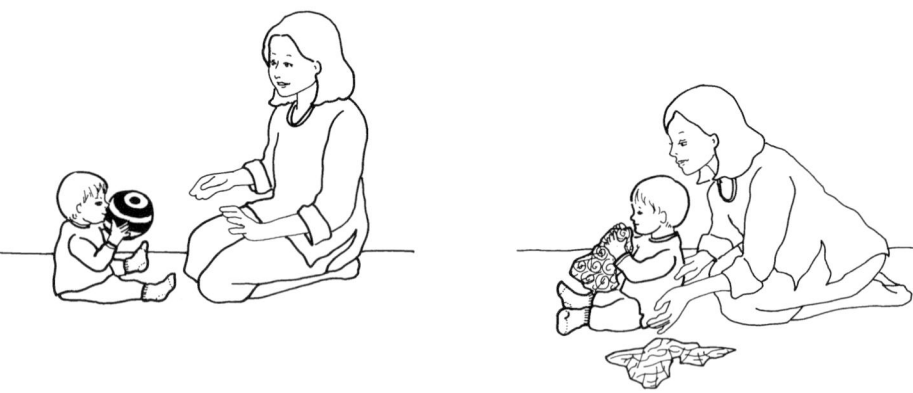

**Hand-to-hand transfer**

As the child performs simultaneous grasping, he begins to transfer an object from one hand to another. While one of the hands holds the object, the other explores it tactilely (Figure 5.5, Activity 131).

**Figure 5.5  Activity 131**
Hand-to-hand transfer

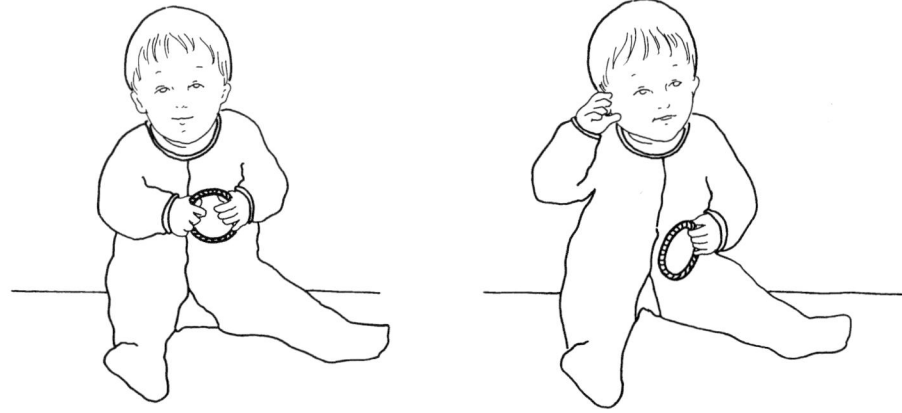

144

**One object in each hand**

While the child is holding an object in each hand, he learns to perform distinct, coordinated movements between the hands. Throughout this process, he develops greater variability in exploring objects (Figure 5.6, Activity 132). Games with music, conducted using broad, bimanual gestures, are alternatives for exercising arm movements.

**Figure 5.6   Activity 132**
One object in each hand

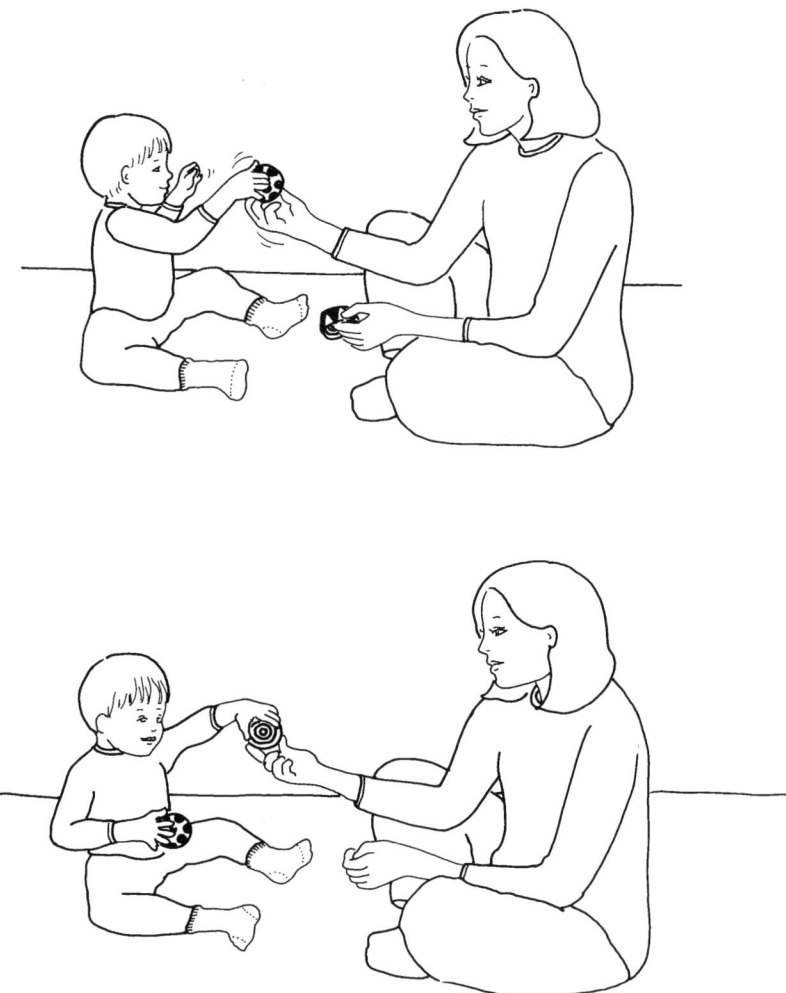

Children with balance deficits may have problems coordinating the manipulation of objects with both hands if they are not adequately positioned. Some are able to free up only one of their hands for handling the object and also need to use their arms for support. Many children will persist in this essentially unilateral hand use for grasping and exploring toys due to sensory deficits or impairments.

**Tearing paper**

More evident progress of the child's development of bimanual functioning is seen in how he performs daily life activities.[13] During the initial stages of bimanual object exploration, give the child pieces of paper for him to tear, or ask him to open a bag of cookies, or help him drink from a cup, for example (Figure 5.7, Activity 133).

**Figure 5.7   Activity 133**
Tearing paper

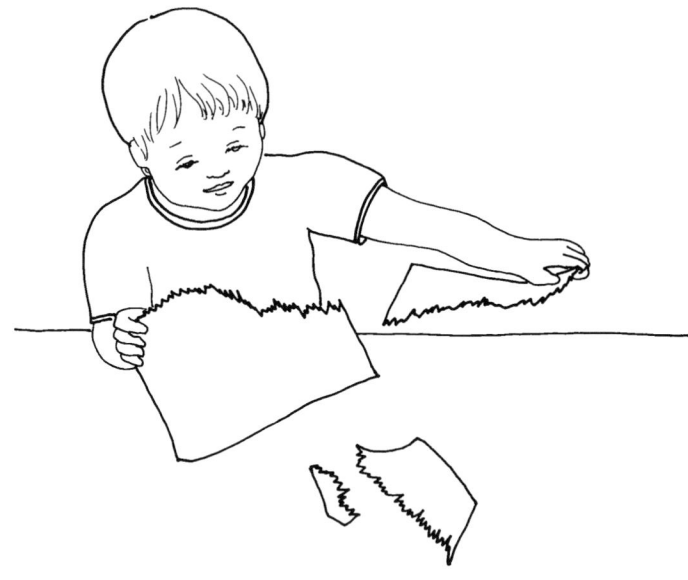

**Twisting and untwisting**

Another alternative is to encourage the child to handle objects of daily living that will require him to move his hands in various directions, such as asking him to open a bottle of juice. This allows him to train manual function while contributing to greater autonomy in everyday living skills (Figure 5.8, Activity 134).

**Figure 5.8   Activity 134**
Twisting and untwisting

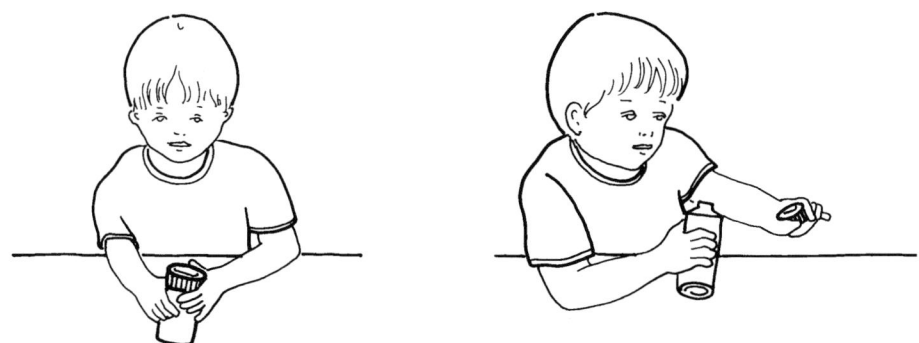

**Releasing objects**

The child, at first, learns to release an object by touching surfaces; voluntary release develops later in infancy and is one of the components of skilled object interaction.[9] You can offer the child sound-making objects of different sizes and weights, and gradually begin to ask him to put the objects in specific places within the context of the situation (Figure 5.9, Activity 135).

**Figure 5.9    Activity 135**
Releasing objects

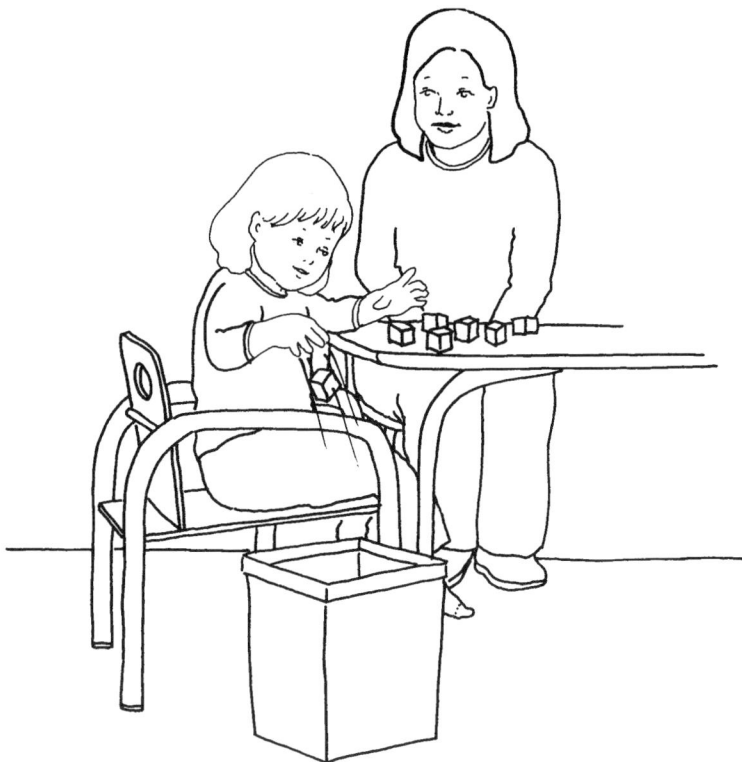

Coordination may be compromised in children with brain injury, resulting in prolonged and uncoordinated replacement and release of the object.[14] In some situations, the child may enlist the help of the other hand to release an object. These natural solutions help make the child's movements more functional and autonomous. Children and adolescents with TBI may also use these tactics, but they are usually transitory.

## Placing and Stacking

Children can make new tridimensional discoveries through tactile recognition of objects. They use their hands to explore depth, proportion, and size. Gradually, they will explore the vertical plane, which will demand different amplitude of arm movements, motor planning, balance, and fine motor coordination.

**Container play**

You can encourage the child to put away and retrieve toys from a large container, progressively increasing the number of objects. Varying their size, weight, and shape will help him gradually learn these differences through tactile sensations, and will also facilitate his adjustment of both anticipatory reaching movements and the release of objects within a container. This type of activity can be incorporated into daily life routines, such as gathering up toys and placing them in a box after the child is done playing with them (Figure 5.10, Activity 136).

**Figure 5.10   Activity 136**
Container play

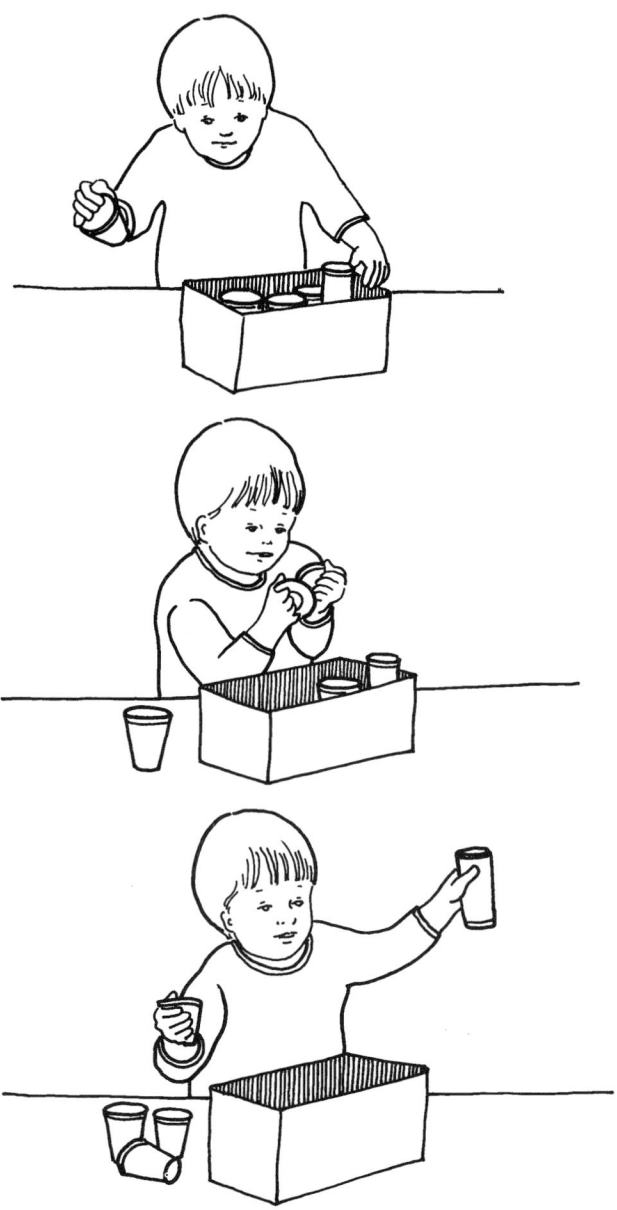

## One inside the other

Replacing and removing objects from a box precedes more precise placing movements, which demand greater selectivity and integration of sensory information.[8] The simple, bimanual act of placing one object inside the other can be stimulated by using objects found in the child's day-to-day life, such as plastic cups or boxes of various sizes (Figure 5.11, Activity 137).

**Figure 5.11    Activity 137**
One inside the other

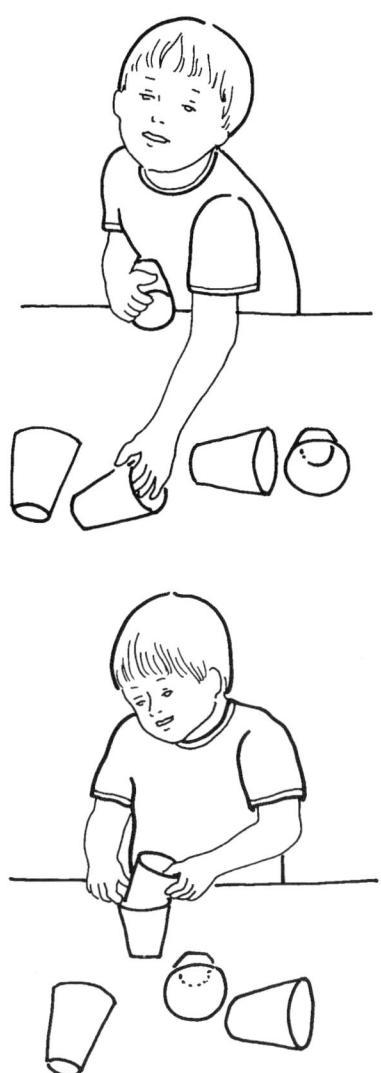

**Ringtoss**

Gradually, insertion of toys that stimulate manipulation on a vertical plane can be added (Figure 5.12, Activity 138).

**Figure 5.12    Activity 138**
Ringtoss

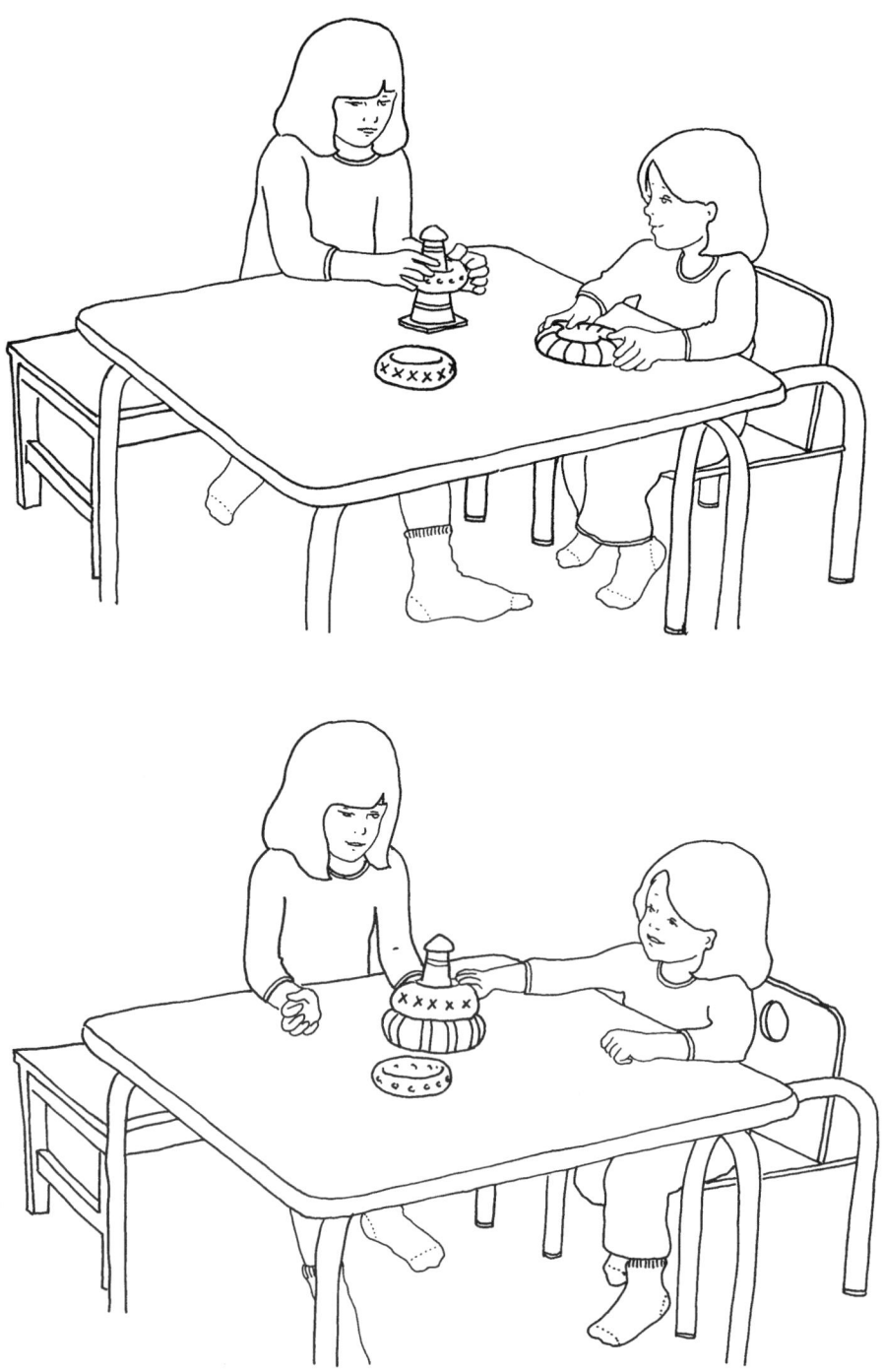

**Stacking blocks and building blocks**

Games of building and stacking allow the child to explore the spatial orientation of the objects through vision and touch. Give the child blocks of different sizes, colors, and shapes and let him use his imagination and creativity to make decisions about how to construct balance (Figure 5.13, Activity 139 and Figure 5.14, Activity 140).

**Figure 5.13   Activity 139**
Stacking blocks

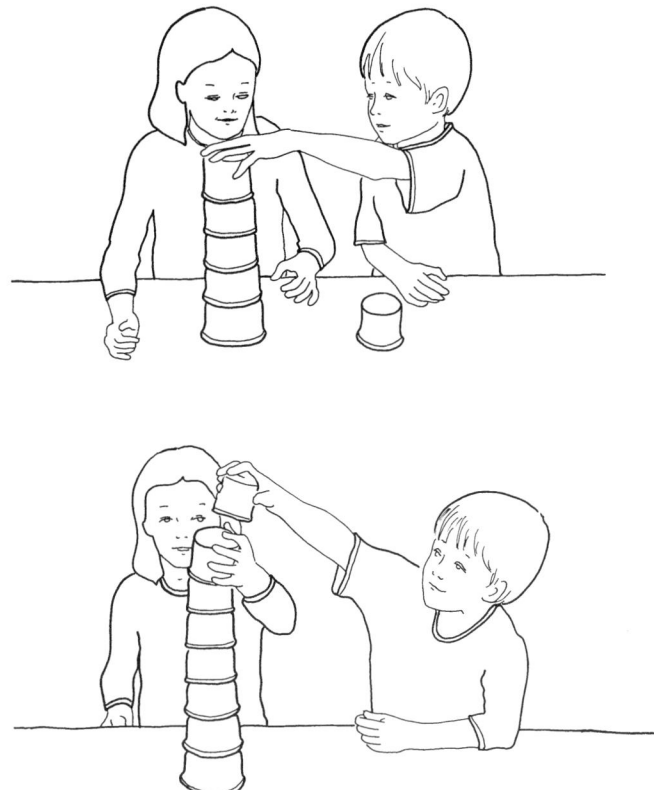

Children with diplegia may have visuo-constructive deficits.[15] After TBI, children may also have difficulties with activities that involve taking things apart, putting them together, or manipulating them in order to achieve the desired results.[16] These difficulties may persist throughout development, leading to poor motivation for activities of this nature.

*Fine Motor Skills*

The ability to use the fingertips to perform isolated finger movements increases the ways in which a child is able to explore objects. Maturation of the pincer grasp and development of perceptive and cognitive abilities help facilitate the execution of functional activities such as handling silverware, buttoning, and tying bows or laces.[24]

**Figure 5.14   Activity 140**
Building blocks

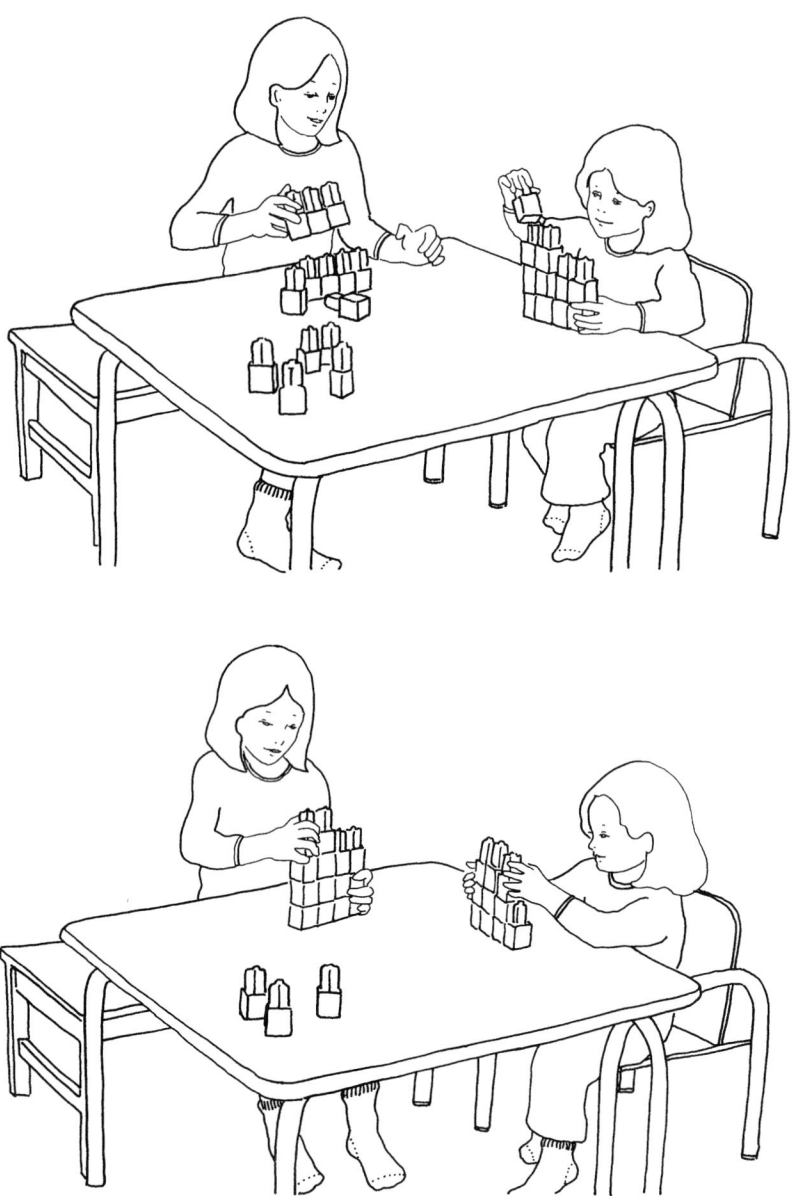

Children with brain injury may have visual disorders that interfere in the fine manipulation of objects. Postural control deficits, spasticity, ataxia, and involuntary movements can, in varying degrees, compromise the pincer grasp in children with CP. For children with palmar grasp patterns, the grasping of small or tiny objects is difficult. Be sure to choose the toys according to the child's grasping abilities. Adapting the objects, especially those used in activities of daily life can facilitate handling and independence in daily life tasks. Many self-care activities require bilateral movements that are sequential and complementary allied with fine, precise movements.[17]

The association between cognitive and motor abilities plays an important role in the development of fine manual skills.[18] Poor interest in objects can compromise the child's development of motor strategies that are necessary for more complex skills.[19]

**Pegboard**

The pincer grasp involves touching the tip of the thumb to the tip of the index or middle finger, a movement that demands neuromotor control and flexibility. Games that involve fitting together small objects of various sizes and shapes can help the child create and experiment with different neuromotor strategies (Figure 5.15, Activity 141). Engaging the child in activities of daily life that include fine placing such as buttoning a shirt or putting on wardrobe accessories (e.g., belt, jewelry, watch) is a way to motivate him to participate in household tasks and develop or improve his fine motor skills.

**Figure 5.15    Activity 141**
Pegboard

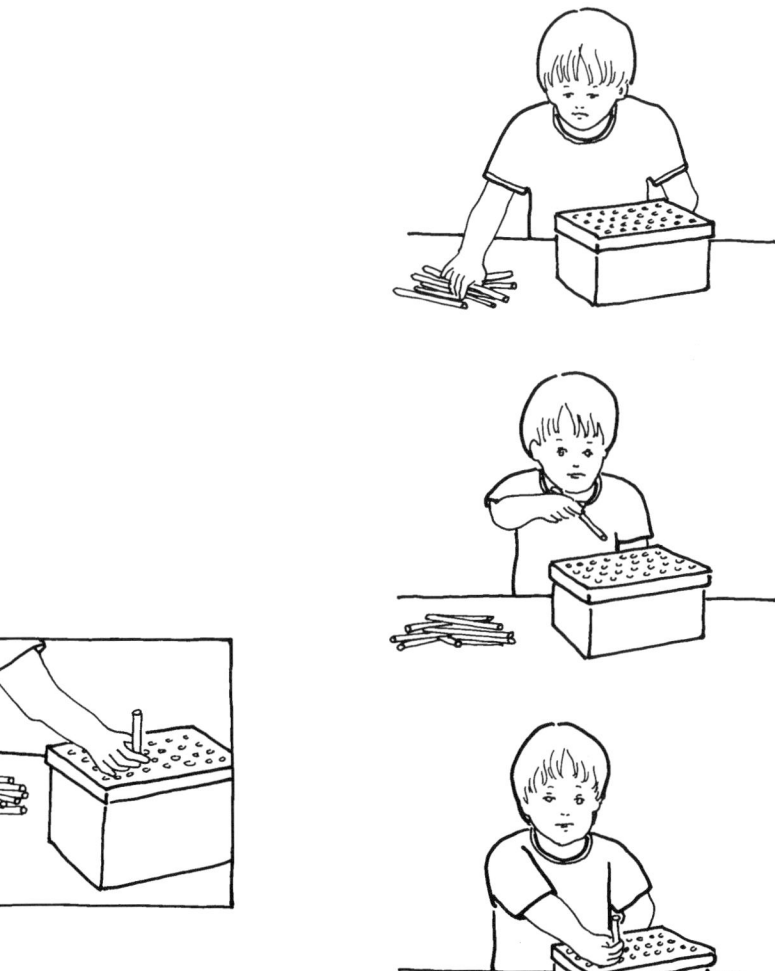

It is particularly difficult for the child with involuntary movements to sustain head and trunk positioning, and stability of the proximal joints of the upper limbs during manual activities. In these cases, adequately positioning and supporting the child's upper limbs on a firm surface can help facilitate the finer distal movements.

## Hand-held electronic games

After the trauma, children with TBI may have fine motor deficits, especially those related to prolonged reaction time, reduced velocity, impairments in coordination and the strength required for manipulation.[20] Initially, electronic games can help motivate the child to apply fine motor skills, sustain his attention and contribute to dexterity in the disassociation of movements between the right and left hands (Figure 5.16, Activity 142).

**Figure 5.16   Activity 142**
Hand-held electronic games

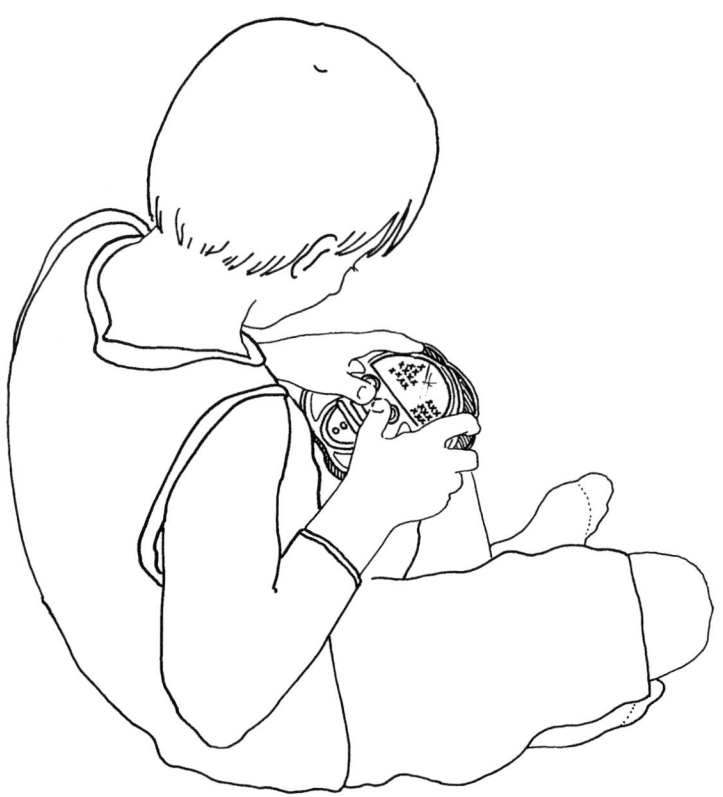

**Fine bimanual placing**

You can help the child execute fine bimanual activities by using the hand with greater placing skill while the other holds the object. Some children can use an opposed grasp pattern (thumb and fingers) with larger objects, but they will not have the dexterity to hold small or tiny ones (Figure 5.17, Activity 143).

**Figure 5.17   Activity 143**
Fine bimanual placing

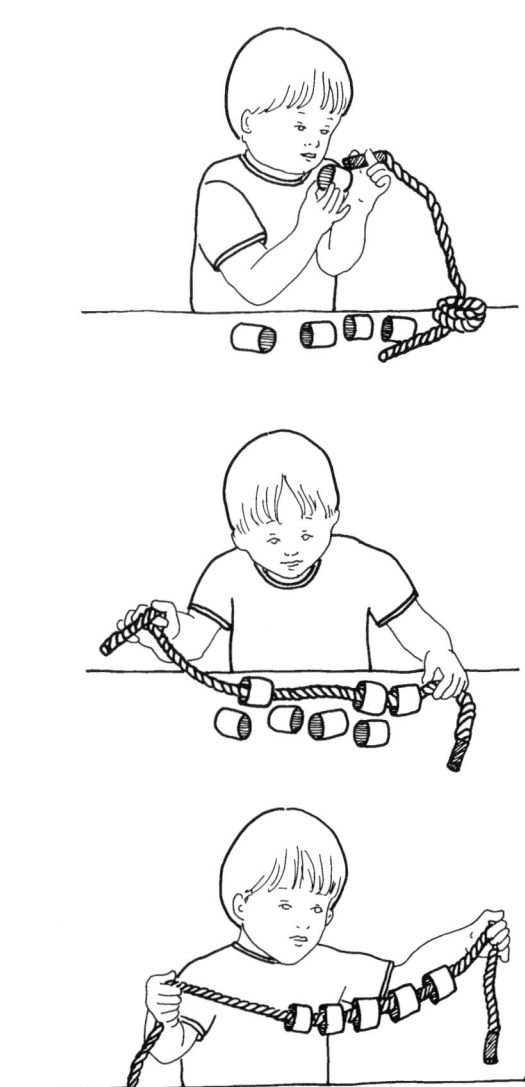

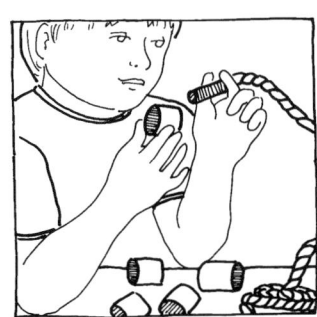

**Stringing small beads**

Engage the child in context-sensitive activities that promote the training of fine, bimanual skills. For example, give him tiny beads to string is an activity that he will likely enjoy and whose final product is rewarding (Figure 5.18, Activity 144).

**Figure 5.18   Activity 144**
Stringing small beads

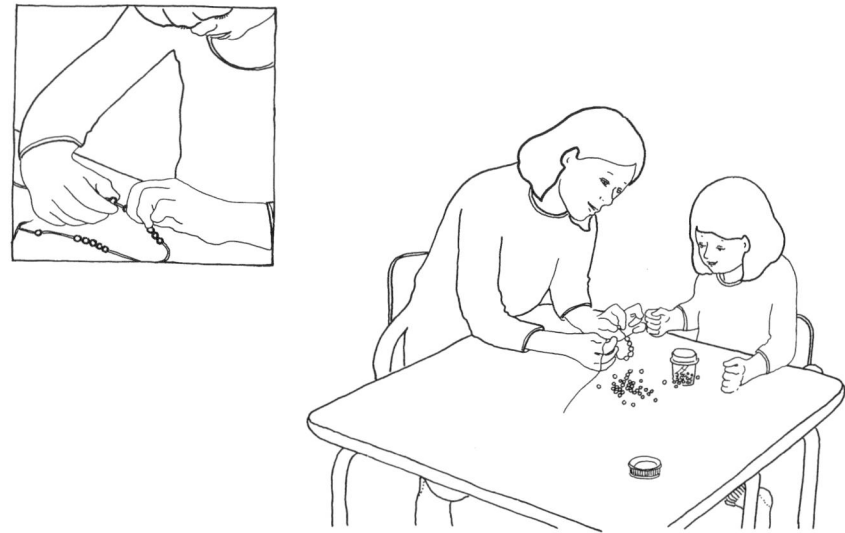

Children with brain injury may develop alternative ways to stabilize and manipulate objects that require both hands. These strategies can often include the use of other parts of the body, which helps improve the child's functionality and independence. Experimenting with various forms of performing a given movement can help the child make adjustments and discover the best way to do the manual activities.

## Sensory Integration and Planning

Sensory input is essential for fine manual dexterity.[21] Contact with an object triggers activity of the neuronal networks, which analyze the sensory input, establish a perception of the external world, then plan and execute movements. Sensory deficits in the hands, in association with motor impairments, may compromise the learning of new skills and the precision and coordination of manual movements.

**Touch recognition**

Stereognosis is the ability to use tactile information to recognize the shape, size, texture, and consistency of an object.[22] The child, in his day-to-day activities, uses these markers, for example, to look for a toy in a box and to adjust the movement of a key in the lock. As with the other senses, tactile sensation develops as the central nervous system matures. Astereognosia, or deficient stereognosis, can be present with CP, especially in children with hemiplegia,[23] as well as those with TBI. You can help the child develop strategies for recognizing an object through tactile input by encouraging him to look for a given item in his school bag, in a dresser drawer and other such contextualized situations. This will allow him to recognize his capacity to identify objects separately with his hands. If necessary, suggest alternatives that could help him in his day-to-day routines, such as using both hands to identify one object (Figure 5.19, Activity 145).

**Figure 5.19    Activity 145**
Touch recognition

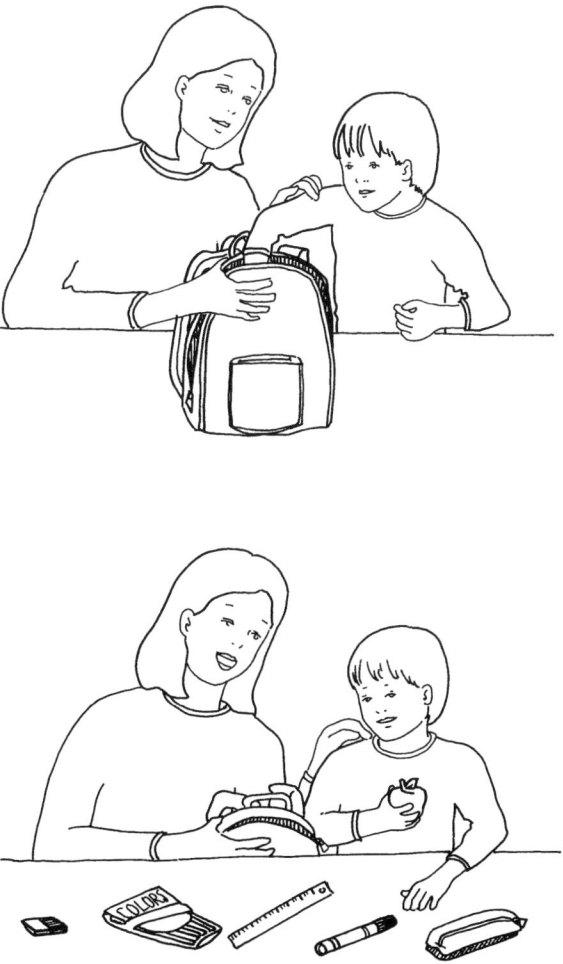

**Tearing and gluing**

Sensory information and the ability to plan and execute a sequence of actions are factors related to the child's manual performance. In cut-and-paste activities, he can use visual input to guide his hand, preparing it for the grasping of paper and the mounting of his collage. By using tactile information, he can regulate the grasping force and the handling of the paper during the pasting (Figure 5.20, Activity 146). In day-to-day life, during leisure moments, encourage the child to play with other children, which may make him more motivated to participate in activities while allowing him to interact and learn with others.

**Figure 5.20    Activity 146**
Tearing and gluing

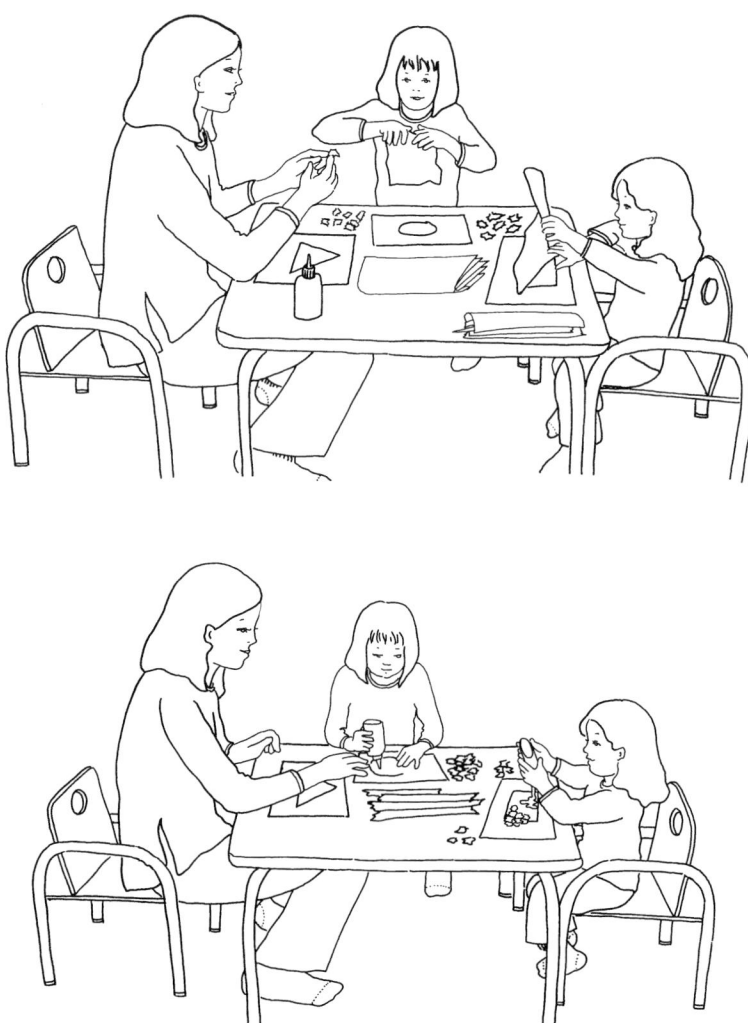

**Cutting with scissors**

Handling a pair of scissors requires separating the motor function of the two sides of the hand, with flexion and extension of the tripod digits acting simultaneously.[9] Initially the child can exercise the simple opening and closing of the blades to train the rhythm of the necessary movements. Encourage him to cut small pieces of paper, then cardboard and, finally, thin sheets (Figure 5.21, Activity 147).

**Figure 5.21    Activity 147**
Cutting with scissors

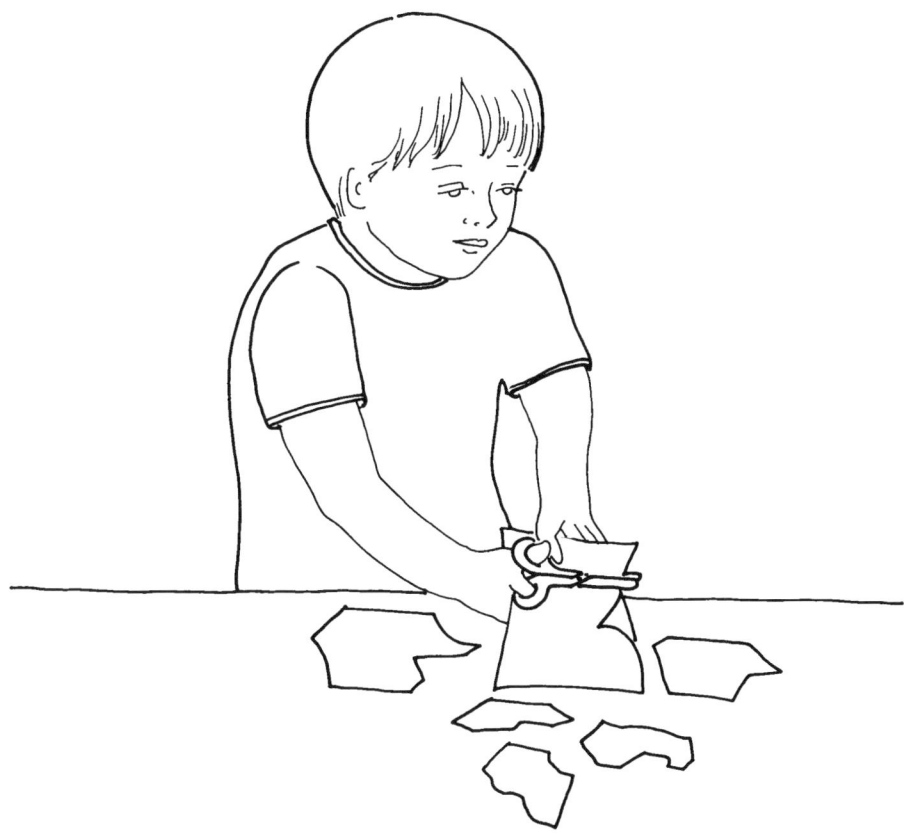

**Folding paper**

Folding exercises motor planning and visuo-spatial abilities. You can encourage the child to perform these activities, beginning with more simple tasks such as folding a piece of paper. Exploring these skills within a familiar context may help him transfer his knowledge to different daily life situations in which this skill is used, such as folding a piece of paper to place in an envelope, or during household chores, such as folding and putting away clothes (Figure 5.22, Activity 148).

**Figure 5.22    Activity 148**
Folding paper

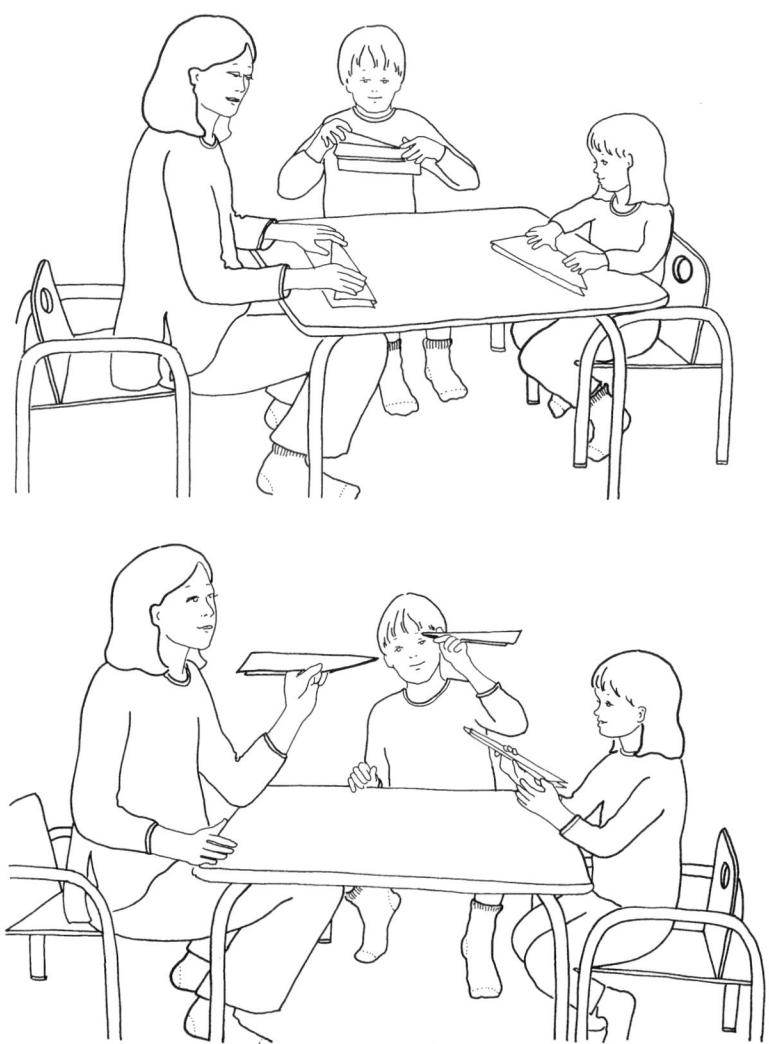

**Turning hands**

Many of the child's activities of daily life, such as washing his face, combing his hair, opening and closing containers, turning the pages of a book or magazine, require pronation-supination movements. Some children with brain injury may have difficulties performing supination movements, with predomination of forearm pronation patterns. In addition to daily life situations, playful activities can help motivate the child to actively and spontaneously perform supination movements during development age. You can draw various figures on the child's palm and act them out with simple gestures, encouraging him to turn the palm of his hand upwards (Figure 5.23, Activity 149). Using puppets for storytelling, sticking pieces of colored paper or tape on the child's palm and encouraging him to open and supinate the hand to remove the paper are also activities that can be used to stimulate this movement.

**Figure 5.23   Activity 149**
Turning hands

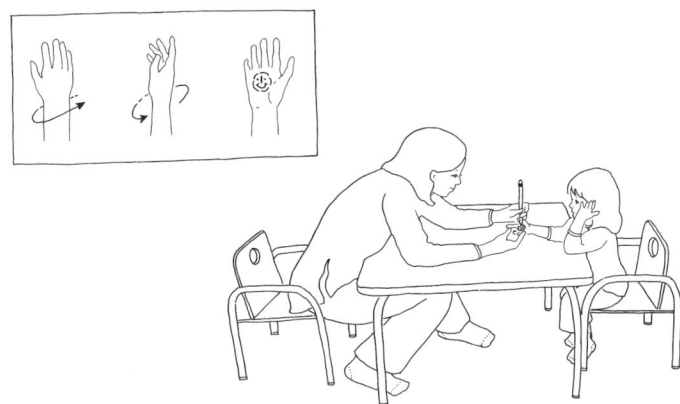

**Turning pages**

When looking at a storybook with the child, at home or in school, teach him to turn the pages, which will help develop arm movements and, gradually, the selectivity necessary for grasping one page at a time. While he learns to handle a book, engage him in language activities that help develop his vocabulary, detail perception of the illustrations, recognition of certain graphic concepts, and others (Figure 5.24, Activity 150).

**Figure 5.24   Activity 150**
Turning pages

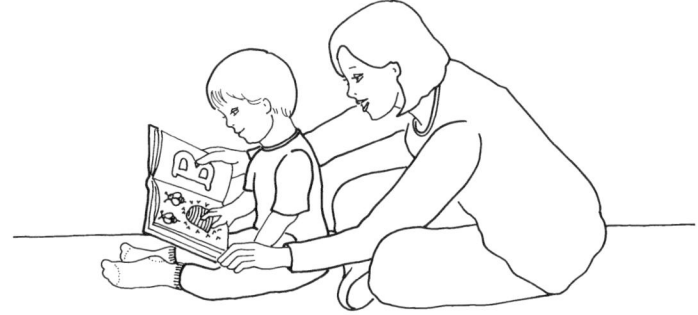

**Playgrounds**

Neighborhood and school playgrounds are special places to children, where they can play and interact with other children. During activities in the playground, the child can explore sensory integration and bimanual coordination, such as putting sand into a pail, using tools for different purposes, digging, understanding the differences between heavy objects and light ones, and exercising planning skills. Playing in the sand can facilitate the development of tactile identification of objects in children with sensitivity deficits (Figure 5.25, Activity 151).

**Figure 5.25   Activity 151**
Playgrounds

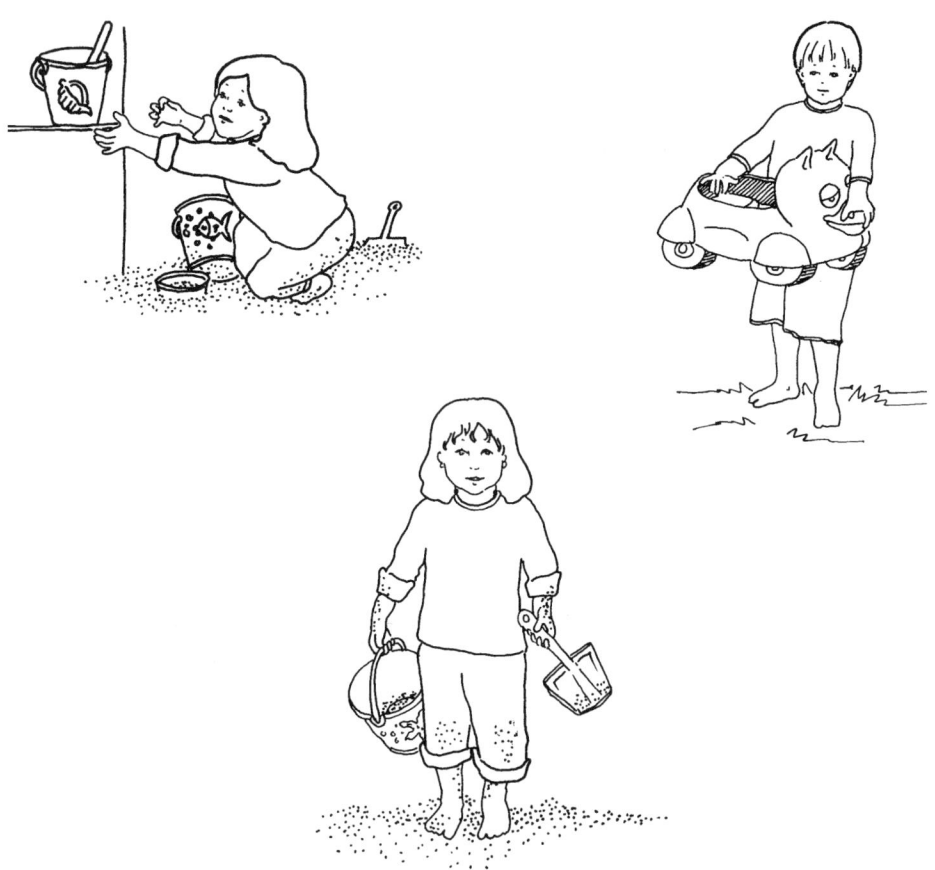

*Graphomotor Skills*

Painting, drawing and molding activities are related to expression and creativity in the child and can be developed, in various levels of complexity, throughout childhood. Studies conducted in different countries and cultures have shown that the evolution of children's drawings progresses through similar stages.[5] On the other hand, children who are not afforded the chance to experience these activities in early childhood may not be able to attain all of the milestones inherent to handwriting and drawing.

**Drawing**

Some children with CP may begin handwriting later than other children; those with TBI may have to relearn graphic functions after the injury. Encourage the child's interest in this activity by positioning his body in a way that will most facilitate his performance. Positioning him at an appropriately sized table so that he has optimum trunk stability and placing a sheet of paper on top of the table in front of him can help improve his performance (Figure 5.26, Activity 152). At first, offer him chunks of chalk or thick crayons, which are easier to grasp; however, variations in how these items are held are to be expected.[23–24] To stimulate free drawing, doodling or scribbling, draw lines on the paper and encourage the child to copy them, which will help him begin using these movements.

**Figure 5.26   Activity 152**
Drawing

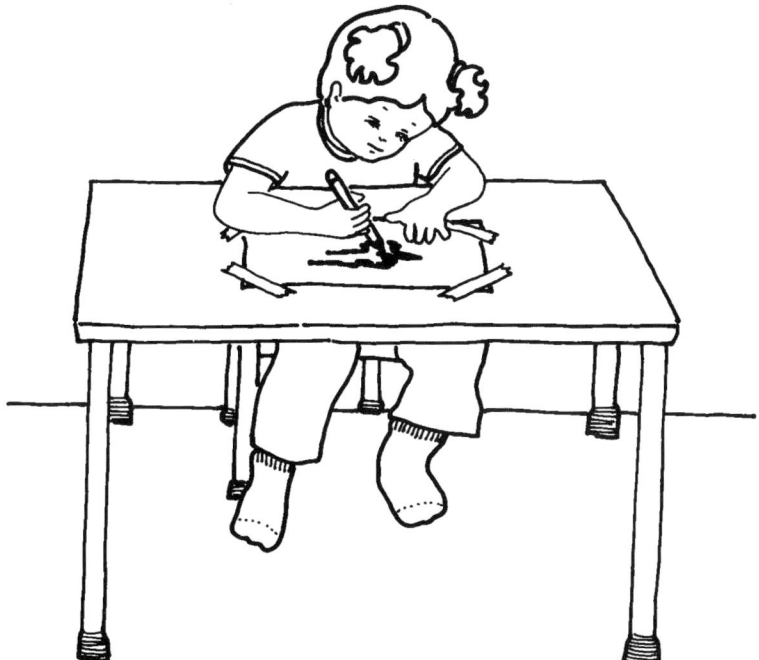

The drawing patterns of children with ataxia are characterized by broad strokes and irregular lines. As their experience grows and they mature, these children develop greater control of the movements but some will require adaptations to assist them.

**Drawing with a computer mouse**

Children with CP and involuntary movements may have considerable difficulties holding a pencil to draw or trace a line.[25] You can help the child discover ways that will best facilitate his attempts at drawing or writing. You may also consider the possible use of alternative means, and how they can impact on the child's future (Figure 5.27, Activity 153).

**Figure 5.27    Activity 153**
Drawing with a computer mouse

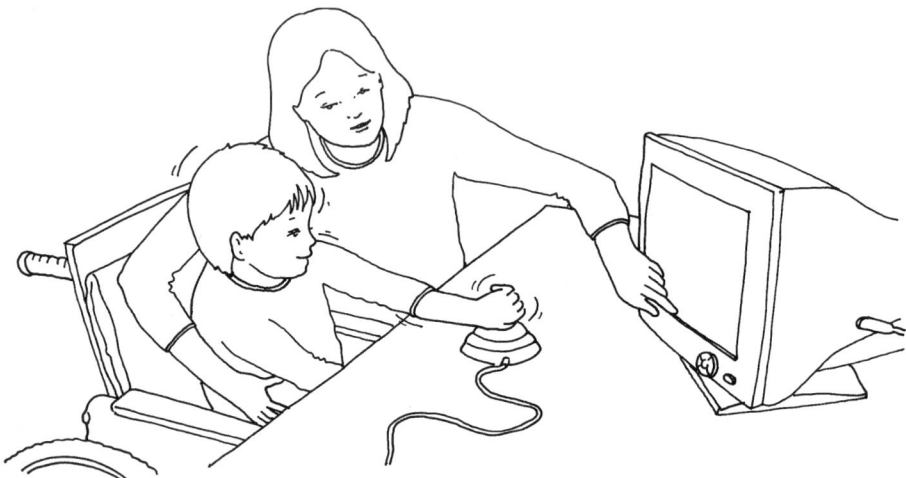

Some children with TBI switch handedness. They may also have shaky, trembling hand movements that often improve during recovery. It is difficult to accept that the child does not have the same level of performance as before the injury, but this may very well be a temporary situation. Allow the child to do what he feels he can, such as holding a pencil with his "best" hand, which will help him regain his skills. Free drawing, doodling or scribbling are of considerable importance to the child during the early phases of post-TBI recovery because it helps integrate perceptual and motor systems.

**Finger painting**

Painting with fingers is a sensory activity that the child can engage in even before he is able to hold a pencil. You can help by spilling some paint onto the paper, slowly sliding his hands through it and helping him make movements in different directions, while talking to him throughout the process. Finger painting is an alternative way of stimulating bimanual sensory activity, and is also indicated for encouraging the expression and creativity of children who have significant difficulties holding a pencil and drawing lines in the early stages of recovery. The first attempts at drawings by children with TBI can be the most difficult, especially for those who switched handedness. In addition to switching handedness, the child may have ataxia, which will further compromise coordinated movements. Finger painting demands less selective movements and can be a means to recovering graphic expression (Figure 5.28, Activity 154).

**Figure 5.28   Activity 154**
Finger painting

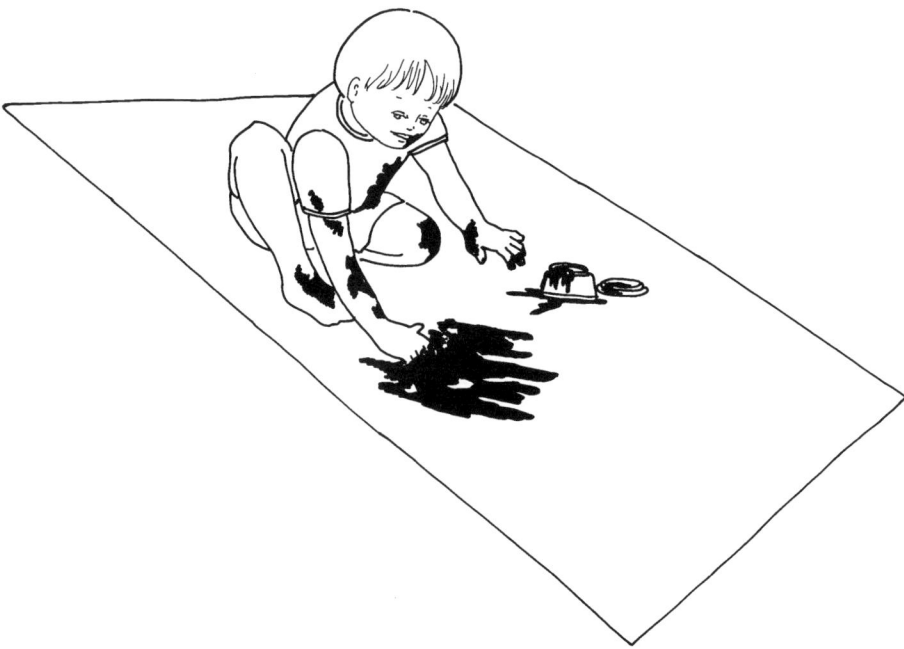

**Modeling clay**

The use of materials with different textures and consistencies promotes the development of stereognostic perception in the child. When the child works with modeling clay, he performs movements that cannot be done with paint. Without even looking at the clay, he is able to feel different shapes and volumes. Similarly, these molding activities can be incorporated into everyday family routines, such as in the preparation of bread or cookies (Figure 5.29, Activity 155).

**Figure 5.29   Activity 155**
Modeling clay

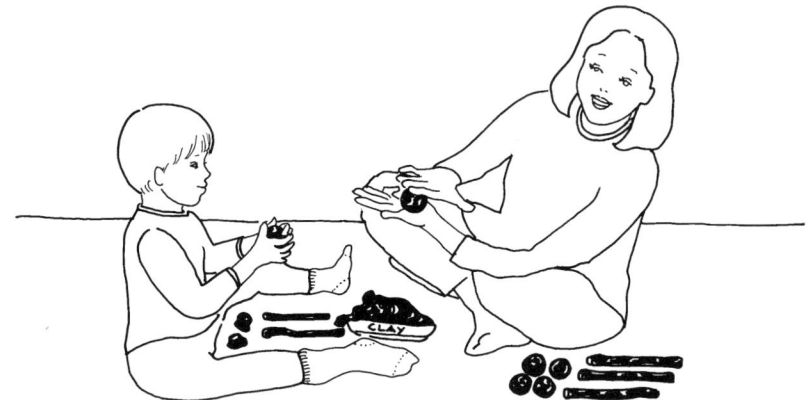

**Paintbrushes**

The use of paintbrushes and paint requires more precise, selective movements. To use them, the child or adolescent should be able to control grasping force and the amount of paintbrush pressure he will apply on the paper. Painting with paintbrushes helps exercise graphic expression and movement coordination. When offering the child a paintbrush, select it according to his grasping abilities; if necessary, the paper should be taped in place. Thicker paintbrushes may be easier to hold, may facilitate directing the gestures required for painting, and, consequently, can help the child develop this skill and exercise his creativity (Figure 5.30, Activity 156).

**Figure 5.30   Activity 156**
Paintbrushes

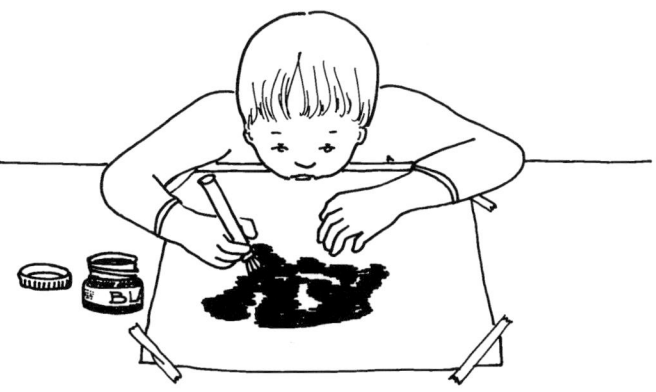

## *Interactive Games*

**Imitating sequential actions**

There are many types of imitation games, and many children naturally engage in these types of activities. To mimic an action, the child must be able to observe and reconstruct a sequence of acts based on an example, integrating visual and kinesthetic information. By being attentive to the importance of these activities to the child's praxic learning, you can take advantage of his natural interest and propose games that explore a series of movements and suggest that he imitate them (Figure 5.31, Activity 157).

**Figure 5.31   Activity 157**
Imitating sequential actions

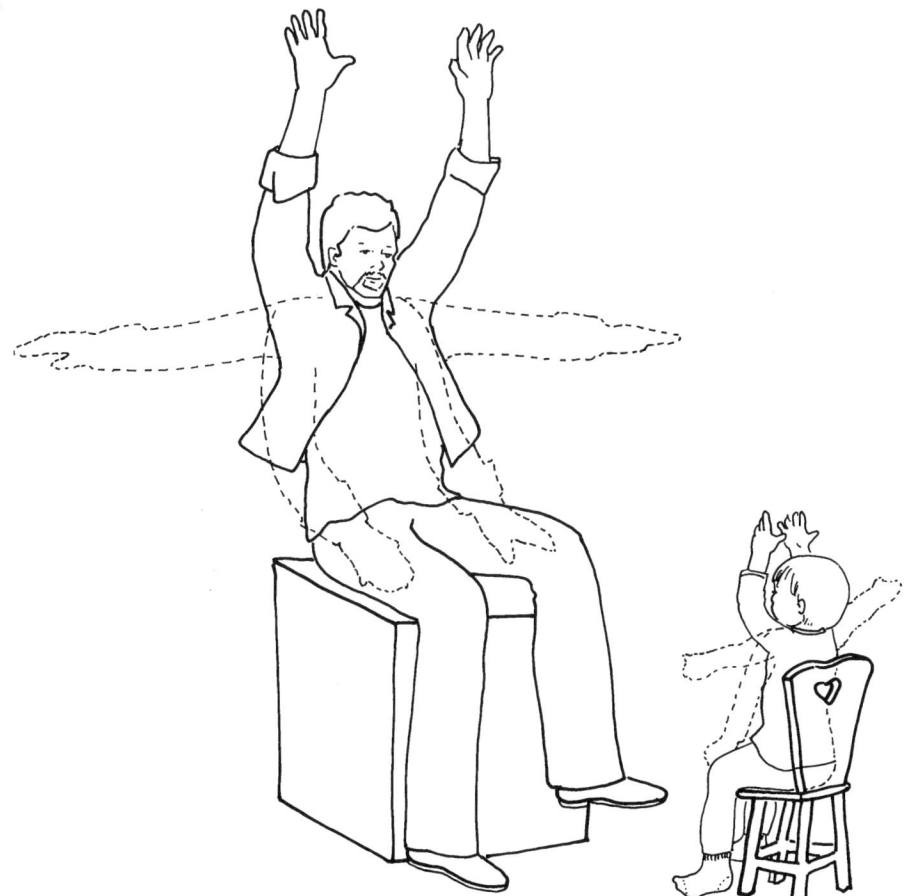

**Throwing a ball**

To throw a ball at a target, the child must coordinate the visual location of the target with the bodily movement required to propel the object, demanding a synchronization of the holding, throwing and releasing movements. After performing this sequence, the child needs to regain his balance. Initially, he may roll the ball along the floor mainly using his wrists and elbows. The direction of these movements may be very imprecise at first. You can stimulate the child to play games with his siblings, cousins or friends. Gradually, as the child develops better coordination, he may be able to use broader, quicker movements to throw the ball through the air with more precision (Figure 5.32, Activity 158).

**Figure 5.32    Activity 158**
Throwing a ball

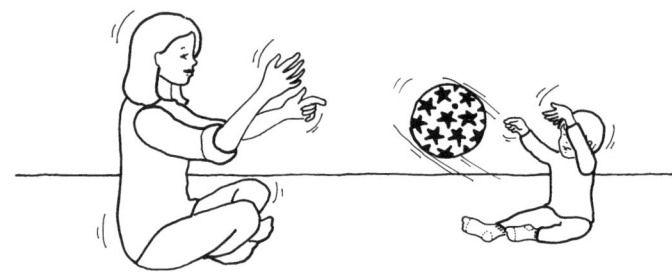

**Sports**

A group game is characterized, above all, by the interaction among players. It is a recreational way to stimulate the development of divided attention and concentration. It also provides the child with different situations that demand the use of his hands and arms. Encourage the child to participate in group games with friends or other members of the family, during leisure time or during more structured situations. For example, in a basketball game, children and adolescents move about in a wheelchair, in various directions through playful activities such as tag. At the same time, they can also be encouraged to engage in games that involve balls of various sizes, textures and weights, with targets that are also at varying distances, heights and which can either be fixed in place or moving. When choosing an activity for the child, remember to consider his interests what he most likes to do, and to discuss these choices and the possible need for adjustments (Figure 5.33, Activity 159).

**Figure 5.33    Activity 159**
Sports

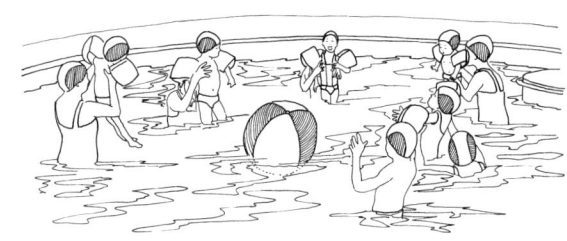

# School-aged Children and Adolescents with TBI

Most children and adolescents who sustain a TBI during school age return to school some months after the injury. Their ability to deal with and perform their functions in this setting should be carefully discussed by everyone involved in their rehabilitation process.

Head injury can affect manual skills acquired prior to the trauma or compromise the acquisition of new ones due to neuropsychological disorders that can also manifest later in the child's development. In addition to neuropsychological deficits, the child and adolescent may present movement impairments in varying degrees and, depending on the location of the injury, a switch in handedness can occur. During the early post-TBI recovery stages, motor deficits are common, especially hemiparesia, as are dysfunctions of the visual field.[12] These initial visuo-motor deficits are often quickly recovered during the first few post-injury months.

Perhaps many of these adaptation problems could be minimized with the involvement of teachers and educators in the student's recovery process. Contextualized proposals that respect the needs of the post-injury student, and that take into account the school's resources, tend to yield better results.

Many of the activities described in the first part of this chapter can be applied to school-aged children and adolescents who have post-TBI visuo-motor coordination disorders. However, the tasks should be adapted to the individual interests and needs of each child or adolescent, considering their level of pre-TBI function and current degree of impairment. Furthermore, in addition to adapting the tasks, the intensity of the activities should be adjusted to accommodate the various stages of the recovery process. Initially, the child and adolescent will tire more easily and perform the exercises more slowly; this is to be expected. It is important to adjust the timing and intensity of the rehabilitation activities.

This chapter presented activities that can help children and adolescents develop manual skills during the first years of life and discover individual, more efficient ways of performing a movement; they can also be used during the post-TBI recovery process. However, it is very important that the children engage in activities that they are interested in and that have been contextualized. This will help children apply their developing skills to their daily life, which will contribute to their learning processes.

# References

1.   Skold A, Josephsson S, Eliasson AC. Performing bimanual activities: the experiences of young persons with hemiplegic cerebral palsy. Am J Occup Ther 2004; 58(4):416–425.

2.   Geppert J. Yes, survive I did. Lancet 2004; 363(9421):1632.

3.   Chester C, Henry K, Tarquino T. Assistive technologies for children and adolescents with traumatic brain injury. In: Ylvisaker M, editor. Traumatic brain injury rehabilitation: children and adolescents. Boston: Butterworth-Heinemann, 1998: 107–120.

4.   Myhr U, von Wendt L, Norrlin S, Randall U. Five-year follow-up of functional sitting position in children with cerebral palsy. Dev Med Child Neurol 1995; 37(7): 587–596.

5.   Cole M, Cole SR. O desenvolvimento da crianca e do adolescente. 4th ed. Porto Alegre, Brazil: Artmed, 2004.

6.   Piaget J, Inhelder B. A psicologia da criança. 19th ed. São Paulo: Difel, 2003.

7.   Piaget J. O nascimento da inteligência na criança. Rio de Janeiro: LTC, 1987.

8.   MacKenzie CL, Iberall T. The grasping hand. Amsterdam: North-Holland, 1994.

9.   Henderson A, Pehoski C. Hand function in children. St. Louis, MO: Mosby, 1995.

10.  Duff SV, Gordon AM. Learning of grasp control in children with hemiplegic cerebral palsy. Dev Med Child Neurol 2003; 45(11):746–757.

11.  Vasta R, Haith MM, Miller SA. Child psychology: the modern science. 2nd ed. New York: John Wiley & Sons, 1995.

12.  Poggi G, Calori G, Mancarella G et al. Visual disorders after traumatic brain injury in developmental age. Brain Inj 2000; 14(9):833–845.

13.  Hanna SE, Law MC, Rosenbaum PL et al. Development of hand function among children with cerebral palsy: growth curve analysis for ages 16 to 70 months. Dev Med Child Neurol 2003; 45(7):448–455.

14.  Gordon AM, Lewis SR, Eliasson AC, Duff SV. Object release under varying task constraints in children with hemiplegic cerebral palsy. Dev Med Child Neurol 2003; 45(4):240–248.

15.  Sans A, Boix C, Lopez-Sala A et al. Visuo-constructive disorders in periventricular leukomalacia. Rev Neurol 2002; 34 (Suppl 1):S34–S37.

16.  Lezak M, Howieson DB, Loring DW. Neuropsychological assessment. 4th ed. New York: Oxford University Press, 2004.

17.  Hung YC, Charles J, Gordon AM. Bimanual coordination during a goal-directed task in children with hemiplegic cerebral palsy. Dev Med Child Neurol 2004; 46(11):746–753.

18.  Dellatolas G, De Agostini M, Curt F et al. Manual skill, hand skill asymmetry, and cognitive performances in young children. Laterality 2003; 8(4):317–338.

19.   Mohan A, Singh AP, Mandal MK. Transfer and interference of motor skills in people with intellectual disability. J Intellect Disabil Res 2001; 45(Pt 4):361–369.

20.   Golge M, Muller M, Dreesmann M, Hoppe B, Wenzelburger R, Kuhtz-Buschbeck JP. Recovery of the precision grip in children after traumatic brain injury. Arch Phys Med Rehabil 2004; 85(9):1435–1444.

21.   Gordon AM, Charles J, Duff SV. Fingertip forces during object manipulation in children with hemiplegic cerebral palsy. II: bilateral coordination. Dev Med Child Neurol 1999; 41(3):176–185.

22.   Krumlinde-Sundholm L, Eliasson AC. Comparing tests of tactile sensibility: aspects relevant to testing children with spastic hemiplegia. Dev Med Child Neurol 2002; 44(9):604–612.

23.   Steenbergen B, van der Kamp J. Control of prehension in hemiparetic cerebral palsy: similarities and differences between the ipsi- and contra-lesional sides of the body. Dev Med Child Neurol 2004; 46(5):325–332.

24.   Case-Smith J, Allen AS, Pratt PN. Occupational therapy for children. 3rd ed. St. Louis, MO: Mosby, 1996.

25.   Clarke M, McConachie H, Price K, Wood P. Views of young people using augmentative and alternative communication systems. Int J Lang Commun Disord 2001; 36(1):107–115.

# 6

# Activities of Daily Life

*Katia S Pinto and Sheila M Denucci*

As children grow and develop, their participation in self-care activities such as eating, bathing and dressing increases. The parents, by establishing daily home routines, encourage their children to perform these activities while providing opportunities for them to develop and practice skills that are necessary for their independence. Children with motor impairment and associated disorders, such as cognitive, sensory or neuropsychological deficits, may have difficulties in activities of daily life (ADL).

The functional gains of a child with cerebral palsy (CP) in ADL follow an order similar to that of a child without neurological deficits.[1] This fact reflects the process of maturation and learning in functional performance. Nevertheless, children with CP may have delayed development of these acquisitions and may experience diminished performance in ADL during adolescence or adulthood; these losses are mainly related to difficulties in mobility and the ability to dress without assistance.[2] Each child, however, is different in terms of his disability. Some individuals with CP are able to achieve independence in self-care, continue their education and have professional careers.

After the injury, children with traumatic brain injury (TBI) may have motor, perceptual or praxic disorders, involving multiple areas, including self-care and mobility.[3] Impaired sitting and standing balance, in addition to ataxia and dysmetria, can make it difficult for these children to change position during transfers, perform tasks, and manipulate objects for feeding and dressing.[4] Hemineglicence, and visuo-spatial perception deficits can lead, for example, to incomplete hygiene of some parts of the body, difficulties manipulating food or decreased wheelchair mobility. Ideomotor apraxia (difficulties performing a task) can cause movements to be fragmented or exaggerated. Children may have problems directing and controlling the speed at which they execute their movements or may even use a part of their body as if it were an object. In cases of ideational apraxia (an interruption in the logical succession of movements needed to carry out complex gestures), the child may commit errors in ordering movements or choosing actions for given tasks, for example, inverting the motions for tying a shoelace or using the wrong piece of silverware for the wrong type of food.

Despite the different impairments, children with TBI usually quickly recover physical function during the first year after trauma. During this period, most of these children attain a level of independence in ADLs that is appropriate to their chronological age.[5]

In order to help the child attain a level of functional independence, intervention should target the skills that are part of the daily home routine; this promotes the child's development. There is a reciprocal relationship between learning how to perform a task and having the opportunity to execute that task in the context of daily domestic routines.[6] The rehabilitation program for the child should be included in the family's everyday life, becoming part of the daily routines established by the family. This setting optimizes the time spent for the development or recovery of abilities and encourages the child's participation.[7] The consolidation of functional abilities is one of the main objectives of a rehabilitation program, which involves learning processes; however, this goal is only attained to the extent that the acquired skills improve the child's day-to-day competence.

## Program of Activities

Different levels of assistance rendered to the child lead to various changes in the family's daily routines, such as allowing the child more time to perform a given task.[6;8] Sometimes, parents tend to help their children more than they should, or even perform the tasks for them. This is understandable because, while children may be capable of a given movement, such as using a spoon, they may take a long time to eat, may become unmotivated and require the family's assistance. On the other hand, although parents are aware of and concerned about their child's needs, there may be other daily tasks that demand their attention, leaving them with little time left over in their day. This can result in parents doing things for their children, rather then spending the necessary time to allow them to do it themselves. However, it is important for families to understand that the experience of doing things on their own, performing ADL at their own pace, will, little by little, prepare these children for more independent living, within realistic expectations. Encouraging children to participate in the activities of their daily life can lead to a greater capacity for, and pleasure in, doing them.

Depending on the impairments of the child with brain injury, adaptations and the use of special aid devices can facilitate the child's performance in daily activities or the care given by the family. When selecting these resources, individual factors, available physical space and the child's context should all be considered, for they influence the functional results.[8] Inappropriate indication of adaptations, without prior assessment of functional repercussions, may occasion more functional damage than gains.[9]

The training of a given skill should proceed from the most simple to the most complex, and the activity should be adjusted to the child's capacity and potential. Children may often find alternative means of improving their performance in a given activity, such as a distinctive way of holding a cup without spilling its contents. Other times, the team and family will have to develop new strategies to help them improve their performance.

This chapter describes the activities carried out with the assistance of the family, which may enhance the capacity of children with CP or TBI to achieve the full extent of their self-potential and adaptation to the environment. The activities described are based on three main themes:

- carrying, positioning, transferring, and mobility
- feeding, eating, and swallowing disorders
- self-care.

Depending on the type of disorder, post-trauma recovery phase, or developmental stage, the family and the treatment team should find the activity level within each category that best corresponds to the child's or adolescent's needs.

## Carrying, Positioning, Transferring, and Mobility

### Carrying child in a forward-facing position

There are strategies that can help facilitate the handling of the child with CP during carrying. The child can be positioned on your lap, facing his surroundings, so he is able to see objects and people around him (Figure 6.1, Activity 160). You can help support the legs and trunk of the child, keeping him in a seated position, which promotes muscle relaxation. This position also stabilizes the pelvis and aligns the head and trunk. Children still developing head control can lean their trunks slightly forward, to free the head from support and train balance.

**Figure 6.1    Activity 160**
Carrying child in a
forward-facing position

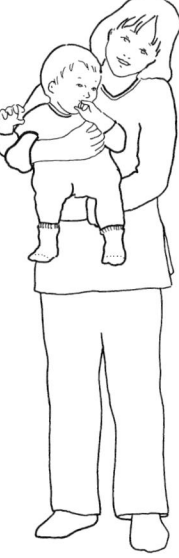
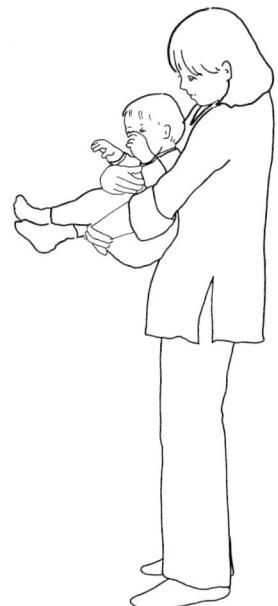

## Carrying child in a tummy position

By carrying the child tummy-down (tummy facing the lap), you can help him adapt to the prone position, which promotes head balance. Elevating the upper part of his trunk while he is in prone encourages cervical extension. If the child does not have head balance, you can support his head with one of your arms (Figure 6.2, Activity 161).

**Figure 6.2   Activity 161**
Carrying child in a
tummy position

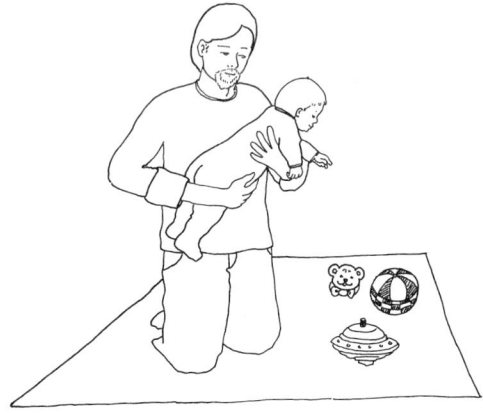

## Carrying child front to front

A child with CP or TBI who has attained head balance can be carried with his legs around your waist (Figure 6.3, Activity 162). This way of carrying relaxes the legs while promoting trunk stability and face-to-face contact. It is important to involve the child when picking him up and encourage him to wrap his arms around your neck. As trunk balance improves, the child can release his hands, and you can reduce the amount of support you are providing. Although small children with TBI may adapt better to the lap, many will require carriages or wheelchairs for transportation, at least during the initial stages of recovery.[10–11]

**Figure 6.3   Activity 162**
Carrying child front to
front

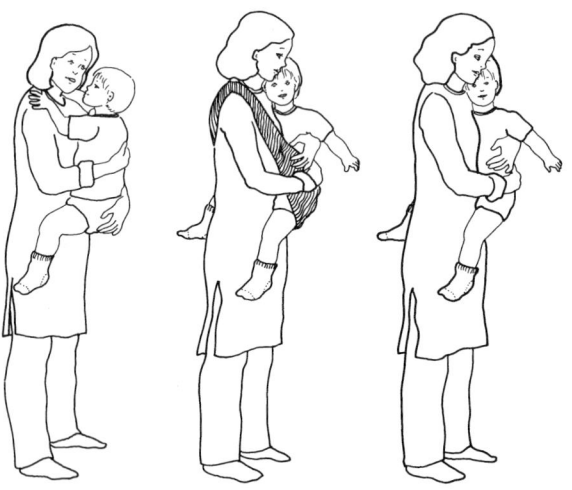

**Corner chair**

Special chairs can be useful for the child in home and school situations. Smaller children without neck or trunk balance can benefit from the corner-chair type seat that allows for regulation of backrest inclination, height and distance from the attached table-board (Figure 6.4, Activity 163). The corner chair with an elevated support base permits foot positioning on the floor, which can contribute to trunk stability.

**Figure 6.4    Activity 163**
Corner chair

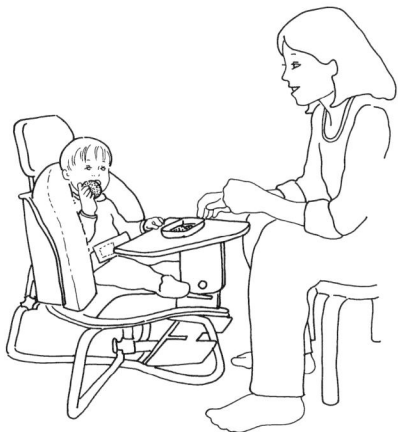

In each particular case, use of the chair can meet various needs that range from clinical goals such as adequate positioning of the child with feeding disorders, to stimulation activities, such as facilitating hand use, better visualization of the child's surroundings and improvement of trunk balance. This resource permits the child greater integration in family life.

**Cut out table**

Older children with trunk control can use a chair with a cut out table that allows them better positioning through upper limb support, helping them reach and handle objects (Figure 6.5, Activity 164). Chairs with armrests can also contribute to trunk stability.

**Figure 6.5    Activity 164**
Cut out table

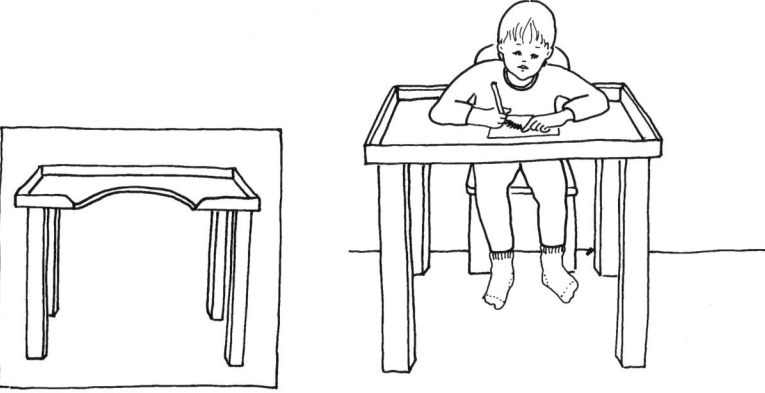

**Adapted wheelchairs**

The use of carriages or wheelchairs also contributes to better positioning of the child during daily life activities.[12] The team and family should select the mobility aid that best adapts to the child's needs and functional level, regulating the incline of the back and headrest to his capacity for cervical or trunk control (Figure 6.6, Activity 165). In more severe cases, chairs and carriages should contain safety straps and lateral head and trunk support, in addition to a reclinable backrest. Anatomical pillows are often required for better positioning of the pelvis and consequent adjustment of trunk alignment. If the child has involuntary movements, padding the chair's metal parts minimizes the risk of self-injury. Simpler adjustments can be made to the baby carriage, such as adding foam rolls and Velcro® straps.

**Figure 6.6    Activity 165**
Adapted wheelchairs

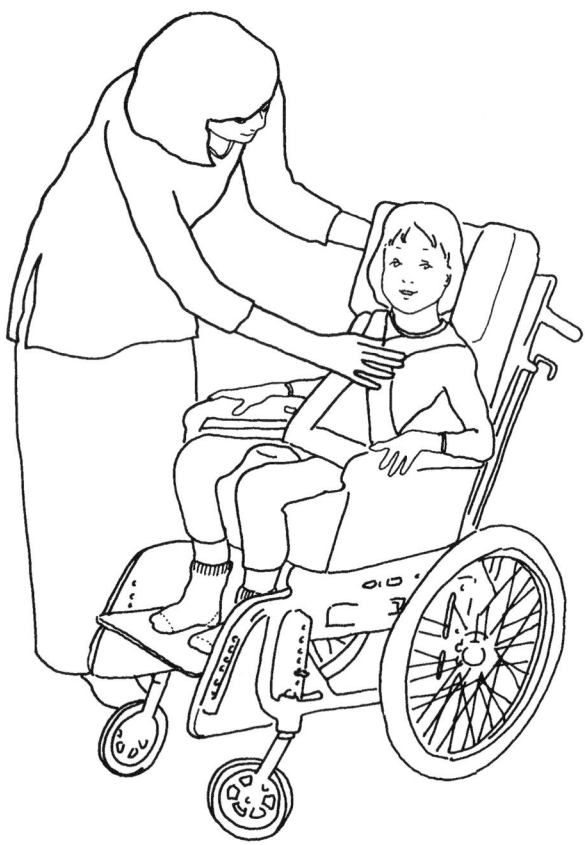

Adequate wheelchair positioning for children who are capable of maneuvering the wheelchair by themselves makes it easier for them to use it, which in turn fosters independence and social integration. Use of removable tableboards on the chairs enables the child to perform manual activities, in addition to providing anterior trunk support.

## Wheelchairs for mobility

The use of wheelchairs is indicated for the locomotion of children without functional gait or with limited mobility. Managing the wheelchair requires the ability to steer, propel, avoid obstacles and make transfers (Figure 6.7, Activity 166). It might be necessary, at first, to show the child how to propel the wheelchair forward, guiding the movement of his hand along the rim of the wheel or teaching him how to maneuver by, for example, braking one wheel and spinning the other. When the child is using the wheelchair at home, on the street or in school, games that explore different paths or passageways can be proposed. The team, together with the family, can help the child discover the bodily adjustments necessary for sustaining wheelchair stability during upward or downward shifting.

**Figure 6.7    Activity 166**
Wheelchairs for mobility

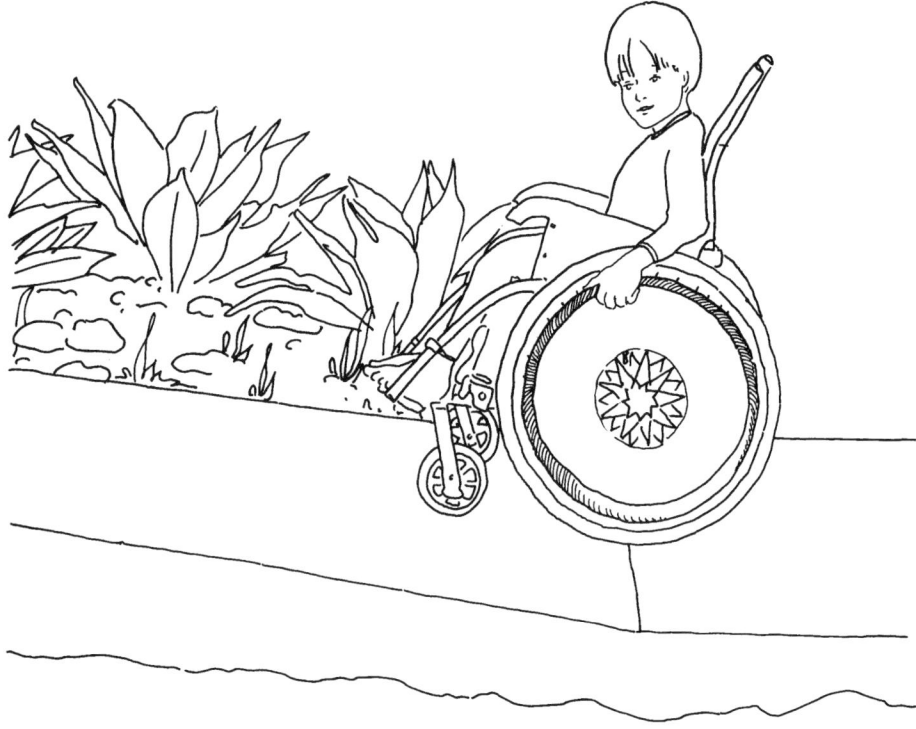

Some children with involuntary movements find alternative ways to propel the wheelchair, such as using the foot for propulsion on the ground. The same may be true for children with TBI in the initial stages of recovery. Motorized wheelchairs may be an option for children with poor motor control or insufficient strength for driving a manual wheelchair.[13]

179

**Stand-pivot transfer**

Using a wheelchair demands, in addition to autonomy, an equally important ability: the capacity to transfer from the wheelchair to the bed or to a chair. Some children with brain injury are independent in their transfers, but many require the help of an adult. Due to impairment of the selective movements of the upper limbs, and of the rotational movements of the trunk, the child with CP may experience difficulties elevating the trunk and transferring himself in the seated position. In these cases, the ability to adopt intermediary positions such as standing makes transfers easier. You can help the child stand, pivot and sit on the bed or chair on the side. The same strategy can be used for transferring to a car (Figure 6.8, Activity 167).

**Figure 6.8    Activity 167**
Stand-pivot transfer

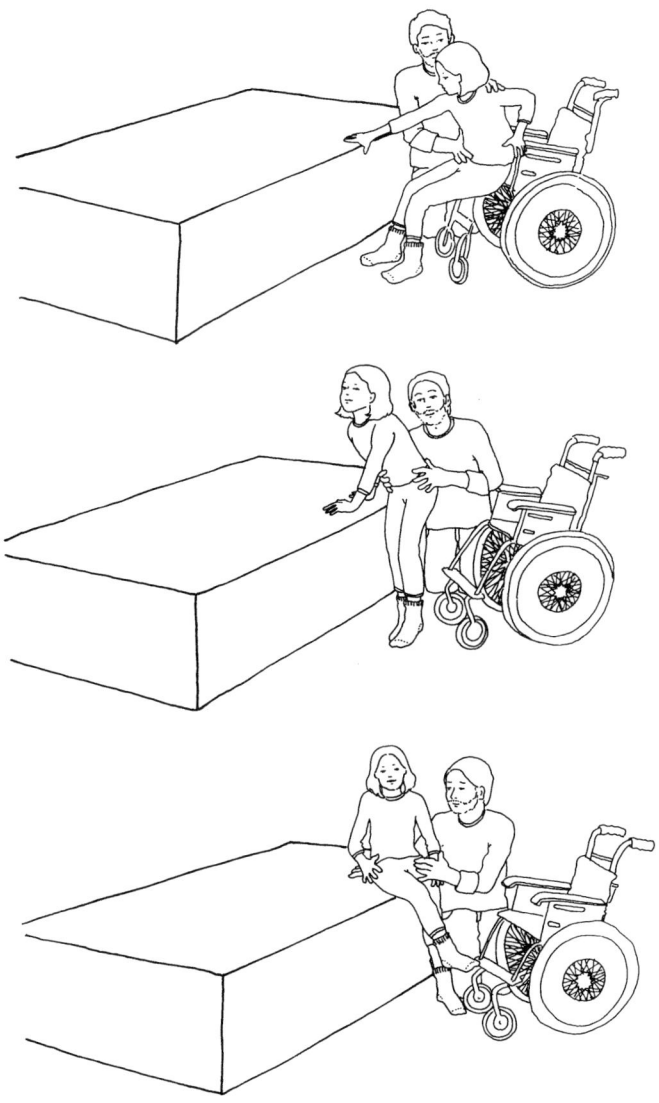

**Climbing up and down furniture**

Weakness in lower limbs and balance deficits can cause the child with TBI to require help during transfer and mobility activities, especially in the first year post-trauma.[4] You can encourage and help the child climb up and down furniture, such as a bed or a sofa, so that he may experience the movements and the sequence of actions involved in the transfers (Figure 6.9, Activity 168). This activity will help him attain balance. Helping the child adopt intermediary positions such as kneeling facilitates the transfer from the floor to the furniture.

**Figure 6.9  Activity 168**
Climbing up and down furniture

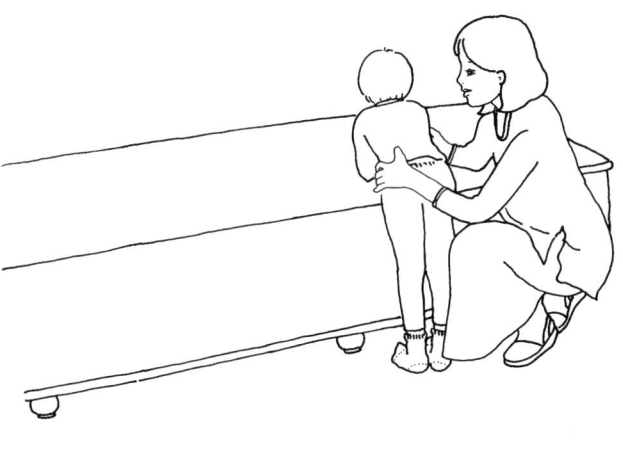

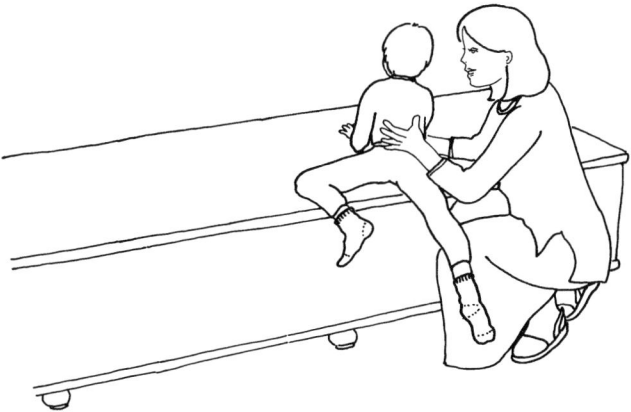

**Anterior walkers (walkers that are pushed with the frame in front of the body) or posterior walkers (walkers that are pulled with the frame behind the body)**

Walkers are recommended for children with balance problems during walking. Initially, with your help, the child can experiment with the walker without moving from place, e.g., leaning against the wall or piece of furniture while participating in games and playing with members of the family. Games such as kicking a ball, dancing, changing trunk position and releasing the hand are activities that can be introduced, gradually adjusting the amount of support and accommodating the shifts in balance. When a child feels confident enough to try walking with a walker, you should help him begin in a straight line and then on irregular terrain with curves and obstacles (Figure 6.10, Activity 169). If necessary, a sheet could be used to support his trunk, providing greater assurance and safety.

**Figure 6.10 Activity 169**
Anterior or posterior
walkers

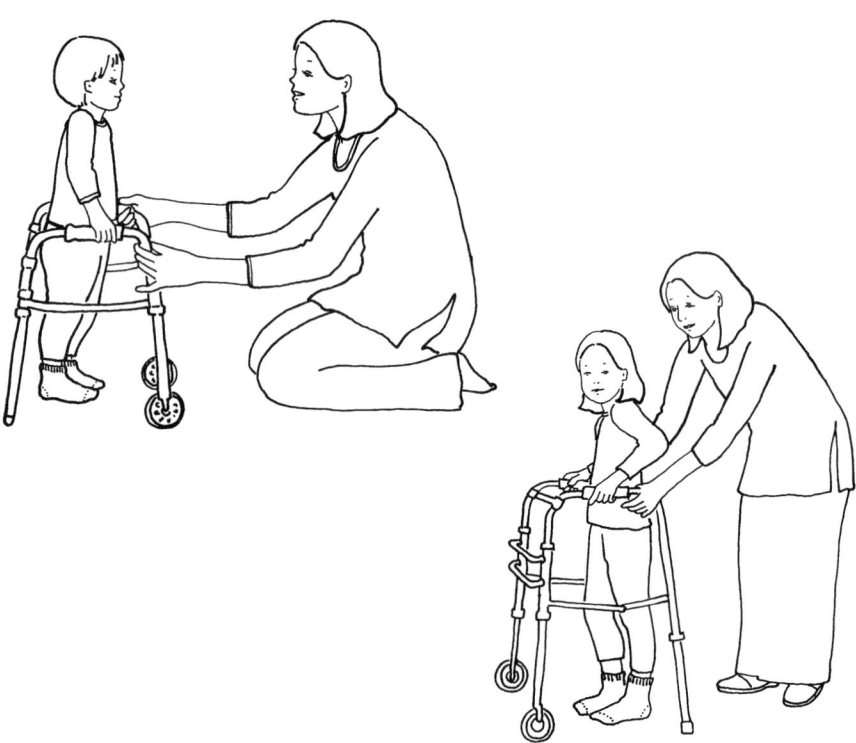

The child's balance deficit should be considered when selecting the type of walker. Children with ataxia or involuntary movements may benefit from the use of an anterior walker with added weights for additional stability. Children with better postural control can use a posterior walker, which fosters trunk extension during gait. Walkers with wheels that rotate can also be used, enabling a child to turn around corners. Children with triplegic or hemiplegic-type CP may require forearm support for stability and grasping. Children with TBI can also benefit from this adaptation, but it is usually transitory.

**Crutches**

Crutches are indicated for children with balance deficits but sufficient strength in the arms to support part of their body weight. Crutches are more versatile and facilitate walking on uneven terrains, and are generally introduced following use of the walker.

When the child is learning to use crutches, he may benefit from practicing on certain types of terrains, such as grass, which can help him maintain his balance, thereby making it easier to keep the crutches firmly on the ground. Gradually, you can help the child experience movements with the crutches, alternating going forward with one leg and the crutch, then performing the same motion with the other leg (Figure 6.11, Activity 170). Family field trips or recreational activities in school in which variations in speed and direction of gait are explored, can help promote the child's agility. If he has trouble grasping, adapted devices should be used to position his hand on the handle of the cane during the initial stages of gait training.

**Figure 6.11   Activity 170**
Crutches

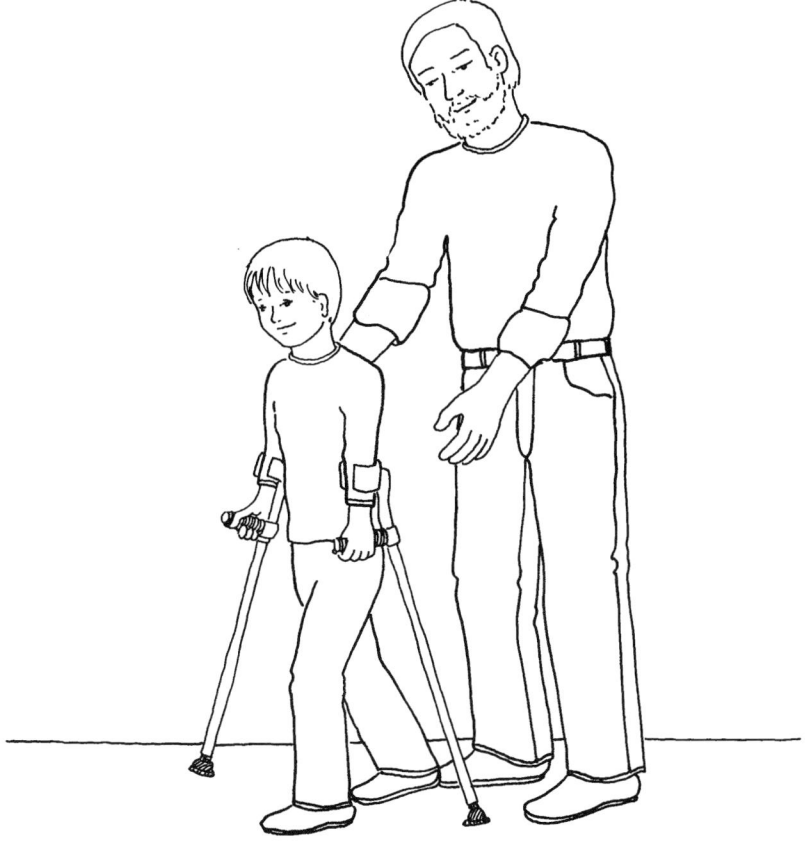

**Mobility aids in school and community**

When indicated, it is important to introduce mobility aids as early as possible into the child's daily routine. At first this process may appear to be difficult and demand a lot of effort on the child's part, especially if he is able to move about faster using other means, such as crawling. Thus, there must be good collaboration among the members of the family, team and school. The goals can be attained by organizing the child's setting and making the necessary modifications such as location of furniture and placement of activities that encourage gait in the child, taking advantage of his natural interest and need to move about at home or in school (Figure 6.12, Activity 171). Visits to the home and school can help the team analyze, together with the family members and teachers, suggestions for changes in the child's surroundings.

**Figure 6.12    Activity 171**
Mobility aids in school
and community

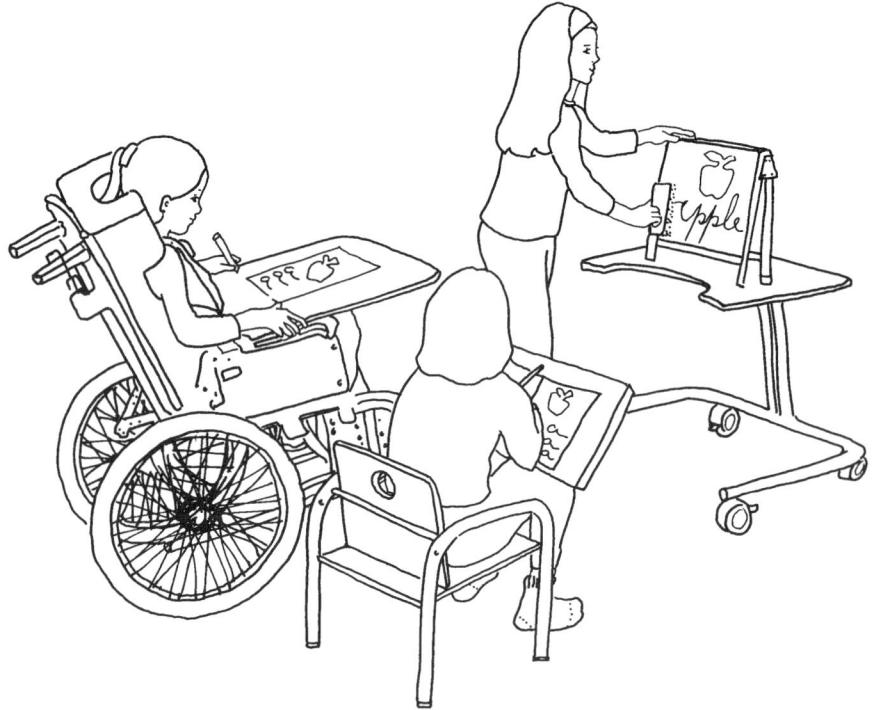

## *Feeding, Eating, and Swallowing Disorders*

During the first few months of life, the child's eating activity is predominantly reflexive, characterized by sucking and swallowing movements. As he matures neurologically, his reflexes become integrated into voluntary movements, which gradually become more complex, evolving to chewing.

Feeding disorders are common in children with cerebral palsy, especially those with quadriplegia and cognitive delays.[12;14] The persistence of primitive reflexes, insufficient oral pressure for sucking, dental arch abnormalities and uncoordinated movements frequently hamper the acts of sucking, biting, and chewing. Children with TBI may also have feeding disorders.

Difficulty swallowing, called dysphasia, is a symptom commonly found in children and adolescents with TBI and severe CP.[15–17] It can affect any part of the digestive tract, altering the transport of saliva and/or nutrients from the mouth to the stomach. Depending on their motor and cognitive deficits, children with CP may have chewing and swallowing disorders throughout their development, as well as other disorders of the gastrointestinal tract, such as gastroesophageal reflux.[18] These problems may manifest as early as the first feedings, such as difficulties sucking (impairment of the sucking reflex). Swallowing difficulties in post-TBI children or adolescents, when present, may be temporary and affect the oral and pharyngeal stages, sometimes involving functions such as sucking and chewing.[19] The degree of impairment can range from mild to acute, depending on the type, location and extension of the brain lesion, and on the amount of time the child remained in a coma or on a respirator.[20–21] After severe trauma, the child's oral feeding capacity may be impaired, creating the risk of food being aspirated into the lungs. Direct feeding of liquid supplements though a nasal-gastric tube, by gastrotomy or by vein may be necessary. The return to oral feeding should be assessed after removal of the respirator, when safe swallowing is again possible. In order for the family and rehabilitation team to begin discussing when and how to begin the stimulation of, and transition to, oral feeding, it may be necessary to first assess the child's or adolescent's ability to swallow his own saliva, observe his swallowing protection mechanisms, e.g., coughing, and perform specific exams that allow for the visualization of swallowing, e.g., videofluoroscopy or nasofiberoscopy. In some cases, this transitional process is gradual, with continued parallel use of enteral or parenteral feeding, because of the child's difficulties consuming an adequate amount of food within a reasonable amount of time. The family should know about the risks involved in oral feeding, which may affect the child's or adolescent's clinical condition by causing respiratory problems, such as pneumonia resulting from aspiration of food into the lungs.[22]

Adequate positioning is one of the most important aspects in dealing with children who have feeding disorders.[23] Alignment of the trunk, head and neck minimizes the risk of aspiration. Wedge-like inclines used in the bed or adjusted wheelchairs may be helpful in positioning larger children during feeding.

## Using inclines

Many children with spastic quadriplegia-type CP present oropharyngeal dysphagia (problems in swallowing) and/or gastroesophageal reflux, which can produce respiratory or nutritional problems.[14] Impairment of the swallowing mechanism can also be present after TBI. Adequate positioning of the child when lying down increases comfort and reduces the chances of respiratory damage caused by aspiration. You can use a foam incline to help keep the child's head and trunk elevated, preferably more than 60 degrees (Figure 6.13, Activity 172). Ensuring that the consistency of the food is adequate for the child and offering it in the proper manner significantly contributes to his nutritional health.

**Figure 6.13 Activity 172**
Using inclines

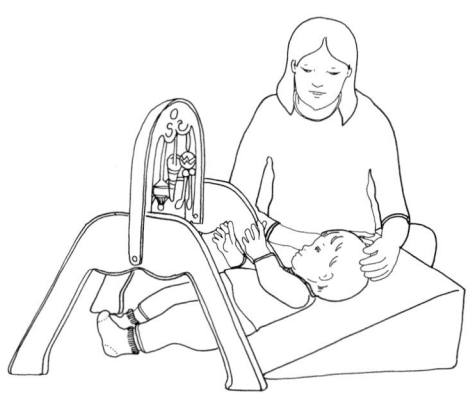

## Elevating head of bed

Elevating the bed frame or the mattress and placing a wooden support under the headboard or head of the crib to keep it elevated are measures that contribute to proper positioning of the child with gastroesophageal reflux. It is important to check that both the head and the trunk are elevated (Figure 6.14, Activity 173). The child can be kept from sliding down in the bed or crib by using a cloth, underwear-like diaper fastened to straps that are tied to the head of the bed.

**Figure 6.14 Activity 173**
Elevating head of bed

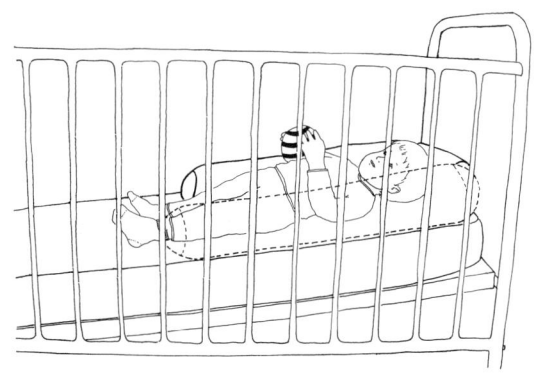

**Feeding child in baby seat**

For smaller children, a baby seat or adaptive seating are recommended. Baby seats are easy to transport and aid the care of the child by affording adequate elevation of the head and trunk during feeding (Figure 6.15, Activity 174). Many parents tend to feed the child while he is semi-lying down in their lap; they feel that, in this position, they can get the child to eat more. These alternatives should be very carefully discussed and analyzed by the team and parents together, for inadequate positioning greatly increases the risk of aspiration.

**Figure 6.15   Activity 174**
Feeding child in baby seat

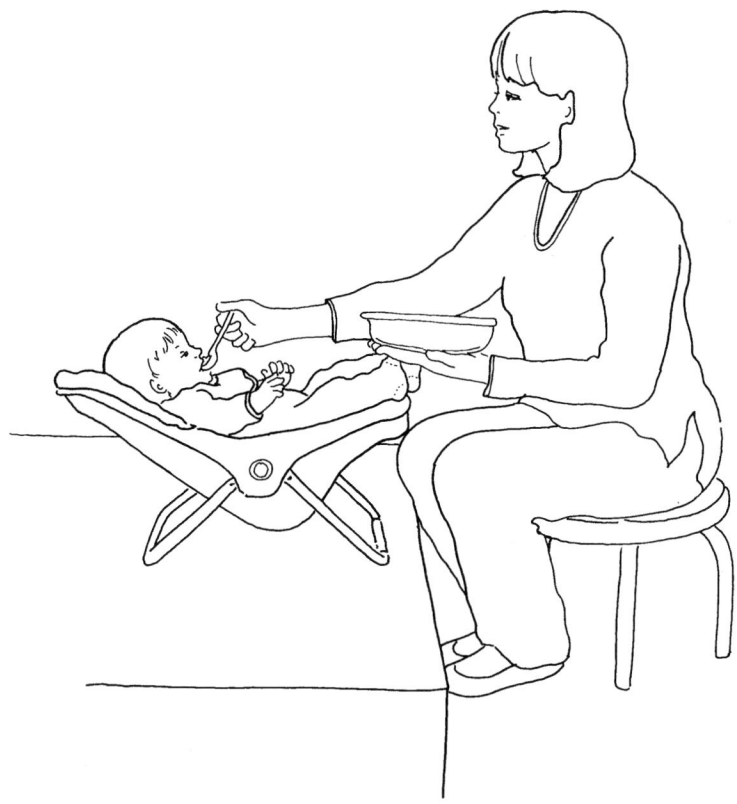

**Feeding child in corner chair**

A corner chair is an alternative type of adaptive seating, indicated for feeding children who are older but still do not have neck or trunk control. The chair's backrest should be reclined, preferably more than 60 degrees (Figure 6.16, Activity 175). The head and trunk should be kept symmetrically aligned, adjusting the head support and the safety straps. In addition to facilitating the task, this position also fosters interaction with the family. You should sit in front of and at the same level as the child, and offer the spoon frontally so that he does not have to perform exaggerated cervical extensions.

**Figure 6.16 Activity 175**
Feeding child in corner chair

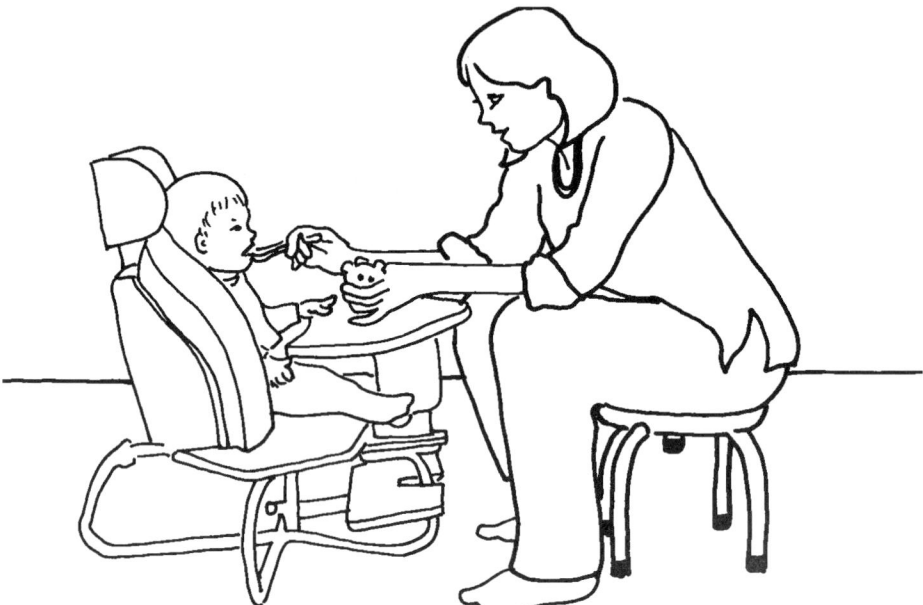

In addition to positioning, the team should assess the child's nutritional needs and physiological patterns and discuss the most appropriate adjustments and adaptations with the family. Consistency of the food, as well as the amount, rhythm and mode of feeding, should also be addressed. Among the choices of eating utensils, the silicon spoon most facilitates the placing of food in the child's mouth, attenuates the effects of the biting reflex, and adapts to the movements of the tongue without hurting him. If the child has problems retrieving the food from the spoon, pressing the spoon onto his tongue or depositing the food in the middle of the tongue can help. The food should be fed to the child slowly, in small amounts, to prevent it from escaping through the oral cavity, and to facilitate his control over propulsion and swallowing.

**Helping child suck on a bottle**

Sucking difficulties in children with CP may result in the capacity to swallow only a very small amount of nourishment, and are oftentimes exacerbated by the escape of food from the mouth. There are several causes of sucking disorders, such as the child's inability to close his lips, tongue movement disorders, insufficient pressure in the oral cavity, or impaired coordination of the sucking, swallowing, and breathing mechanisms.[24] When bottle-feeding a child, you can apply more pressure on the nipple while holding his cheek muscles with your index finger and thumb. If the child has problems closing his lips, provide additional support under the jaw to help him close his mouth (Figure 6.17, Activity 176).

**Figure 6.17   Activity 176**
Helping child suck on a bottle

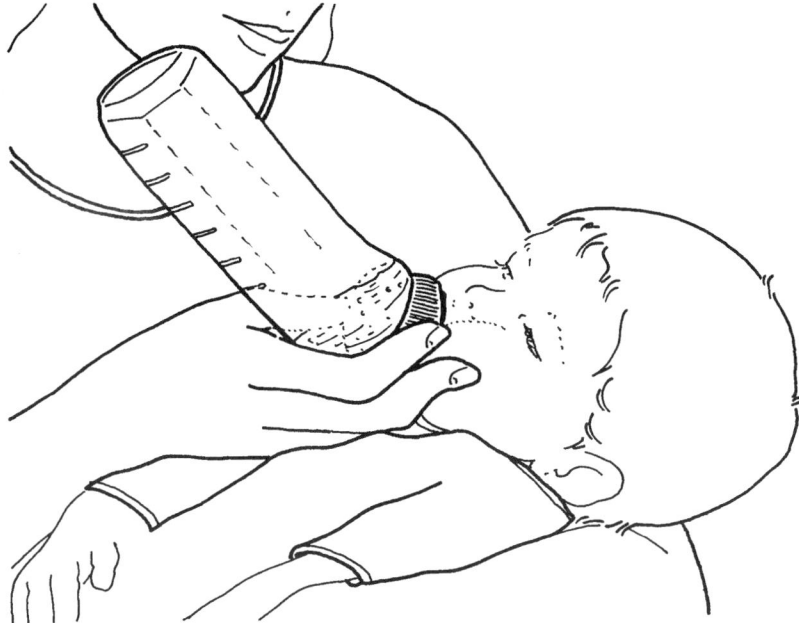

There are a great variety of nipples for bottles, made from different types of materials and molded in various formats. Using the nipple that best meets the child's needs can help facilitate sucking. For some children with impaired sucking, who tire more easily, the use of latex nipples may best because they offer less resistance and facilitate the sucking movement. On the other hand, silicone nipples may be more effective for children who have strong sucking mechanisms, but find it difficult to pause during suction. It is important to be attentive to the size of the nipple hole. A larger opening can help food flow, but can also make it difficult for the child to control his swallowing, thereby increasing the risk of choking.

*Learning to chew*
Chewing is a function that develops with other oral motor skills. When chewing, the child coordinates the movements that open and close the jaw

while the tongue works to gather all of the food distributed throughout the oral cavity, which will then be swallowed. The parents naturally modify the consistency of their children's food throughout their development (liquid – paste – solid). Nevertheless, some children with severe CP are not able to attain the chewing phase and may not be prepared to eat solid foods. On the other hand, because of the chewing and swallowing problems exhibited by children with CP or in the early post-TBI recovery stages, parents may feel apprehensive about changing the diet from liquid to paste-like or solid foods. In these circumstances, it is important to discuss the possibility of modifying the consistency of the child's food and the strategies that can help facilitate the transition process. Based on the level of the child's development and oral-motor coordination, he can be fed paste-like foods such as soups, with small pieces of cooked vegetables, which will expose him to new textures.

There are a number of activities that can help foster the learning and rehabilitation of chewing mechanisms in children and adolescents with CP and TBI. You can try giving them the food item in a little sack made from gauze. Hold the end of the sack and place it in the child's mouth, between his teeth, and allow him to chew so that he can taste the flavor, then encourage him to repeat the movement. By doing this, he safely practices chewing and saliva-swallowing coordination without risk of swallowing food.

When the chewing mechanisms are impaired after TBI and in some cases of CP, several reflexes, such as biting, may be exaggerated. It should be remembered that the grip is a reflex, in other words, it is an involuntary action. Massaging the area with circular movements by starting at the ears and gradually working down towards the mouth and chin can help the child relax these muscles and eventually open his mouth. Using silicone spoons with long handles, with depth and size appropriate to the child or adolescent's needs can facilitate feeding and help minimize the risk of hurting the inside of his mouth.

*Swallowing and breathing*
The act of swallowing is coordinated with the act of breathing. When this coordination is not harmonious, problems such as choking followed by coughing can occur, and the habit of eating with the mouth open can develop. Some children with brain injury are unable, while breathing, to make the brief pauses necessary for chewing and swallowing the food. Consequently, they bite, chew with their mouths open, swallow and breathe, all at the same time, increasing their risk of choking.

When feeding a small child, it is important to observe whether he is pausing to breathe. If he is not, remove the bottle from his mouth or wait more time between spoonfuls, which will help pace his chewing and swallowing to match his breathing.

**Holding a baby bottle**

A small child can be placed on your lap during feeding. Recline the child onto a cushioned support, propped up in an aligned position while you help him hold his bottle with both hands (Figure 6.18, Activity 177). This position fosters face-to-face contact and the reaching for, and holding of objects.

**Figure 6.18   Activity 177**
Holding a baby bottle

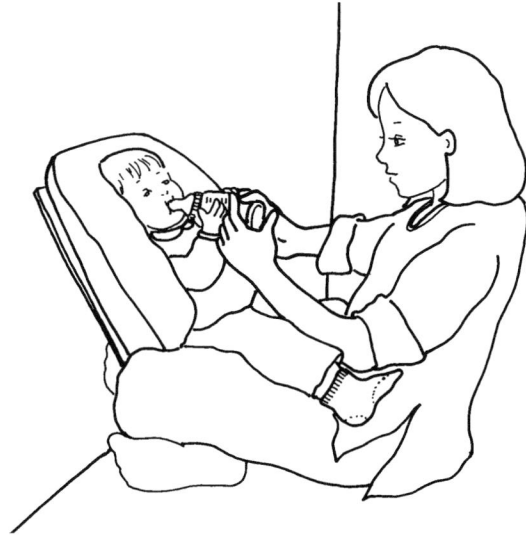

**Eating with hands**

As the child's ability to chew and swallow develops, the introduction of solid food can begin. Children with cervical balance and hand grasping can be taught to bring food to their mouths using their hands. According to the movements that each child is able to make, you can promote the development of grasping with fingertips by offering food in small pieces (Figure 6.19, Activity 178). In some cultures, this form of eating is common, even in adulthood.

**Figure 6.19   Activity 178**
Eating with hands

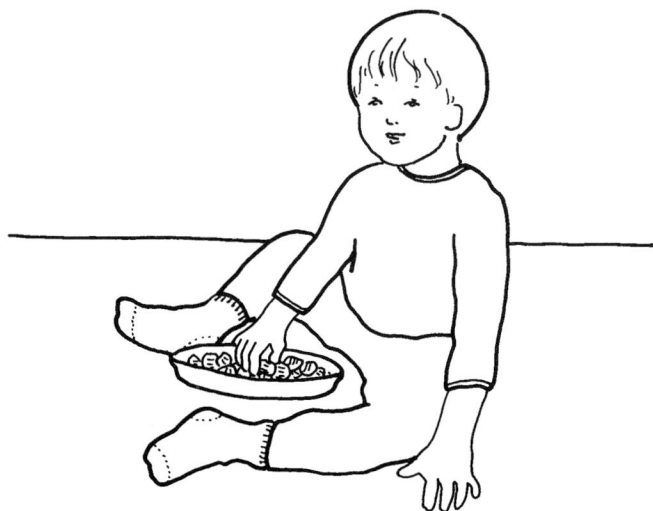

191

**Feeding self with spoon**

During the stages in which the child is learning to eat you can help him bring the spoon to his mouth by supporting his arm. In cases of hemiplegia, help the child use his impaired arm to steady the plate, keeping it within his sight (Figure 6.20, Activity 179). Be attentive to whether the child's exertion in performing a movement worsens the hypertonia of the impaired hand or triggers associated reactions that affect his ability to perform this activity. In these cases, adapted eating utensils can be used to facilitate his independence.

**Figure 6.20    Activity 179**
Feeding self with spoon

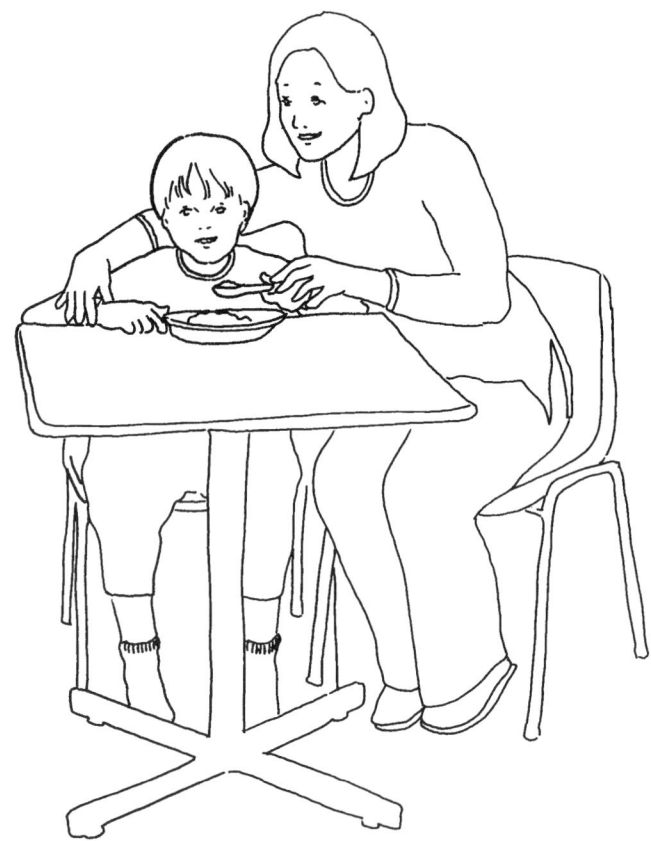

**Use of adapted cups**

Cups with straps facilitate the child's grasping, and use of special caps/lids or straws help reduce the amount of dribble from the mouth or the likelihood of spills during eating.

**Use of adapted plates**

Plates with raised or perforated borders, with or without internal divisions, supported on a non-slip surface, make it easier for the child to manipulate food, especially if he has uncoordinated movements or lack of bimanual function.

## *Self-care*

Perceptual and praxic disorders can interfere with the self-care activities of children with TBI. These children may have difficulties sequentializing their movements or they may neglect an area of their face when washing, or not recognize the function of the items used for self-care tasks. Helpful strategies include dividing the activity into stages, helping children gradually perform each stage, and helping them identify the objects and their functions.

### Face washing

In the face washing activity, it is very important to encourage the child to participate in all the stages of the process: opening and closing the faucet, using soap, washing all parts of his face, drying up with a towel (Figure 6.21, Activity 180).

**Figure 6.21    Activity 180**
Face washing

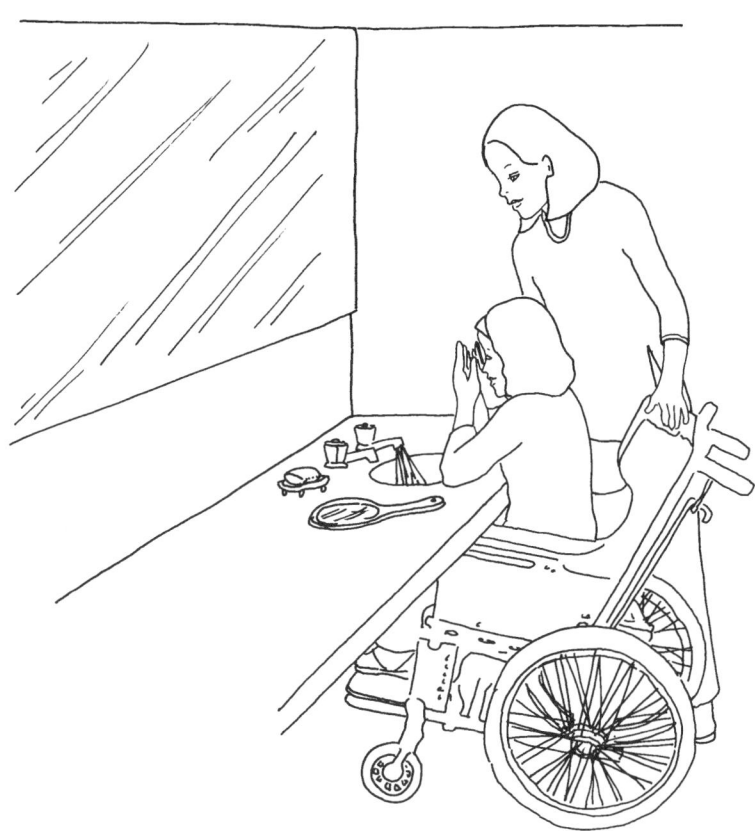

**Hair care**

During hair care, the child may find it easier to use larger combs or brushes, with thicker, lighter handles. Mirrors placed at an appropriate height and angle also permit the child to accompany his progress (Figure 6.22, Activity 181). Children with difficulties grasping may require handle enlargers or Velcro to secure these items in their hands. It is essential that the child participate in the activity, sometimes assisted, at other times experimenting with his own way of combing his hair.

**Figure 6.22    Activity 181**
Hair care

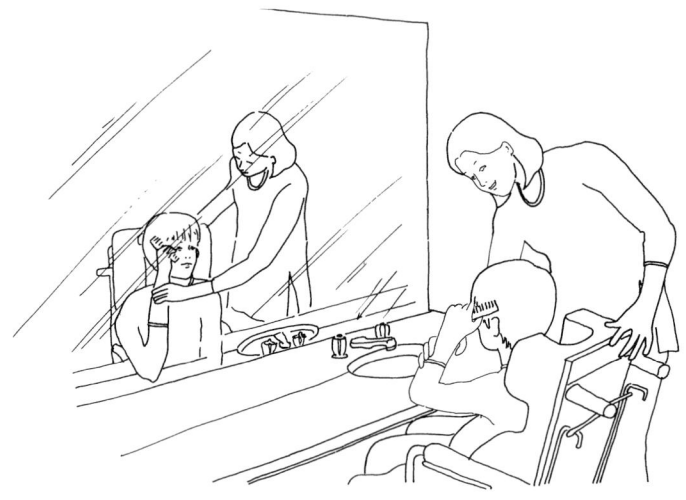

**Teeth brushing**

You should sequentialize the task, using a toothbrush of adequate size for the child's oral cavity (mouth) (Figure 6.23, Activity 182).

**Figure 6.23    Activity 182**
Teeth brushing

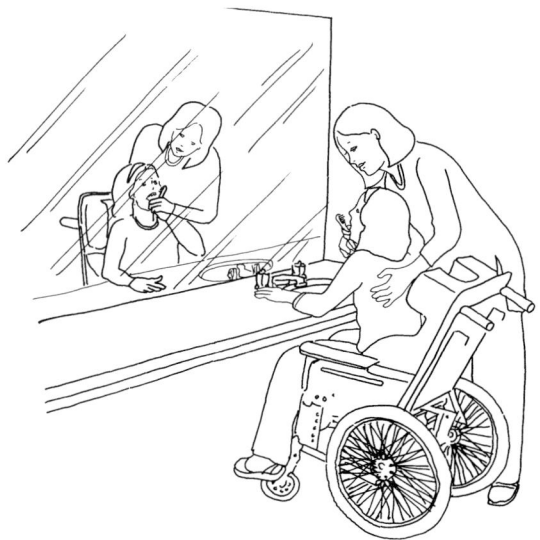

## Baby bath

When a baby is taking a bath, it is beneficial to allow him to play with the water, listen to your voice as you name the parts of his body, and perceive the sensation of objects with different textures; these actions contribute to the development of the infant's first movements and notions of body image, which will later promote his ability to bathe independently. Exploring tactile sensations with the hands, using sponges, soaps, oils, creams and towels can be done during hygiene care (Figure 6.24, Activity 183).

**Figure 6.24    Activity 183**
Baby bath

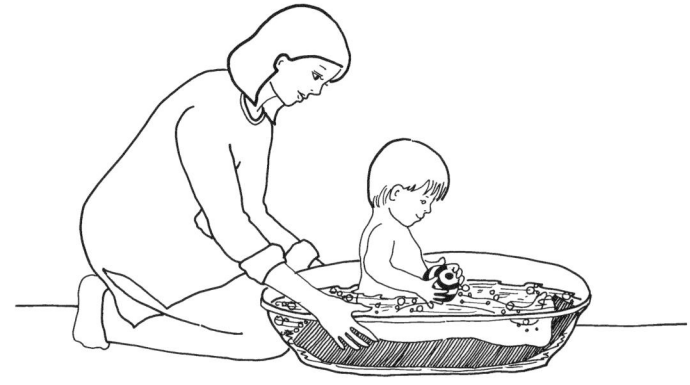

## Self-bathing

Older children who are able to sit without support, but who do not have standing balance, can use chairs during the bath or shower. Children who are already able to stay in the standing position but still have balance deficits can use railings for support during the bath (Figure 6.25, Activity 184). Sponges with straps for the hands or with long handles help the child reach lower or back parts of his body. Firmly secured liquid soap dispensers and shampoo bottles contribute to the child's independence. Towels should also be within easy reach.

**Figure 6.25    Activity 184**
Self-bathing

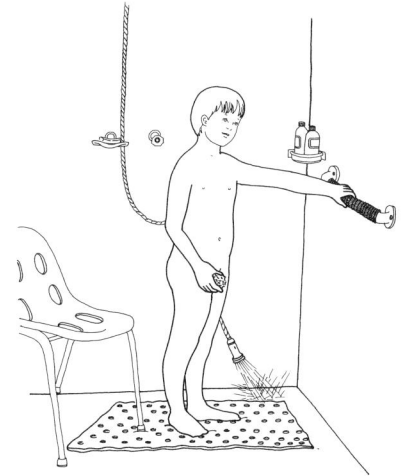

**Using bath chair**

Older children with severe impairments can be more easily maneuvered in bathing or hygiene chairs (Figure 6.26, Activity 185). Children with TBI in the initial stages of recovery may also require these chairs, albeit often temporarily. The child's sense of safety and security is very important during the bathing.

**Figure 6.26   Activity 185**
Using bath chair

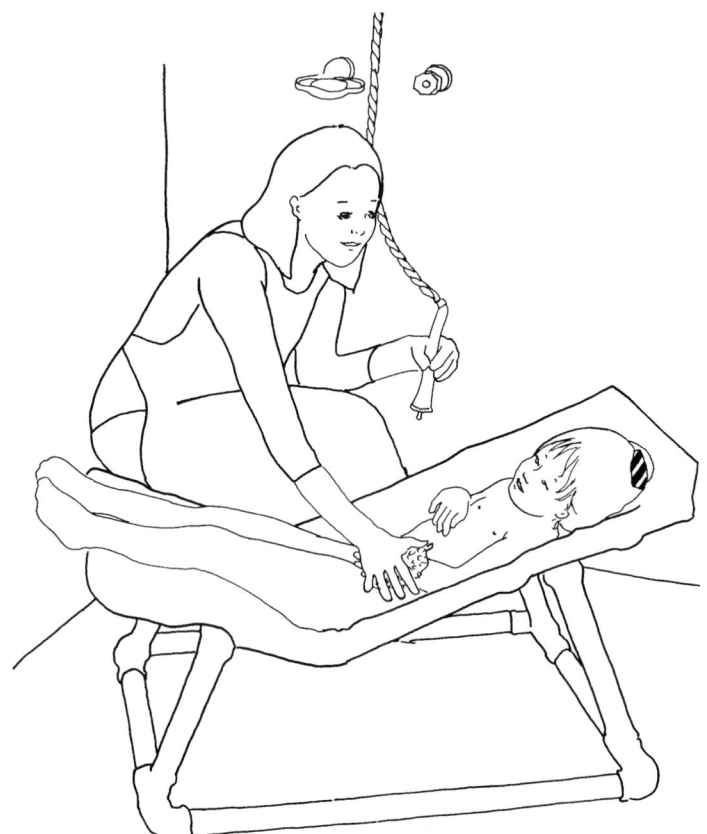

*Dressing*

Children usually learn to undress before they learn to dress. The honing of fine coordination skills and spatial-temporal orientation contributes to independent dressing. Guiding their arms and legs, and removing socks and shoes, are ways for children to cooperate during wardrobe changes. It is important to encourage the child with brain injury to participate early on in activities related to dressing and undressing. In addition to fostering the development of motor skills, these activities involve elements of body image and spatial association that influence motor behavior. You can help the child recognize parts of his body, asking that he lift his arms, lower his head, place his foot into the pant leg, among other tasks. Giving the child the opportunity to choose his own clothes, exploring the characteristics of each piece with him such as color, front/back, types of accessories, are important for the recognition and learning of new concepts.

You can help the child to discover positions and movements that facilitate independence in dressing activities, such as elevating the pelvis in the supine position to put on shorts, or leaning against the wall while getting dressed.

Knowing about the types of appropriate children's clothing and shoes can contribute significantly to the child's independence in dressing. Looser clothing made out of light materials, fastened with Velcro or large buttons, are easier for the child to manage. Wardrobe accessories should be simplified, such as elasticized waists instead of buttons and snaps. Clothes for daily wear, especially school clothes, should not contain ribbons, bows or small buttons because they make the child rely on others for putting on those articles.

*Toilet training*
Self-sufficient toileting involves the attainment of various skills: knowing when to go to the bathroom, going to the bathroom, removing articles of clothing from the lower limbs, using the toilet and cleansing after toileting.

In order to begin toilet training, it is important to first understand the child's voiding pattern.[25] For two weeks, you should register the number of times the child voids. This report should list information such as time and frequency, and will govern the planning of when and how often to bring the child to the bathroom. Based on this report, you can begin to toilet train, at first teaching the child how to void in the toilet or potty seat.

The difficulties in toilet training a child with brain injury depend on the impairment of muscle tone, range of motion, motor coordination, and neuropsychological factors, such as initiative, memory, and continuity. Small children may benefit from potty seats or reducer rings, which diminish the size of the toilet seat, thereby providing a degree of stability in the seated position and generating a sense of safety and security. Some strategies that can help the child remain in position for the required amount of time include using the wall for trunk support and engaging in playful activities during potty training.

Adapted toilet seats may provide greater safety and autonomy for the child who does not yet have trunk control. Railings on the walls next to the toilet afford safer support for the child and can be of assistance when transferring to the wheelchair or standing position. These railings can also serve as support when putting on or taking off clothes.

## The Return Home of the Child or Adolescent with TBI

The adolescent or school-aged child should return to school as soon as it is deemed possible. Being back in the school environment promotes socialization with other children and adults in different settings and may contribute to the development of his potential in various activities of daily life. The family and the team should talk with the teachers about the program that is being carried out with the school-aged child or adolescent, and his potential for independence, so that they may give continuity to the activities begun at home. It is important, at this stage, that the child or adolescent not be exposed too early to situations that are too complex for him to master. There are tactics that can promote the child's participation in school, such as bringing snacks from home that are already cut into small pieces, wearing pants with elastic waist bands, or clothing that does not contain buttons or hooks that are difficult to handle. The school plays an important role in shaping, supporting and encouraging the child's abilities, helping to prepare him for a more independent life.

Effective, directed treatment with meaningful activities for the family can be provided in the child's or adolescent's natural, familiar setting through the reestablishment of daily routines.[26] While this chapter has described techniques that support the child's daily life, the same strategies can also support the needs of the adolescent who is recovering from a TBI. It is important to adapt the activities to the capacity, potential, and interests of each age group. A more engaged participation in grooming activities, for example, is expected among adolescents because of the physical, emotional, and social changes inherent to that age group. Strategies designed to promote independent home-care functioning can also be used with adolescents. Skills involving planning, problem-solving, self-protection and temporal orientation can be explored while the teenager carries out household chores such as helping to prepare a snack or breakfast, cleaning a room or taking out the trash. Home-care routines, although similar to self-care routines, usually involve more complex tasks such as use of various types of materials and tools, and can also help the adolescent see the need to plan and come up with different solutions for problems or day-to-day situations.

Autonomy reinforces an individual sense of achievement and competence, in addition to broadening the possibilities of developing habits and skills that could later be applied to other life experiences.

# References

1.  Mancini MC, Fiuza PM, Rebelo JM et al. Comparison of functional activity performance in normally developing children and children with cerebral palsy. Arq Neuropsiquiatr 2002; 60(2-B):446–452.

2.  Strauss D, Ojdana K, Shavelle R, Rosenbloom L. Decline in function and life expectancy of older persons with cerebral palsy. NeuroRehabilitation 2004; 19(1):69–78.

3.  Garcia PM, Sanchez CA. Perceptive and praxic impairments in traumatic brain injury patients: significance in activities of daily living. Rev Neurol 2004; 38(8):775–784.

4.  Duong TT, Englander J, Wright J, Cifu DX, Greenwald BD, Brown AW. Relationship between strength, balance, and swallowing deficits and outcome after traumatic brain injury: a multicenter analysis. Arch Phys Med Rehabil 2004; 85(8):1291–1297.

5.  Dumas HM, Haley SM, Fragala MA, Steva BJ. Self-care recovery of children with brain injury: descriptive analysis using the Pediatric Evaluation of Disability Inventory (PEDI) functional classification levels. Phys Occup Ther Pediatr 2001; 21(2–3):7–27.

6.  Kellegrew DH. Constructing daily routines: a qualitative examination of mothers with young children with disabilities. Am J Occup Ther 2000; 54(3):252–259.

7.  Ketelaar M, Vermeer A, Hart H, Petegem-van Beek E, Helders PJ. Effects of a functional therapy program on motor abilities of children with cerebral palsy. Phys Ther 2001; 81(9):1534–1545.

8.  Ostensjo S, Carlberg EB, Vollestad NK. Everyday functioning in young children with cerebral palsy: functional skills, caregiver assistance, and modifications of the environment. Dev Med Child Neurol 2003; 45(9):603–612.

9.  Nicholson JH, Morton RE, Attfield S, Rennie D. Assessment of upper-limb function and movement in children with cerebral palsy wearing lycra garments. Dev Med Child Neurol 2001; 43(6):384–391.

10. O'Flaherty SJ, Chivers A, Hannan TJ et al. The Westmead Pediatric TBI Multidisciplinary Outcome study: use of functional outcomes data to determine resource prioritization. Arch Phys Med Rehabil 2000; 81(6):723–729.

11. Dumas HM, Carey T. Motor skill and mobility recovery outcomes of children and youth with traumatic brain injury. Phys Occup Ther Pediatr 2002; 22(3–4):73–99.

12. Barks L. Therapeutic positioning, wheelchair seating, and pulmonary function of children with cerebral palsy: a research synthesis. Rehabil Nurs 2004; 29(5):146–153.

13. Bottos M, Bolcati C, Sciuto L, Ruggeri C, Feliciangeli A. Powered wheelchairs and independence in young children with tetraplegia. Dev Med Child Neurol 2001; 43(11):769–777.

14. Furkim AM, Behlau MS, Weckx LL. Clinical and videofluoroscopic evaluation of deglutition in children with tetraparetic spastic cerebral palsy. Arq Neuropsiquiatr 2003; 61(3A):611–616.

15. Duong TT, Englander J, Wright J, Cifu DX, Greenwald BD, Brown AW. Relationship between strength, balance, and swallowing deficits and outcome after traumatic brain injury: a multicenter analysis. Arch Phys Med Rehabil 2004; 85(8):1291–1297.

16.     Morgan A, Ward E, Murdoch B. Clinical characteristics of acute dysphagia in pediatric patients following traumatic brain injury. J Head Trauma Rehabil 2004; 19(3):226–240.

17.     Morgan A, Ward E, Murdoch B, Kennedy B, Murison R. Incidence, characteristics, and predictive factors for dysphagia after pediatric traumatic brain injury. J Head Trauma Rehabil 2003; 18(3):239–251.

18.     Puyuelo-Sanclemente M, Poo Arguelles P, Basil Almirall C, Le Metayer M. A fonoaudiologia na paralisia cerebral. São Paulo: Santos, 2001.

19.     Morgan A, Ward E, Murdoch B. Clinical progression and outcome of dysphagia following paediatric traumatic brain injury: a prospective study. Brain Inj 2004; 18(4):359–376.

20.     Garg BP. Dysphagia in children: an overview. Semin Pediatr Neurol 2003; 10(4):252–254.

21.     Rosenthal M, Bond MR, Griffith ER, Miller JD. Rehabilitation of the adult and child with traumatic brain injury. 2nd ed. Philadelphia: FA Davis, 1990.

22.     Wilkinson TJ, Thomas K, MacGregor S, Tillard G, Wyles C, Sainsbury R. Tolerance of early diet textures as indicators of recovery from dysphagia after stroke. Dysphagia 2002; 17(3):227–232.

23.     Gisel EG, Tessier MJ, Lapierre G, Seidman E, Drouin E, Filion G. Feeding management of children with severe cerebral palsy and eating impairment: an exploratory study. Phys Occup Ther Pediatr 2003; 23(2):19–44.

24.     Gangil A, Patwari AK, Aneja S, Ahuja B, Anand VK. Feeding problems in children with cerebral palsy. Indian Pediatr 2001; 38(8):839–846.

25.     Rugolotto S, Sun M. Toilet training. Pediatrics 2004; 113(1 Pt 1):180–181.

26.     Pace GM, Schlund MW, Hazard-Haupt T et al. Characteristics and outcomes of a home and community-based neurorehabilitation programme. Brain Inj 1999; 13(7):535–546.

# 7

## The Role of the Orthopaedic Surgeon in Brain Injury: Working in a Family-based Context

*Aloysio Campos da Paz Jr*

As early as 1743, Nicholas Andry first coined the word "orthopaedics" in his book, *Orthopaedia: Or, the art of correcting and preventing deformities in children: by such means as may easily be put into practice by parents themselves, and all such as are employed in educating children.*[1]

Orthopaedic surgeons have been treating children with varying types and degrees of motor dysfunction since the onset of this specialty.[2–5] While the rehabilitation of a child with physical disabilities often requires the participation of various professionals from different fields, the orthopaedic surgeon plays an important role when aspects of the treatment focus on motor dysfunction or functional deformity.[6] It is also true that an orthopaedic surgeon's practice and activity cannot often be transferred to the family. Thus, within the perspective and goals of this context-sensitive, family-based rehabilitation program, which counts on the interrelated group efforts of multidisciplinary professionals, the orthopaedic surgeon must strive to incorporate the family into the decision-making process. This entails transferring to them the necessary information, permitting the fullest extent of their participation in a process that has historically precluded intervention of the family, who is uniquely qualified to provide data on their growing, developing child.[7–16]

Since the impact of brain injury on the musculoskeletal system of children with cerebral palsy (CP) is different from that in children with traumatic brain injury (TBI), this chapter will discuss CP and TBI in separate sections, to allow for clearer discussions about the specificities of the orthopaedic surgeon's involvement in each of these two pathologies.

## Cerebral Palsy

Children with CP often begin to receive medical assistance at birth and continue throughout the various stages of their life. The interventions that are done early on an infant or child will impact on their future.[7–9;17] Thus, in order to determine the most appropriate conduct and approach to a child with CP it is important to determine what is essential now, based on the child's present condition and on the changes brought by time, a process that requires team effort by the rehabilitation professionals and the family.

## The Limits of Surgery

Frequently, the orthopaedic surgeon on the rehabilitation team of a child with CP first sees the child in the early developmental stages. In most cases, this child has developmental delays and/or altered muscle tonus, with its attendant consequences. While consulting with the family at the beginning of the program, the surgeon may hear variations on two questions: "Will my child walk?" and "How will his 'deformities' be corrected?" Helping to give the family clear, honest answers to these important questions is one of the first aspects of the orthopaedist's role in the family-team approach to rehabilitating a child.

Orthopaedic surgeons often have a strong tendency to surgically intervene because, historically, they have been taught to correct deformities and are trained to do so. This may lead towards an excess of surgical procedures. It is necessary, then, to have an understanding of some basic developmental concepts.

One of these basic concepts is that children are still growing and, as they grow, they will change; in some cases, they will be unable to walk or will have difficulties doing so.[18–20] Given this reality, a surgeon should exercise caution when suggesting surgical intervention, so as not to precipitate unnecessary invasive measures. A significant number of children have combined disorders due to cortical lesions and injury to the basal ganglia and brain stem. Over time, involuntary movements may gradually manifest and, as a consequence, the positioning of an extremity may also change. For example, a child who has a foot turned inward may come to have a foot turned outwards.

Surgical procedures cannot be universally applied to all children with CP.[9] Strategy comes before technique. The concept that surgery or orthopaedic measures should be fundamentally related to the developmental process of a child with brain injury led in 1994, to a study that permitted the assessment of whether spastic children had the necessary conditions for walking: "Walking prognosis in cerebral palsy: a 22-year retrospective analysis".[20] This study permits the preview, with reasonable accuracy, of each child's walking potential, thereby helping to prevent unnecessary surgical procedures. Every surgical procedure should aim at enhancing the child's quality of life or improving the child's ability to walk.[21–22] This is because we are dealing with the consequences of a change in the normal interaction of joint motion. A shift from biomechanics to pathomechanics.[23–24] Experience has shown that no deformity is fully corrected and in fact may even be over-corrected.[25] Therefore, the aforementioned joint interaction is affected for better or for worse, depending on the measure that is adopted. This is the key to a good outcome and highlights the importance of clinical or, if possible, technologically assisted gait evaluation.[26]

If spasticity is a generalized phenomenon that may be present in each segment of the locomotor system, capable of triggering countless consequences, then we cannot be guided exclusively by the need to correct deformities alone. In other words, all children are individuals with their own lesion-associated characteristics and specific developmental stage, and should be respected as such within their own complex form of growing. This is associated with the fact that the muscle imbalance generated by the damage to the brain is not synchronized with the rate of bone growth, which is defined by genetic and environmental factors and the consequent phenomena that occur in the developing cartilagenous plates of the bone extremities.[27] The bone grows in disaccord with the development of a spastic muscle group. This is one of the main issues that an orthopaedic surgeon must understand when considering surgical intervention in CP.

## The Differences Between Function and Aesthetics: the Emphasis on Performance

The poliomyelitis epidemics and the high incidence of congenital lesions and trauma produced an orthopaedic culture that was focused on the prevalence of the resultant deformities.[28]

For years, the main concern was to correct the physical form in an effort to attain the aesthetic stereotypes imposed by society, with little regard for the basic fact that individuals are not the same. Poliomyelitis generated a surgical practice based on muscle transplants (transposing the insertion of a tendon in order to obtain a change or strengthen a function), tenotomies (the sectioning of a tendon from a muscle complex that is shortened, leading to a deformity), arthrodesis (fixating bones to gain stability, generally in the feet) and osteotomies (the sectioning of a long bone in order to change its alignment and improve function).[28-40]

What made sense in the treatment of spinal cord injury caused by the polio virus was extrapolated, often without any critical analysis, to the surgical treatment of CP. The focus was on the consequences of the brain damage, but with little or no understanding of the impact of different types of brain injury on the growing, changing child. At that time, surgery rarely took neurodevelopment into account. Measures that could have helped children adapt to and live within the family and the community, and that valued their learning potential, independently of how it was manifested, were not considered. The fact that the most important thing was to attain a positive objective was frequently annulled by the prejudice against *being* different or *doing* things differently.[8-9]

Since then, there has been tremendous progress in the field of neurosciences and neuroradiology. Within our context-sensitive, family-based approach, there have been important gains produced by the alliance between neuropsychology and various surgical subspecialties, lending new insights into the child's neurodevelopment. In orthopaedics, advancements in both technology and research have changed how we rehabilitate a child with CP. For example, gait analysis allows, through simple observation, an understanding of the pathomechanics of walking. This "simple" observation is buttressed by the capacity for precise documentation that the movement laboratories afford nowadays, which can range from simple recordings and analysis in slow-motion home video to sophisticated movement labs with digital technology, force plates, and dynamic electromyography.[41]

Movement analysis allows us to record and assess the *before* and the *after* of interventions, and permits us a more informed and knowledgeable basis for making surgical decisions founded on data derived from the body in motion.[42–43]

Nevertheless, it is essential that the data obtained in these laboratories be analyzed together by those who will intervene; decisions should not be made based on reports alone. In this family-based approach, input from the entire multidisciplinary team and the family should be considered so as to make the best decisions regarding the child's present and future conditions. For the child with CP who is able to walk, any surgical intervention, even the most simple, will benefit from prior documentation of the child's locomotion. We are evaluating a function that is often performed in a multitude of ways, depending on each child and his potential. This documentation gives us a base for comparing the child's condition before and after the intervention. One example is if a child's equinism (walking on tiptoes) is corrected, a reduction in walking speed will occur (a simple chronometer can register this fact). Aesthetically, the result may lead us to believe that a child has improved because he is now able to place his heel on the floor, but from a functional viewpoint his gait is slower and requires greater energy expenditure. Due to issues of this nature, decisions about surgery should involve the family's input and, if possible, the child's. Even simple recording of the child's movement can be beneficial in explaining his condition to the family, who will be afforded the opportunity to see, in slow-motion replay, how the child's gait is affected.

## Timing

Although there are a number of necessary surgical interventions that will bring unquestionable functional improvements to the child with CP, they are nonetheless usually elective in nature and should be subjected to deliberation to determine the best time, if ever, to perform them. Conferring with the rehabilitation team and the family will help point towards the best route to take, based on the various particulars of each child's rehabilitation process, not the least of which is the child's cognitive development. For example, interrupting the school activities of a diplegic child so that he can undergo a surgical procedure is, in a way, to interfere in his development and learning, and possibly delay one of the final objectives of rehabilitation, namely, his autonomy, social skills and acquisition of cognitive milestones. The parents and rehabilitation professionals should use the time prior to (or in lieu of) the surgery to emphasize the child's potential, strengths and ability to attain an objective, independently of how he is able to do it.

## Issues that will Permit the Parents to Critically Evaluate the Rehabilitation of their Child with Cerebral Palsy

When the parents consult with the orthopaedic surgeon on the rehabilitation team, they should consider discussing the following questions:

- When would be the best time to intervene if at the moment the deformity is not getting worse?
- Will what is being done now have to be repeated throughout my child's development and growth?
- Will my child be able to engage in activities of daily life in the same way that he does now? For example, today, although his feet are equinus, he is able to run. Will he maintain this ability or will he have to "limp quickly" if submitted to corrective surgery?
- Will full correction of plantar flexion performed today on a boy be as effective on a girl, who may one day grow up to wear high heels?
- Is surgery urgent, or can it wait?

## Concepts and Principles

Movement, especially that which results in gait, is done through a systematic interaction of all the joints of the human body throughout the various stages of neurodevelopment. This harmonious interaction is characterized by a constant transformation of potential energy into kinetic energy, resulting in function. In a child with CP and spasticity, this harmony is disrupted and compensatory mechanisms develop that lead to new relationships among the joints.

These new relationships define the transition from biomechanics to pathomechanics. Depending on the injury, the disorganization of brain commands in CP is characterized by hemiplegia, diplegia, triplegia or, quadriplegia with or without involuntary movements. These involuntary movement disorders need to be identified, because when they are present the sequence of events in the child's neurodevelopment is often different from what occurs in the spastic child without any of these conditions, and because unpredictable changes in the interactions among the deformities can result. An equinus varus foot (positioned downwards and inwards) may, during growth, evolve into valgus (turned outwards) with new pathomechanical interrelationships.

Furthermore, it is not uncommon to find children with quadriplegia and involuntary movements who have cognitive levels that, with the communication technology available nowadays, require added focus on educational support and assistive gait devices rather than on surgical procedures.[45]

When dealing with a multiplicity of anomalous positionings, a possible measure is examination of the child under sedation. This can allow us to obtain information about whether or not the deformity has already been structured by muscle shortening resultant from prolonged spasticity, or if only the latter prevails. Sedation makes it possible to correct the change in form if it is due to spasticity alone. At the same time, a myoneural blocking,[46] after electrical stimulation to precisely determine the neuromotor point, followed by the use of a cast and, later, a plastic splint, can prevent tendon lengthening consequent to prolonged spasticity.

In some cases lengthening a tendon may be necessary to enable gait with less energy expenditure. This is because, given the mobility of the subtalar joints (those that join the bones below the ankle), energy is lost due to increased inversion and consequent reduced impulsion at each step during the support phase. When the child touches the floor during the support phase, there is an accentuation of foot inversion. Consequently, because of the constant systematic interaction of the calcaneous soil, subtalar, ankle, knee and hip joints, the lower limb goes into full external rotation.[47] Pathomechanical factors make the injection of energy into the ground relatively gradual, with a loss of energy at various systemic levels in the cranial caudal direction. Therefore, the reversibility of these phenomena during the take-off phase demands use of all the energy that was lost during stance, resulting in heightened slowness.[48] Nonetheless, a tendon lengthening should be avoided before first determining exactly what the child has in terms of spasticity and to what extent the equinism is associated with a musculotendinous shortening. Due to loss of plantar flexion strength, lengthening beyond what is necessary triggers reduction of impulsion, secondary flexion of the knee and hips, with greater energy expenditure and increased limping.[9,49] Therefore, myoneural blocking that reduces triceps' spasticity should precede lengthening of the Achilles tendon. A certain degree of plantar flexion should be maintained in order to facilitate locomotion by projecting the center of gravity forward. A child who undergoes a hyperextension of the ankle will have more difficulties walking after the correction of equinus.

Another situation in which myoneural blocking should precede surgery is in cases of adduction deformities, for which surgery is performed to enable better gait or, in the case of quadriplegics, to facilitate hygiene and wheelchair positioning. In the presence of spasticity, better interaction among the joints and improved function can be obtained by transposing a muscle insertion or a tendon section. We should also remember that we are dealing with generalized spasticity, with a predominance of several muscle groups. A simple sectioning or transposition will not yield complete joint balance, it will only decrease the effects of the dominance of one group over another. We are, in reality, seeking a "balance among the spasticities".

Any surgery in CP is usually elective and rarely an emergency procedure. When it is impossible to conduct a movement study through dynamic electromyography, successive exams with time intervals can consolidate information that will lead us to act with greater assurance. The orthopaedist should, in these cases, bring to the team and the family the necessary balance in the decision-making process that is oftentimes impacted by the anxiety of all those who are involved with the child.

# Traumatic Brain Injury

## Acute Care

Children and adolescents who have sustained TBI, in contrast to CP, do not always have motor sequela.[50] In this section we will address how injury to the motor cortex, cerebellum or basal ganglia affects a locomotor system that often had already attained a level of neuromotor development that was subsequently interrupted or altered due to neurotrauma.

Preventive orthopaedic care should begin immediately following a trauma to the brain, while the child is still in the acute stages. This immediacy helps minimize deformities that could, due to spasticity, negatively interfere in the rehabilitation process and render the use of devices such as splints either ineffectual or downright impossible. To begin with, adequate positioning of the child in the intensive care unit (ICU) is essential, to avoid accentuated extensor or flexor patterns.[51] Determining and implementing the correct positioning is an exhausting task, frequently disregarded when more urgent attention must be given to keeping the respiratory pathways clear so as to prevent life-threatening complications.[52-53] Mobilization and relaxing activities are beneficial, so long as the patient's every reaction is observed and respected, such as increased heart rate and respiratory frequency caused by pain. This may prevent the risk of triggering, through forced passive movements, complications secondary to musculotendinous lesions that can induce heterotopic ossification.[54] However, it is not easy to physically manipulate a child who has been through trauma. He may reject these attempts at proper positioning due to pain, a situation that is exacerbated by occasional mishandling. The child may also not be able to communicate and express how he is feeling when submitted to unpleasant or painful manipulations. Furthermore, in cases in which the accident produced fractures, management of the child may be even more complex. All this can generate situations that are difficult for the rehabilitation team and the family.[55] It is important to remember that the patient is a child who suddenly, due to the injury, is required to live in a new setting that, to him, is often hostile and unpleasant. The efficacy of many of the methods used during the first stages of post-TBI recovery is debatable and thus should be carefully assessed so that the best approach is selected for each individual child, based on his condition. For example, there is the risk that a splint is masking the progression of a deformity and the fact that forcing a position when the child has spastic muscles can generate pain or discomfort and increased spasticity.

During the initial stages, the child is often treated within a nosocomial focus. Concrete difficulties associated with life-saving attitudes hinder a more amenable and ludic process aimed at functional recovery that would enhance short and long-term results and lessen the discomfort that many children face at this time. Orthopaedic surgeons must play an active role in ensuring that any and all efforts made towards avoiding and reducing motor sequelae are the most suitable for each individual child. Their involvement should not be limited to simply treating multiple fractures frequently associated with these cases, for they have an important role to play in the team that is working together towards improving the condition of the child who has sustained a TBI.

## The Journey from the ICU to Home and School

Once the acute phase has passed and the child has left the ICU, a new chapter in the natural history of TBI begins. In this transition, orthopaedic surgeons should accompany the child and evaluate his evolution with the resources available to them, rather than wait to be called upon only when the team is questioned by the parents as to why their child's frequent complaints of pain, difficulties positioning, and limited joint movements have not yet been corrected.

When dealing with the sequelae of TBI, the orthopaedic surgeon's approach should consider the child's behavioral changes, recurrence of joint pain, and communication difficulties associated with speech and writing impairments. This demands a close interaction with neuropsychologists and therapists, but especially with the child and his family, for there to be a thoroughly deliberated assessment of the "if" and the "when" of any surgical intervention. Orthopaedic surgeons must not be seen as passive and often distant "consultants" involved in occasional surgical procedures. On the contrary, they must be actively engaged in evaluating and dealing with the consequences of the brain trauma on the child's central nervous system.

## Functional Diagnosis as an Aid to the Decision-making Process

Present-day, advancements in the field of movement analysis, which permits study of the physics of gait, motor coordination of the upper limbs and balance, allows for an evaluation of the activities of daily life to be better quantified and, consequently, compared throughout treatment. Nevertheless, if we consider the historical evolution of movement analysis,[57–62] this resource, if not fully available, may be accomplished by simple home video recordings, to the benefit of the recovering child.

The goal is to assess the *before* and the *after* of any attempts to improve function. The sequence of events during the child's treatment should be registered dynamically, while the child is in motion. For example, if a plastic splint stabilizes the child's wrist and permits better use of his hand in activities of daily life, does this justify surgical intervention to substitute the splint for an arthrodesis to provide internal stabilization?[63-64] This is the type of question that should be discussed with the family and the entire rehabilitation team, and data from the movement lab can provide valuable information for reaching a decision.

Many children with brain injury have spastic hemiplegia, and can benefit from the practice of bimanual activities in which they use the impaired limb as an aid to attaining their functional objective. Herein lies one of the orthopaedist's fundamental roles in brain injury: strengthening the team, interacting with the family and stressing that the most important thing, for the child, is attaining the functional objective, independently of how it is done. This requires that orthopaedic surgeons shift their focus from purely surgical intervention to a non-surgical attitude that gives greater emphasis to the physiopathology of TBI, its natural history and consequences.[56] Returning to the philosophical bases that fundament this idea: what is relevant is *if* the objective can be attained, not necessarily *how* it is attained.

## Principles and Concepts

The obstacles that must be overcome in order to improve function in children with traumatic brain injury are associated with various causes:

- Deformities acquired through lack of correct positioning and/or failures in the administration of adequate care during the acute stages when the child is still in the ICU.
- A tendency to seek the most "normal" joint relationships through continuous use of devices such as splints. Splint immobilization can increase muscle imbalance by atrophying muscle groups that have been overcome by their spastic antagonists. A child with a limb that is immobilized after a fracture often presents muscle atrophy from disuse upon removal of the plaster cast. The same can happen to a child with TBI, with the aggravating presence of spasticity that may "lock" a joint, and the reduction of joint motion after prolonged plaster immobilization.[5]
- Osteoarticular lesions resultant from incorrect manipulations that generate pain and can cause heterotopic ossification due to tissue trauma.
- The presence of a muscle imbalance generated by brain commands that have been impaired due to trauma. A change in form impacts on the entire locomotor system by generating the need for new compensatory positionings and actions.[23]

- Spasticity. This is a diffuse phenomenon that can be present in all the muscles of all the affected segments. The interference of a muscle group can lead to the predominance of an antagonist one, causing new deformities that are difficult to correct.
- Finally, it is necessary to stress that about one-third of these children either change the patterns of the sequelae or evolve to practically normal motricity skills.

All of these concepts are based on the fact that in pathomechanics, as in biomechanics,[23;66] all of the joints interact, enabling movement and consequently, gait. They form a complex that permanently transforms potential energy into kinetic energy. Ignoring this fact and analyzing a joint without the understanding that we are dealing with an interactive system can lead to a functional disaster.

## Comments

In TBI, the most frequent motor disorder is hemiparesia or hemiplegia. Plantar flexion with foot inversion is common, leading to impaired gait. One of the positions typical of mixed hemiplegia can be seen rendered in a classic painting, with controversial interpretations, by the artist Guiseppe de Rivera (1642):[67] the foot is in equinovarus, the knee is flexed and the upper limb with an extended elbow, forearm in supination and hand in palmar flexion. This position could be a consequence of the muscle imbalance that results from post-TBI changes in muscle tonus.

Some children frequently have ataxias that may require the use of assistive devices for walking. Initially, these children need to use wheelchairs and, after a variable period of training, can begin using walkers.

In spastic children the upper limbs may exhibit palmar deviation in the hands, thumb "in the palm" and extension or flexion of the fingers impeding grasping and requiring better positioning of the wrist and thumb with the aid of a splint. If these measures are successful, they can be substituted by surgical fixation of the wrist and positioning of the thumb in opponent.[63;68] These measures often facilitate written communication through either the use of devices that enable grasping or the use of computer keyboards, especially in children with aphasia.

The possibility of heterotopic ossification is a complex problem because in the child it can develop without any expressive symptoms and progress silently in the initial phases.[54;69] Joint stiffness requires periodic measurement of alkaline phosphate levels, which, if elevated, can reveal excessive osteoblastic activity. In these cases, radiological studies of the involved segments are indicated.

The role of the orthopaedic surgeon on the rehabilitation team of a child who has sustained a TBI is still being established. To the extent that surgeons' constant participation grows and allows them to acquire experience, they will be better able to discuss treatment principles and techniques in conjunction with the multitude of information provided by the various specialists and the family who care for the child within this context-sensitive, family-based approach.

# And Lastly . . .

It is important to bear in mind that, when faced with the possibility of a surgical procedure, it is the parents' right to voice all of their doubts, hear all of the available answers, and then discuss the information so that they can reach a decision about if and when they will accept the surgical intervention. Furthermore, a good rule of medicine dictates that a second opinion is always beneficial. Whenever possible, the child or adolescent should be allowed to participate in the decision-making process, to the best of their abilities. Our experience over the years has taught us that when an explanation is clearly given in plain, simple language, children with good cognitive functioning will be able to understand what is probably going to happen as a result of our intervention. They can make drawings and diagrams that can be extremely accurate. Asking them to express, either with words or drawings, what they understood and what they think about the matter not only makes this approach more humane but also enables more effective participation on the part of the children and their families.

To accomplish this, a simple technique for specialists, after they have finished their joint discussions with the team and family, is to give the child and the parents a sheet of paper with these two questions for them to answer:

- *What did I understand?*
- *What do I still want to know?*

As in everything else in life, we must remember that people do not always listen to what we say but rather, what they want to hear. As Hypocrates said, "Whenever a doctor cannot do good, he must be kept from doing harm."[70] An erroneous explanation can sometimes do more damage than an ineffective surgery.

There are many aspects of their practice that orthopaedic surgeons cannot transfer to the family, as can be done with exercises that involve motor function or cognitive development; nevertheless, orthopaedic surgeons should be actively involved in informing the rest of the team and parents, conferring with the therapists about possible physical potentials and obstacles to the stimulation of a given motor function, and accompanying the child throughout all the stages of the rehabilitation and developmental process.

# References

1. Andry de Bois-Regard N. Orthopaedia. Philadelphia: Lippincott, 1961.

2. Lovell W. Pediatric orthopedics. Philadelphia: Lippincott, 1978.

3. Ombrédanne L, Mathieu P. Traité de chirurgie orthopédique. Paris: Masson, 1937.

4. Tachdjian M. Pediatric orthopaedics. Philadelphia: WB Saunders, 1972.

5. Wenger D, Rang M. The art and practice of children's orthopaedics. New York: Raven, 1992.

6. Bleck EE. Physically handicapped children: a manual atlas for teachers. New York: Grune & Stratton, 1975.

7. Campos da Paz Jr A, Miranda S, Grandi M. Uma atitude diante da paralisia cerebral. Rev Bras Ortop 1980; 15(2):45–47.

8. Campos da Paz Jr A, Nomura AM, Braga LW, Burnett SM. Speculations on cerebral palsy. J Bone Joint Surg 1984; 66B(2):283.

9. Campos da Paz Jr A, Burnett SM, Nomura AM. Cerebral palsy. In: Duthie RB, editor. Mercers's orthopedic surgery. London: Arnold, 1996.

10. Trueta J. Studies of the development and decay of the human frame. London: William Heinemann, 1968.

11. Braddock CH, III, Edwards KA, Hasenberg NM, Laidley TL, Levinson W. Informed decision making in outpatient practice: time to get back to basics. JAMA 1999; 282(24):2313–2320.

12. Frymoyer JW, Frymoyer NP. Physician–patient communication: a lost art? J Am Acad Orthop Surg 2002; 10(2):95–105.

13. Herndon JH, Pollick KJ. Continuing concerns, new challenges, and next steps in physician–patient communication. J Bone Joint Surg Am 2002; 84-A(2):309–315.

14. Maruishi M, Mano Y, Sasaki T, Shinmyo N, Sato H, Ogawa T. Cerebral palsy in adults: independent effects of muscle strength and muscle tone. Arch Phys Med Rehabil 2001; 82(5):637–641.

15. Rosenbaum P. Cerebral palsy: what parents and doctors want to know. BMJ 2003; 326(7396):970–974.

16. Strauss D, Ojdana K, Shavelle R, Rosenbloom L. Decline in function and life expectancy of older persons with cerebral palsy. NeuroRehabilitation 2004; 19(1):69–78.

17. Geppert J. Yes, survive I did. Lancet 2004; 363(9421):1632.

18. Bleck EE. Locomotor prognosis in cerebral palsy. Dev Med Child Neurol 1975; 17(1):18–25.

19. Bottos M, Feliciangeli A, Sciuto L, Gericke C, Vianello A. Functional status of adults with cerebral palsy and implications for treatment of children. Dev Med Child Neurol 2001; 43(8):516–528.

20. Campos da Paz Jr A, Burnett SM, Braga LW. Walking prognosis in cerebral palsy: a 22-year retrospective analysis. Dev Med Child Neurol 1994; 36(2):130–134.

21.     Campos da Paz Jr A. Tratando doentes e nao doencas. Brasilia: SarahLetras, 2002.

22.     Davids JR, Ounpuu S, DeLuca PA, Davis RB, III. Optimization of walking ability of children with cerebral palsy. Instr Course Lect 2004; 53:511–522.

23.     Kapandji IA. The physiology of the joints: annotade diagrams of the mechanics of the human joints: lower limb. 5th ed. Edinburgh: Churchill Livingstone, 1987.

24.     Sutherland DH. The evolution of clinical gait analysis part l: kinesiological EMG. Gait Posture 2001; 14(1):61–70.

25.     Kay RM, Rethlefsen SA, Ryan JA, Wren TA. Outcome of gastrocnemius recession and tendo-achilles lengthening in ambulatory children with cerebral palsy. J Pediatr Orthop B 2004; 13(2):92–98.

26.     Gage JR. The role of gait analysis in the treatment of cerebral palsy. J Pediatr Orthop 1994; 14(6):701–702.

27.     Lieber RL, Steinman S, Barash IA, Chambers H. Structural and functional changes in spastic skeletal muscle. Muscle Nerve 2004; 29(5):615–627.

28.     Campos da Paz Jr A, Ramalho Jr A, Jabur D, Cafalli F. Poliomielite. Saude no Brasil 1983; 1(1):41–54.

29.     Sharrard WJW. Paralytic deformity in the lower limb. J Bone Joint Surg 1967; 49B(4):731–747.

30.     Westin W. Tendon transfer about the foot, ankle, and hip in the paralysed lower limb. J Bone Joint Surg 1965; 47A(7):1430–1443.

31.     Sharrard WJW. Muscle paralysis in poliomyelitis. Br J Surg 1957; 44:471–480.

32.     Blount WP, Clarke GR. The classic: control of bone growth by epiphyseal stapling: a preliminary report, Journal of Bone and Joint Surgery, July, 1949. Clin Orthop Relat Res 1971; 77:4–17.

33.     Paluska DJ, Blount WP. Ankle valgus after the Grice subtalar stabilization: the late evaluation of a personal series with a modified technic. Clin Orthop Relat Res 1968; 59:137–146.

34.     Asirvatham R, Watts HG, Rooney RJ. Rotation osteotomy of the tibia after poliomyelitis: a review of 51 patients. J Bone Joint Surg Br 1990; 72(3):409–411.

35.     McCall RE, Lillich JS, Harris JR, Johnston FA. The Grice extra-articular subtalar arthrodesis: a clinical review. J Pediatr Orthop 1985; 5(4):442–445.

36.     Grice DS. Further experience with extra-articular arthrodesis of the subtalar joint. J Bone Joint Surg Am 1955; 37-A(2):246–259.

37.     Grice DS. An extra-articular arthrodesis of the subastragalar joint for correction of paralytic flat feet in children. J Bone Joint Surg Am 1952; 34 A(4):927–940.

38.     Gross RH. An evaluation of tibial lengthening procedures. J Bone Joint Surg Am 1971; 53(4):693–700.

39.     Robin GC. Fractures in poliomyelitis in children. J Bone Joint Surg Am 1966; 48(6):1048–1054.

40.     Campos da Paz Jr A. Alongamento de tibia: metodo de Anderson. Rev Bras Ortop 1967; 2(2/3): 75–87.

41.     Chambers HG, Sutherland DH. A practical guide to gait analysis. J Am Acad Orthop Surg 2002; 10(3):222–231.

42.     Cook RE, Schneider I, Hazlewood ME, Hillman SJ, Robb JE. Gait analysis alters decision-making in cerebral palsy. J Pediatr Orthop 2003; 23(3):292–295.

43.     DeLuca PA, Davis RB, III, Ounpuu S, Rose S, Sirkin R. Alterations in surgical decision making in patients with cerebral palsy based on three-dimensional gait analysis. J Pediatr Orthop 1997; 17(5):608–614.

44.     Koman LA, Smith BP, Shilt JS. Cerebral palsy. Lancet 2004; 363(9421):1619–1631.

45.     Bottos M, Gericke C. Ambulatory capacity in cerebral palsy: prognostic criteria and consequences for intervention. Dev Med Child Neurol 2003; 45(11):786–790.

46.     Tilton AH. Management of spasticity in children with cerebral palsy. Semin Pediatr Neurol 2004; 11(1):58–65.

47.     Campos da Paz Jr A, Souza V. Talipes equinovarus: pathomechanical basis of treatment. Orthop Clin North Am 1978; 9(1):171–185.

48.     Hawking S. On the shoulders of giants. London: Running Press, 2002.

49.     Sutherland DH, Davids JR. Common gait abnormalities of the knee in cerebral palsy. Clin Orthop Relat Res 1993;(288):139–147.

50.     Laurent-Vannier A, Brugel DG, De Augustine M. Rehabilitation of brain-injured children. Childs Nerv Syst 2000; 16(10–11):760–764.

51.     Palmer M, Wyness MA. Positioning and handling: important considerations in the care of the severely head-injured patient. J Neurosci Nurs 1988; 20(1):42–49.

52.     Fuhrman BP, Zimmerman JJ. Pediatric critial care. 2nd ed. St. Louis, MO: Mosby, 1998.

53.     Greenwald BM, Ghajar J, Notterman DA. Critical care of children with acute brain injury. Adv Pediatr 1995; 42:47–89.

54.     Kluger G, Kochs A, Holthausen H. Heterotopic ossification in childhood and adolescence. J Child Neurol 2000; 15(6):406–413.

55.     Savage R, DePompei R, Tyler J, Lash M. Paediatric traumatic brain: a review of pertinent issues. Pediatr Rehabil 2005; 8(2):92–103.

56.     Johnson DA, Rose D. Prognosis, rehabilitation and outcome after inflicted brain injury in children – a case of professional developmental delay. Pediatr Rehabil 2004; 7(3):185–193.

57.     Gage JR. Gait analysis in cerebral palsy. London: MacKeith, 1991.

58.     Inman V. Human walking. Baltimore, MD: Williams & Wilkins, 1982.

59.     Muybridge E. The human figure in motion. New York: Dover, 1955.

60.     Muybridge E. Animals in motion. New York: Dover, 1957.

61.     Perry J. Gait analysis: normal and pathological function. Thorofare, NJ: Slack, 1992.

62.    Sutherland DH. The development of mature walking. London: MacKeith, 1988.

63.    Zancolli EA. Surgical management of the hand in infantile spastic hemiplegia. Hand Clin 2003; 19(4):609–629.

64.    Tubiana R, Masquelet AC, McCullough CJ. Atlas of surgical exposures of the upper and lower extremities. London: Martin Dunitz, 2000.

65.    O'Suilleabhain P, Dewey RB, Jr. Movement disorders after head injury: diagnosis and management. J Head Trauma Rehabil 2004; 19(4):305–313.

66.    Perry J. The use of gait analysis for surgical recommendations in traumatic brain injury. J Head Trauma Rehabil 1999; 14(2):116–135.

67.    Sullivan EJ. Ribera's the boy with the clubfoot: image and symbol. In: Simons G, editor. The clubfoot: the present and a view of the future. New York: Springer, 1994: xiii–xv.

68.    Rayan GM, Young BT. Arthrodesis of the spastic wrist. J Hand Surg [Am] 1999; 24(5):944–952.

69.    Citta-Pietrolungo TJ, Alexander MA, Steg NL. Early detection of heterotopic ossification in young patients with traumatic brain injury. Arch Phys Med Rehabil 1992; 73(3):258–262.

70.    Hippocrates. In: Lyons AS, Petrucelli II RJ, editors. Medicine: an illustrated history. New York: Abradale, 1987: 206–217.

# 8

# The Family of the Child with Brain Injury

*Marc A Forman*

The diagnosis of cerebral palsy (CP) or traumatic brain injury (TBI), and its consequences, in a child generates a fundamental change in the family. While there has been much written about the need for "evidence-based medicine", i.e., treatments and interventions which have a proven basis and scientifically based evidence to support them, we cannot forget the need for "narrative-based medicine", listening carefully to patient and family "stories" in order to best care for our patients and families. Narrative-based medicine is not new. It has recently been rediscovered.[1] Luria previously described the importance of integrating "classical science" with "romantic science", which is the science of the case history, the biography, the patient's story.[2]

So we begin with a story about a child and his family, and then discuss the problems and obstacles which confront the family, the doctors, and other rehabilitation team members who provide care. Throughout the chapter we offer suggestions which we hope in some degree will mitigate the psychological burden for both, as well as offering strategies to help the family in the rehabilitation process.

## Luis B.

He was a much-wanted child, the second in his family. Jorge, his father, was a carpenter; Mariana, the mother, was a housewife and part-time cafeteria worker. Jorge helped with the care of their older daughter, Anna, age 6, a good student in a primary school, but most of this responsibility was carried out by Mariana. When Mariana became pregnant, after several years of trying without success, both parents were happy and excited. They had saved some money, had a modest apartment, and a small but adequate space for the new baby. Jorge quietly hoped that the baby would be a boy, and had fantasies of helping him to learn how to play football. He was an avid fan of the local football club, and envisioned going to the stadium with his son, both wearing the colors of the team. Mariana's pregnancy was uneventful, except toward the very end when she developed a slight fever, which she thought was probably a flu that she had caught from one of her fellow workers. Labor and delivery were easier than with the first child; Luis weighed 2.3 kg and appeared to be a normal, healthy baby. As a newborn Luis was more difficult to feed than had been his sister and much patience was required to feed him because of his slow sucking at the nipple. However, he slept well and responded with smiles to the attention of his parents and sister. Mariana became concerned when he was almost 2 years old; he was not walking, and said only a few words, which were difficult to understand. Jorge thought that his wife was probably exaggerating Luis's problems, but agreed that they should go to the local health clinic for another visit and to talk to the pediatrician there. The pediatrician examined Luis, and referred them to another doctor, a specialist at the local university hospital. This doctor also examined Luis, asked for some tests to be done, and had Luis seen by yet another specialist. Three visits later, the first specialist brought the parents into his office, and said that Luis had CP, might or might not walk, and could be mentally delayed. Jorge said nothing, and seemed to be frozen; Mariana said "No, no" and began to cry. Neither parent was able to ask any questions; they wanted to ask "Are you sure?", but did not know whether they should.

## Giving "Bad News"

The diagnosis of a child's handicap may be apparent immediately at birth, if the child has an obvious genetic syndrome or catastrophic birth injury. More typically, as in CP, the child's handicapping condition becomes more manifest over time, as delays in motor and/or cognitive development occur. A third circumstance occurs when the child is quite normal, and then becomes handicapped after a TBI. Whenever the diagnosis can be made, parents should know as soon as possible, and not be "protected" by keeping them uninformed. The diagnosis, and as much of the prognosis as can be known at the time, should be given by the physician in an empathic manner, in a private setting, not in a busy hospital corridor, at the bedside, or in front of students on rounds. Parents who are informed early and promptly when the diagnosis is evident are more likely to be active participants in the treatment process. The physician cannot expect that the parents will be able to assimilate the information in one sitting. Parents will be anxious, will not hear all the words, will not know how to respond, will be essentially overwhelmed, and perhaps even immobile. They may easily forget, want to forget, not comprehend, ignore, etc. what the doctor has said. Unfortunately, many physicians have been poorly trained in the art of communication, despite many revisions in medical school curricula in an attempt to correct this deficiency. Faults persist, in which the physician is too abrupt, uses language too technical to comprehend, and expects the parents to be understanding and compliant. Doctors need to heed the advice of the American novelist-physician, Walker Percy: "If you listen carefully to your patients, they will tell you not only what is wrong with them, but also what is wrong with you".[3]

There is yet another obstacle which confounds communication between family and doctor. There are circumstances in which the diagnosis or the prognosis is not clear and firm at a particular moment in time. For example, in the instance of the child with CP, delays in motor and cognitive development may first appear to be of unknown origin, which the parents and physicians hope will resolve. As delays and deficits persist, the diagnosis may still remain unclear, despite repeated exams and tests. In other words, the doctor and the family each confront a period of uncertainty. Neither the parents nor the physician are comfortable or secure in the toleration of uncertainty. The parents want to know what is the matter with their child, and what can be done to remedy it. The doctor has been trained and socialized to act, to decide, to do. Yet if the doctor acts prematurely in making the diagnosis, the diagnosis could be wrong. Diagnoses are often part of a longitudinal process, rather than a cross-sectional event. The younger the child, the higher the risk for a diagnosis to be incorrect. The doctor is challenged to keep a trusting relationship with the parents throughout this uncertain time, as well as over the long-term future, by sharing as much information as he or she knows at the time, and telling the parents that they will be informed as soon as the correct diagnosis is clarified. This doctor, who gives the initial diagnosis, becomes at that moment, a critical person in the family's life. The physician who relates the diagnosis is also often a member of a multidisciplinary team, including a functional therapist, psychologist, speech and language therapist, social worker and teacher. The family's ongoing relationship with this treatment team will be discussed later in this chapter.

In the case of a normal child who then suffers a TBI, the family and the treatment team also face a prolonged period of uncertainty about the extent of the damage and ultimate outcome. Families in these circumstances must deal with a more sudden shock, with even less preparation over time than those families who have had a longer period of chronic stress about the possibility of CP in their child.

## The Response of the Parents

After receiving "bad news" about diagnosis and prognosis regarding CP or TBI, parents can be expected to have a host of strong feelings and beliefs as they attempt to cope with this life-altering experience. And one parent may respond differently from the other, creating even more stress for the couple and family. Denial, of course, is a common initial response. The parents may question the doctor's diagnosis of their child, but often between themselves, rather than confronting the doctor directly. They may seek other opinions, go to other hospitals and centers, hoping against hope for a more favorable assessment. The physician may wish to encourage the family to seek another opinion. It is important that the doctor does not view the decision of the parents to seek another opinion as a personal rejection and narcissistic injury. The doctor should "leave the door open" so that the family can return for follow-up care should they choose to do so. Unfortunately, there are parents who, in their desperation, will be exploited by others who promise a "cure", often at considerable expense of time and money, leading to more disappointment and sadness for the family. If the original doctor is aware that the parents are following such a route, he or she should not be reluctant to caution them about the consequences of unproven and false treatments.

One or both parents may develop a pervasive sadness, similar to the mourning of a child who has died. For the family of the child with CP, their child has not truly died, but they have lost the "ideal" child of their fantasies, the child whom Jorge wanted to teach football, or as Taylor writes, they have lost "the potential for lovely ordinariness" of the child.[4] For the family of the child who had been normal and who sustains a TBI, they have lost the child whom they knew, with the full range of his or her personality. Yet even the sadness at such losses poses yet another burden for the parents, because they may feel guilty at being sad for the "lost" child as the "real" child, in the "here and now", is alive and requires more of their care. Pervasive depression and withdrawal in one or both of the parents further complicates care for the child, for the handicapped child needs even more stimulation and attention from parents than does the normally developing child. Care often needs to move beyond ordinary or good enough to extraordinary.

Anger towards the giver of the "bad news" is common. The doctor, and the team, who gave the diagnosis should not have a personal response to this anger. It may be expressed directly by the parents, but often it will be indirectly covered up by ongoing noncompliance with the treatment recommendation. Or it may be more positively channeled into the family's demand for the appropriate medical, educational and rehabilitative services for their child. Anger may be directed against the self, with the emergence of self-blame and guilt. Mother may think that her son's CP might not have occurred if she had only stopped working during her pregnancy and "taken better care" of herself; father may have fearful unconscious guilt related to hostile, completely unacceptable feelings towards his own handicapped child. Guilt surrounding the circumstances which resulted in TBI to the child may become overwhelming for the family, especially if the child was injured in an accident which might have been preventable. But even if not preventable, the parents may have a magical view that if they had only done something different in their lives, the trauma would not have occurred.

As the care of the handicapped child proceeds, the sheer, chronic, unremitting drudgery of lifting, carrying, feeding, transporting to the medical visits, adds a truly physical, fatiguing weight to the parents' already demanding burden. The doctor and the team must be aware of, and sensitive to, all of these emotional and physical factors if they are to work effectively with the family.

# The Family and the Team: Principles of Engagement and Counseling

During the initial diagnostic phase, once the family's feelings have been acknowledged by the team in a sensitive and understanding manner, and as the parents begin to feel more at ease in asking questions, it is often useful to give the family written and/or illustrative information about the disorder, including drawings and videotapes. During this period, and at times of any later crises, the team should not view the anxious, grieving parent as a "patient" who requires psychiatric or psychological intervention. A crying parent is not a psychiatrically disturbed parent, but rather a parent with an understandable, normal psychological reaction to personal trauma. If the doctor and the other members of the rehabilitation team have been appropriately empathic and informative, the family will, and certainly should be, dealing with the same professional team, as much as possible over the long term.[5] By "long term" we may be talking about a lifetime, beginning when the diagnosis is made in childhood, and continuing into adulthood, as developmental challenges and tasks change. For example, as we will discuss later in the chapter, adolescence presents issues and problems different from childhood. In adult life, questions of employment and vocational training become important, as well as the possibility of an independent life wherever feasible. While there certainly will be personnel changes on the team over time, continuity of care is not only desirable, but also essential for the interests of the child and family. The parents, and then the child as he or she grows older, should have the opportunity to develop, and maintain, a positive relationship with a team in which questions are asked and answered, suggestions are made, advice and support are given. Repeated shifts of patients and families from one caregiver team to another only undermine the long-term view of the needs of the child and family. Because the team will generate much information and revisions of the treatment plan as time proceeds, it may be useful for the team to identify a lead clinician to collate the information for the parents, rather than have them deal with each team member for pieces of information. Certainly there should be periodic meetings with the family, child and entire team as treatment proceeds. Team members should continue to listen to the parents' point of view, be flexible and willing to negotiate and change strategies when necessary, and always attempt to offer practical suggestions and advice.

Similarly, and whenever possible, given a child's age and level of cognitive development, he should become an active participant with the team in his own care. Drawings, dolls and play materials can be used to give the child information about his disability. The more a child knows about the nature of his handicap, the more questions he can ask of the team, the more likely will be his compliance with treatment. In addition to the work with the family described above, some handicapped children, especially those with normal or mildly delayed cognitive ability, can benefit from a cognitive behavioral psychotherapy to assist improvement in self-esteem. Children with handicapping conditions are particularly vulnerable to impaired self-esteem, especially those children who retain sufficient cognitive capacity to recognize the difference between them and their non-handicapped peers. Emphasis needs to be placed on strengths and assets. Children with more moderate learning difficulties can profit from an applied behavioral analysis therapy program aimed at targeted behaviors of frustration and aggression if present. Given their understandable desire to help the child as much as possible, parents may need to be cautioned not to overindulge the child, but to allow for as much independent functioning as possible within the limits of the handicap. Parents should feel free to impose a regular routine, as well as mild, non-physical discipline and consequences for problematic behaviors. For those children with persistent problems of aggression, hyperactivity or depression, pharmacotherapy is often indicated, using the medications in the same manner as they are used with non-handicapped children. Stimulants can be helpful for problems of inattention and hyperactivity; fluoxetine and mood stabilizers for affective symptoms, and low dose, atypical neuroleptics for severe impulsivity and aggression.[6] But the treatment team must approach the issue of medication cautiously and give the family adequate and appropriate information about the use of medication for specific target symptoms as an adjunct to the overall rehabilitation program. Otherwise, the family may have the impression that they are not carrying out their own responsibilities in an effective manner.

The transition into adolescence presents further difficulties for the child and family. As handicapped children grow older, they tend to fall further and further behind the developmental trajectory of their age-mates. The normative adolescent steps toward increased independence, such as driving, dating, career planning, etc., may be foreclosed to seriously handicapped adolescents. The expression of normal sexuality and the pursuit of sexual interests becomes a problem for adolescents and their families. Handicapped adolescents who require care for their personal hygiene sustain a necessary, but unfortunate, violation of privacy. Masturbation may be difficult to carry out in a more secluded setting. Historically, there has been a social bias about sexuality in handicapped people, i.e., handicapped individuals are presumed either to be non-sexual, or if they have learning disabilities, to be at risk for sexual promiscuity. (Only relatively recently has the practice of involuntary sterilization of learning disabled females been outlawed in some countries.)[7] A member of the team should consider tactfully raising the taboo topic of sexuality with the adolescent and the family. Once this issue is raised, both the adolescent and the family may feel relieved at having the opportunity to discuss sexuality as a normative fact of life. The discussion should also go on to include suggestions about social activities in which the adolescent boy or girl can meet other adolescents with handicap, as well as opportunities for the development of dating relationships. As will be more fully described below, participation in support groups with other handicapped adolescents can provide a useful forum for both the sharing of information, as well as the commonality of difficulties, and lead to opportunities for meeting others, decreasing social isolation and increasing self-esteem. Throughout this period, adolescent patients should be active participants in their health care and have direct access to team members, without having to necessarily be monitored exclusively through their parents.

Support groups for parents, patients, and siblings are an important component of the counseling process. These groups can be psychoeducational in nature, providing the participants with information about the pathology, giving practical management suggestions, allowing the participants to learn from each other's experience and diminishing the social stigma attached to handicap. Groups may be organized according to the particular type of brain injury with which the child is afflicted, or according to the degree of cognitive and functional impairment across a heterogeneous mixture of pathologies. The groups may be either open, with a rotation of topics over an 8–12 week period, which the member can join at any time in the cycle and stay for the full series; or support groups can be closed, in which there is a fixed membership over an indefinite, but prolonged period of time. The latter tend to create more intensive feeling and more emotional dependency, which may serve as a substitute for the lack of family support. It is important, however, to keep in mind that, in any type of support group, talking and emotional release is not enough. The members are not to be viewed as psychiatric patients who are participating in "group therapy", but as individuals who share a commonality of individual experiences. Practical suggestions and advice need to be offered by the leaders, and the members should be encouraged to relate their own solutions to problems. Often it is helpful to have a parent, patient, or sibling as a co-leader of the group, together with one of the team professionals.

## Impotence and Omnipotence

In many instances the team will be faced with an omnipotence/impotence paradox and potential conflict. The parents, in trying to take care of their handicapped child, may feel impotent and helpless. They cannot resolve the handicap, and cure their own child despite their best efforts. The parents are "arbitrary victims in an unfair lottery".[8] Feeling impotent, the parents turn to the physician and the team, whom they may feel are omnipotent. After all, it is the team members who are experts, who are the trained, all-knowing helpers who possess all of the medical knowledge. The team members wear the clinic or hospital uniforms, which symbolize wisdom and authority. Yet, in especially complex cases, the team members may, in turn, also feel impotent. They cannot cure or reverse the handicap, and the parents' pleas may reinforce the team's feelings of helplessness. In these circumstances, team members first need to acknowledge the presence of such feelings, to actively discuss them within the team, and to understand that their feeling of impotence is also what the family faces. The team then needs to establish particular targeted, implemental objectives for the family and patient, e.g., an altered brace, a new posture for feeding, a different educational strategy. The team should also establish reasonable deadlines by which the objective should be achieved, and assist the parents on working on these specific targets. The team and the family need to have visible accomplishments, even if slowly reached, in order to have a better sense of confidence in the rehabilitation work.

# Noncompliance

Team members may also be faced with the problem of noncompliance on the part of the family. Family members, parents and grandparents, may not follow the team's recommendations, either by directly refusing them – which is uncommon – or more likely, by passively agreeing to the recommendations but then not carrying them out. Noncompliance may continue even after the team has re-educated the family about the recommendations, emphasized the importance of the treatment plan over and over again, solicited questions from the family and made essentially every reasonable attempt to gain the family's cooperation and participation in the treatment plan. In these situations, rather than to continually repeat the same instruction to the family, the team needs to gently confront the family's noncompliance. For example, to say directly to the family:

> We have made these recommendations many times, and we have explained the reasons for them many times, but still you seem to have difficulty in accepting them and following the plan. Could you tell us why, so that we can better understand what we each should be doing? We need your help.

Noncompliance is the family's indirect, and at times unconscious, way of maintaining its own integrity. The family may feel that they know the child best and what is best for their child. Families who feel impotent in the face of handicap may also inappropriately use noncompliance as an expression of disguised anger toward both the team and the handicap. Faced with noncompliance the team needs to consider those various possibilities, and to open up this area for discussion with the family. As the family is able to share reasons for noncompliance and resistance with the team in a trusting manner, the family then becomes more of an empowered partner, so that effective treatment may proceed.

# The Effect of the Handicap on the Marriage and Siblings

While there is little doubt that the presence of a handicapped child increases parental stress, there does not appear to be any significant increase in marital separation and divorce.[9] Similarly, studies fail to show a consistent trend in lowered self-esteem or impaired social competence in the siblings of handicapped children. Nevertheless, team members have to be sensitive to the impact of handicap on family functioning, as statistical data do not necessarily reflect what is happening in a particular family. Some parents are drawn closer together in the need to care for the handicapped child. For others, the handicap could undermine an already fragile relationship. Some siblings participate in the care of their handicapped brother or sister. Anecdotally, it is reported that a higher than expected percentage of siblings with a handicapped brother or sister pursue careers as health professionals. Alternatively, some siblings may have angry feelings directed toward the handicapped sibling and/or the parents, as they feel that their own needs are being neglected, and they may have guilty wishes that the child had never been born. Ambivalence is quite normal and to be expected. In their work with the family, team members should ask questions about the family's support system, about whether the extended family is providing help, and about whether the parents are able to have some relief from caretaking and time for themselves and their own leisure interests. Team members should inquire about the emotional health of the siblings, their social activities and school performance, alert the parents to potential problems, and decide whether any further intervention is required.

The rehabilitation team should be prepared to give anticipatory guidance about the possibility of the development of what has been referred to as "the Vulnerable Child Syndrome".[10] In this syndrome, the parents, already having endured the trauma of having a handicapped child, may anxiously expect that their next baby, although quite normal, may suffer the same fate. Parents may then become excessively indulgent and overcautious about this child, creating anxiety in the child and reinforcing the notion that this is a very fragile being. Team members can provide a very useful preventive intervention in alerting to expectant mother and father to this risk, and advising them to treat the new baby as normally as possible.

# The "Acceptance" of Handicap

Rehabilitation team members are often taught to expect that, at some intermediate point in their work with families, the family, as well as the patient, will learn to "accept" the handicap. This acceptance usually connotes a more comprehensive understanding of the diagnosis and prognosis, and more adequate compliance with the treatment interventions. Acceptance also connotes a more quiescent and peaceful emotional state about the handicap. Further, a dictionary definition of "accept" is "to receive, esp. willingly; to approve; to agree to".[11] However, this view is not congruent with the reality of the handicap for the child and family, and they should not be held to this goal by the team. As one mother of a severely handicapped child with TBI said to me, "My life will never be the same. It has changed forever." Another mother of a child with severe CP said, "I cannot accept my son's condition. I am more angry as the years go by. He asks me whether he will be able to get married someday and where will he be able to go on his honeymoon. I don't know how to answer him."

She thinks that the inability to accept is a fault and that she should be more resigned.

Acceptance of handicap not only relates to the child and family's attitude, but also it can be a subtle condition of acceptance by the team. "Good" patients and families are those that accept; "difficult" patients and families are those that cry, are angry, and pose difficult questions for the team. Many families learn to live with the handicap, but not necessarily to accept it. Furthermore it is important that the team recognize that the resistance to, or failure to, accept, is not necessarily related to noncompliance with treatment. Paradoxically, families may not accept the implications of the diagnosis and prognosis, but continue to come for visits and adhere to the treatment recommendations. Parents may not accept that their wheelchair-bound child will never walk, or they may not come to terms with this eventuality for many years, but they still may adhere to all of the treatment proposed. For them, acceptance is equivalent to the abandonment of hope, a hope that has served to motivate their participation in the rehabilitation program. For the families of handicapped children, hope and denial are closely linked. Denial often serves a positive and protective purpose. Not full and complete denial, to be sure, which precludes the family from seeking help and which further impairs the child's potential for any improvement in functioning. But intermittent, partial denial, from time to time, or even at different moments of the day, can fuel the family's willingness to endure and allow hope to continue.

# Conclusion

For the family there is no conclusion. Their story continues over time as they and their child face new burdens, needs, and challenges. The story may extend into the next generation, as brothers and sisters may be required to be involved in the care of a seriously handicapped sibling after parents die. Similarly, but admittedly less burdensome, the work of the rehabilitation team does not have a definite endpoint. Team members must continue to listen and learn, to guard against unrealistic expectations, to negotiate objectives and strategies with the family, to forge alliances and to support one another when the tasks are difficult and the progress is slow. The team's contact with the family may become more intermittent as time proceeds, or some new personnel may take over as the patient ages, but unlike the practice of acute care, the job never seems to be quite finished. The work of the team, like that of the family, can last a lifetime.

# References

1.  Charon R. The patient–physician relationship: narrative medicine: a model for empathy, reflection, profession, and trust. JAMA 2001; 286(15):1897–1902.

2.  Luria AR. The making of mind: a personal account of Soviet psychology. Cambridge, MA: Harvard University Press, 1979.

3.  Percy W. Love in the ruins: the adventures of a bad Catholic at a time near the end of the world. New York: Avon, 1981.

4.  Taylor DC. Mechanisms of coping with handicap. In: McCarthy G, editor. Physical disability in childhood. Edinburgh: Churchill Livingstone, 1992: 53–64.

5.  Freeman RD, Pearson PH. Counseling with parents. In: Apley J, editor. Care of the handicapped child. London: Heinemann, 1978: 35–47.

6.  Daruna JH, Forman MA, Boris NW. Psychiatric considerations of central nervous system injury. In: Behrman RE, Kliegman RM, Jenson HB, editors. Nelson textbook of pediatrics. Philadelphia: Saunders, 2004: 71–72.

7.  Field MA, Sanchez VA. Equal treatment for people with mental retardation: having and raising children. Cambridge, MA: Harvard University Press, 2000.

8.  Forman MA, Hetznecker W. The physician and the handicapped child: dilemmas of care. JAMA 1982; 247(24):3325–3326.

9.  Hirst M. Dissolution and reconstitution of families with a disabled young person. Dev Med Child Neurol 1991; 33(12):1073–1079.

10. Green M, Solnit AJ. Reactions to the threatened loss of a child: a vulnerable child syndrome. Pediatric management of the dying child, part III. Pediatrics 1964; 34:58–66.

11. Webster's new world dictionary of the American language. New York: Simon and Schuster, 1984.

# 9

# School Success after Brain Injury: Behavioral, Social, and Academic Issues

*Mark Ylvisaker and Timothy Feeney*

Behavioral and social difficulties are unfortunately common in developmental disabilities and following traumatic brain injury (TBI) in children. These difficulties may combine with cognitive impairments to create a major obstacle to successful school integration. Historically, the dominant approach to behavioral intervention has been to organize consequences in such a way as to modify the behavior in a positive direction; the dominant approach to social interactive difficulties has been to provide the child with decontextualized language/social skills training. For a variety of reasons, both of these traditional approaches have been questioned in their application to children with acquired brain injury and developmental delays. Positive Behavior Supports offer an alternative to traditional contingency management. This approach highlights the organization of antecedent supports to facilitate behavioral self-regulation and the role of everyday people in the child's life as they work to create satisfying behavioral habits by setting the child up for success. Context-sensitive social skills coaching offers an alternative to traditional social skills training. In this chapter we will offer a rationale for the alternative frameworks and describe associated intervention and support procedures. The chapter ends with considerations for supported education and discussion of decision making around a continuum of supports for students with chronic disabilities. Although the chapter focuses specifically on students with traumatic or acquired brain injury, many of the intervention themes are also relevant for children with congenital developmental disabilities.

## Behavioral/Self-regulatory Intervention

### Outcome Following TBI

Estimates[1,2] of new persisting behavior disorders (i.e., those not predating the injury) among children with severe TBI range from approximately 35% to 70%. Most studies suggest that persisting behavior problems after the injury are common.[3-7] Frequency of behavioral difficulties is increased by the frequent finding that *pre-injury* behavioral disorders are themselves a predictor

229

of TBI.[5,8,11] Reported behavior problems include both externalizing symptoms (e.g., disinhibition, aggression, immature behavior (relative to age expectations), rigidity, awkward social interaction) and internalizing symptoms (e.g., depression, lack of initiation, social withdrawal).

Contrary to the popular belief that children recover well from injuries acquired at an early age, persisting behavior disorders following TBI tend to be more common and more severe in younger children.[12-16] Woodward and colleagues[17] found that the younger children in their study were more impaired than the older children. Similarly, Michaud and colleagues[15] identified a dramatically increased likelihood of special education placement for behavior disorders if the child had the injury as a preschooler. Pediatric TBI that occurred beyond the preschool years was less predictive of a subsequent behavioral diagnosis. Animal studies have similarly shown that many functions related to the frontal lobes (vulnerable in closed head injury)[14,18] are more severely affected if the injury occurs at a young age.[19] For these reasons, the escalating behavior problems of the children described below were cause for great concern.

This concern was compounded by the finding that the profile of cognitive and behavioral functioning often worsens over the years after pediatric TBI, rather than improving, as parents, teachers and others understandably expect. Behavioral outcomes later in childhood and into the adult years tend to be worse than predicted shortly after the injury.[2,20] Long-term follow-up studies of children with relatively "pure" prefrontal injuries have, with few exceptions, documented an evolution of increasing behavior problems over the years after their injuries.[1,21-26] Eslinger and colleagues[27] reviewed the nine available long-term case studies of children with isolated prefrontal injury and concluded that impairment of "social executors" is the most consistent and critical theme with this population, and that delayed social difficulties may continue to emerge through adolescence. With these findings as background, a primary goal of intervention for these children is to prevent the predicted behavioral deterioration from occurring.[28-31]

The case studies described in the next section combined behavioral with cognitive, executive function, and communication-focused interventions. The relation between cognitive and behavioral outcomes after pediatric TBI is unclear in the research literature. Max and colleagues[32] found a positive correlation, whereas other investigators have found at most a weak correlation.[33-34] Brown and co-workers[5] found a correlation early in recovery, but not later.

A possible explanation for the discrepancies is that the cognitive impairments commonly associated with frontal lobe injury (e.g., difficulty with complex organizational and planning tasks,[35-36] difficulty processing abstract and indirect language,[37] and impaired strategic behavior under novel or stressful circumstances[38]) are often not assessed by follow-up test batteries, but are required for successful school performance. Indeed, a hallmark of prefrontal injury is reasonable performance during office-bound testing and apparently good overall recovery, despite reduced effectiveness in demanding educational, social, and vocational contexts.[22,39-43] The children in the case studies were judged to have cognitive and executive function deficits in the classroom, particularly in the areas of organizing and planning. These difficulties exceeded expectations based on psychoeducational testing and substantially contributed to the children's behavioral difficulties. Cognitive difficulties in an increasingly demanding school context predictably lead to frustration and behavior problems, particularly for children with relatively significant inhibition impairment.

Environmental variables have an impact on outcome, creating a rationale for environmentally based interventions focused on school and family routines. For example, child outcome and family adjustment are reciprocally related. Positive/negative child outcomes increase the likelihood of positive/negative family adjustment; similarly positive/negative family adjustment increases the likelihood of positive/negative child outcomes. This predictable dynamic has recently been established in the research literature.[44-46]

Wade and colleagues[47] further reported that a family-centered problem-solving intervention yielded statistically superior outcomes, compared to a standard intervention control group, in the following areas: knowledge of TBI, problem-solving skills, family relationships, and child behavior (as reported by the parent). The positive effect sizes for internalizing symptoms in the child, depression/anxiety, and withdrawal were all reported to be large. Thus, interventions directed at collaborative family problem solving – and by logical extension, collaborative school staff problem solving – may be of benefit for the adults, but more important, of substantial benefit for the child with chronic impairment after brain injury. With this large outcome literature and growing intervention literature as background, one of the hypotheses underlying our work with children with brain injury is that extended support for families and school staff, in the form of education, case management, ongoing training, and collaborative problem solving, contributes to improved child outcomes.

## Intervention

The procedures that Wade and colleagues[47] taught to parents were consistent with the theory and practice of Positive Behavior Supports (PBS), which has evolved since the early 1990s as an alternative to traditional applied behavior analysis (ABA). Table 9.1 outlines the critical differences between these approaches. Feeney and Ylvisaker[28-29] demonstrated the effectiveness of PBS procedures with three adolescents and two young school-age children with TBI. The case illustrations offered below used PBS procedures, combined with support-oriented cognitive and executive function intervention procedures.

| Table 9.1<br>Contrasting themes: traditional applied behavior analysis and positive behavior supports | |
|---|---|
| Traditional ABA | Positive behavior supports |
| **Focus and goals** | |
| Focus on specific behaviors, with the goal of increasing the frequency of positive and decreasing the frequency of negative behaviors. Focus on external control of behavior via systematic manipulation of consequences. | Primary focus on lifestyle change satisfactory to the individual and important others in that life. Secondary focus on specific behaviors. Focus on internal control of behavior and behavior change via manipulation of antecedents, including both remote and internal antecedents to behavior. Often combined with cognitive and executive system intervention. |
| **Assessment** | |
| Functional behavior assessment, ideally conducted by behavior specialists in analogue (i.e., experimentally controllable) environments. | Functional behavior assessment, ideally conducted in natural environments and involving collaboration among staff, family, and the individual. Assessment of background setting events (including general lifestyle, internal states of the person, and environmental facilitators and barriers) is mandatory. |
| **Intervention modalities and methods** | |
| Primary use of **contingency management** (i.e., systematic and planned manipulation of consequences), designed to increase (positive and negative reinforcement) or decrease (extinction or punishment) specific behaviors. Procedures include differential reinforcement of low rates of target behaviors or of alternative behaviors; token economy procedures, extinction procedures (e.g., ignoring negative behaviors, time-out); response-cost procedures (e.g., losing points for negative behavior). Less focus on antecedents, typically immediate antecedents (e.g., specific provocation, environmental conditions, instructions/demands, etc). Often primary use of extrinsic reinforcers (e.g., food, stickers, tokens) not logically and naturally related to the targeted behavior. | Primary focus on **control of antecedents**, including both remote (e.g., negative events at an earlier time) and internal (e.g., sense of loneliness, perceived failure, physical pain) setting events, with the goal of making background setting events as positive as possible. Assurance of adequate amount of choice and control, engagement in meaningful activities, positive momentum before difficult tasks, positive communication from communication partners, positive communication alternatives to negative behavior, natural and logical rewards for positive behavior. |
| **Organization of intervention** | |
| Specific behaviors often taught in a sequential manner: acquisition, then stabilization/fluency, then transfer/generalization. | Specific behaviors often targeted in natural settings and in the context of natural activities from the outset (with support); thus transfer/generalization facilitated from the outset. |
| **Setting, content, providers** | |
| Intervention often provided in "behavior management" settings (e.g., segregated classroom, clinic, residential center); intervention largely delivered (at least in the acquisition stage) by behavior specialists. | Intervention ideally provided in natural (home, work, school) community settings, with primary providers being those people who are natural communication partners in those settings (e.g., family members, work or school staff, peers), supported by specialists. |

For individuals with TBI, positive, antecedent-focused procedures are theoretically preferable to traditional contingency management for the following reasons, each of which is associated with reduced efficiency of contingency management:

- ventral frontal lobe injury is associated with weak response inhibition and inefficient responses to feedback/consequences[48–50]
- dorsal frontal lobe injury may include initiation impairment
- right hemisphere frontal lobe injury (in conjunction with limbic system damage) impairs social perception
- a history of failure and frustration may lead to oppositionality, which also reduces the effectiveness of contingency management.

Many children and adolescents with brain injury manifest some combination of these four conditions, thereby rendering consequence-oriented behavior management relatively ineffective. The frontal lobe themes have also been highlighted in discussions of a variety of developmental disabilities, including ADHD, autism, fetal alcohol syndrome, and others.

The following two case studies illustrate the combined behavioral, cognitive, communication, and executive function interventions that we have found useful for many children and adolescents with brain injury. Ylvisaker and Feeney[31] offer procedural elaboration, theoretical support, and further case illustrations of this everyday, context-sensitive, antecedent support-oriented intervention framework.

## Case Illustration: Young Child

Mark was a 7-year-old boy who was injured at age 5 in an automobile–bicycle accident.[29] His injuries included multiple skull fractures associated with a TBI involving focal right frontal injury. Following more than two months of combined acute hospitalization and inpatient rehabilitation, he was discharged to home, receiving home-bound instruction and therapies for the remainder of the school year. There was no pre-injury history of neurologic, developmental, learning, or behavior problems.

At the time of his injury, Mark was in a half-day kindergarten program and was described by his teacher as a bright child who had no difficulty with the curriculum. He was said to be socially mature and had many friends. His supportive family included two working parents, both with a high-school education, and three siblings.

At two years post-injury, Mark was enrolled in a first-grade class and evidenced significant physical disability, typically using a wheelchair for mobility in the school. His dysarthric speech was intelligible only to familiar listeners. Memory and general information processing efficiency were impaired, interfering with classroom instruction and learning. However, once information was well understood, he retained it well. Planning and organizational difficulties were evidenced by extremely disorganized personal spaces and frequent forgetting of things and classroom routines. His WISC-III full scale IQ was reported as 79.

Despite the help of a one-to-one paraprofessional aide, Mark had difficulty meeting the academic and interpersonal demands of his class, largely because of his severely slowed processing and memory and organization problems. With significant academic accommodations and schedule changes, he managed most of the adapted demands of the classroom teacher. However, behavioral challenges emerged during this first year back in school, almost two years post-injury. When confronted with tasks that were cognitively or physically challenging, Mark responded with physical aggression, including hitting and throwing objects at people. Initially he hit only his aide, but subsequently he also hit peers who were near him when he was acting out. This resulted in increasing social isolation, emerging attitudes of helplessness and self-pity, and many removals from the classroom. Mark generally accepted help when he recognized the need for it; however, in the absence of this recognition, he responded to assistance with intense and sustained aggressive behavior. The behavior plan in place prior to the experimental intervention was reactive: first, time-out from classroom activities, proceeding to exclusion from preferred activities, and finally removal to the principal's office in the event of persisting negative behaviors.

Mark's revised intervention plan did not include specific extinction procedures designed to eliminate the challenging behaviors. Rather, the following positive supports were added to his daily routine with the goal of making the challenging behaviors unnecessary and inefficient. The intervention plan included elements derived from a functional behavior assessment (completed collaboratively with staff and family) and elements based on theory and experience with children with TBI. The components were combined (versus tested singly) because Mark's behaviors were serious (jeopardizing his classroom placement) and because the components that were not specifically derived from the functional behavior assessment fit comfortably into classroom routines and were considered good classroom practices.

- *Daily Routine: Negotiation and Choice:* Daily routines were analyzed collaboratively and decisions about the minimum amount of work to be accomplished and plans for achieving the goals (within limits set by general classroom routines) were made collaboratively with the student. Specific time demands (e.g., "You must finish these ten problems in five minutes") were eliminated from the routine, because they had previously evoked oppositional behavior.
- *Positive Momentum:* Staff ensured that the plan included relatively easy tasks with a guaranteed high level of reinforcement before difficult work was introduced, and if possible, a student-preferred activity preceded

every mandated activity. Thus "positive momentum" was created prior to potentially stressful tasks.

- *Reduction of Errors:* In addition to eliminating time demands and negotiating amount of work to be completed, instructional staff were trained to provide sufficient modeling and assistance so that Mark would experience few errors (which historically evoked negative behavior and interfered with learning). Thus instruction was consistent with the principles of "errorless learning" which has been shown to be important for individuals with significant memory impairment.[51]

- *Escape Communication:* Because the functional behavior assessment indicated that most occurrences of challenging behavior served to communicate a need to escape a task or place, Mark was taught positive communication alternatives (e.g., "I'm done" or "I'm finished"). Staff were trained to encourage these alternatives at natural transition times and when the students began to appear anxious or upset, and to reward his use of positive escape communication.

- *Adult Communication Style:* Instructional assistants were trained to (1) increase their frequency of supportive and reinforcing interactions with the student, (2) anticipate his difficulties and offer assistance or model escape utterances, and (3) avoid "nagging" (as perceived by him).

- *Graphic Advance Organizers:* Because of significant organizational impairment, the student was provided with photograph cues. In some cases one photograph was sufficient to orient the student to the task; in others, a sequence of photos was used to guide the student through organizationally demanding tasks. Staff worked with the student to choose the content of the photographs, which could include him engaged in the activity with or without staff, critical materials, important places, and the like (e.g., Mark took a photo of his cubby to represent, "Hang up your coat and put your backpack away"). The photos were placed in small binders that could be hidden in a fanny pack or pocket.

- *Goal–Plan–Do–Review Routine:* Mark was given a graphic "map" that represented the general sequence of activities from an executive function perspective: Goal (i.e., "What are you trying to accomplish?"); Identification of difficulty level (i.e., "Is this going to be hard or easy?"); Plan (i.e., "How do you plan to get this done? What do you need? What are the steps? How long will this take?"); Review (i.e., "What were you trying to accomplish? How'd it work out? What worked for you? What didn't work? What was easy? Difficult?"). These interactions with staff were brief and collaborative (versus a performance-oriented quiz).

Success of this support-oriented intervention depended crucially on effective participation of the everyday people in Mark's life. Staff training included the following components:

- Participation with the consultant in the functional behavior analysis was critical in training staff and securing compliance with the intervention plan.

235

- The consultant provided school staff with brief orientation and training in each component of the intervention.
- Specific training-to-mastery was provided in the use of photograph prompts and of escape communication.

Maintenance of treatment gains was facilitated by training for the following year's school staff and by training for parents. The parents were trained to implement the goal–plan–do–review routine for both typical and unplanned activities in the home. In addition, they were taught to support Mark and respond to his behavior in a manner similar to that used in school.

Frequency of aggressive behaviors during this intervention study is represented in Figure 9.1. During the week of baseline observation (A), Mark's frequency ranged from eight to eleven episodes per school day. Four of the five days, the frequency was ten or eleven episodes (dramatically higher than that of the other students in the classroom). During the first intervention phase (B), frequency decreased to zero in the last four days. Frequency increased to six or more episodes during the return to baseline and then rapidly returned to low levels when the intervention was again implemented.

Intensity of aggressive episodes was also tracked. During the baseline condition, the mean rating on the disruption elements of the Aberrant Behavior Checklist[52] was approximately three (moderately severe problem). Mean

**Figure 9.1**

Frequency of aggressive behaviors during baseline and treatment conditions: Mark

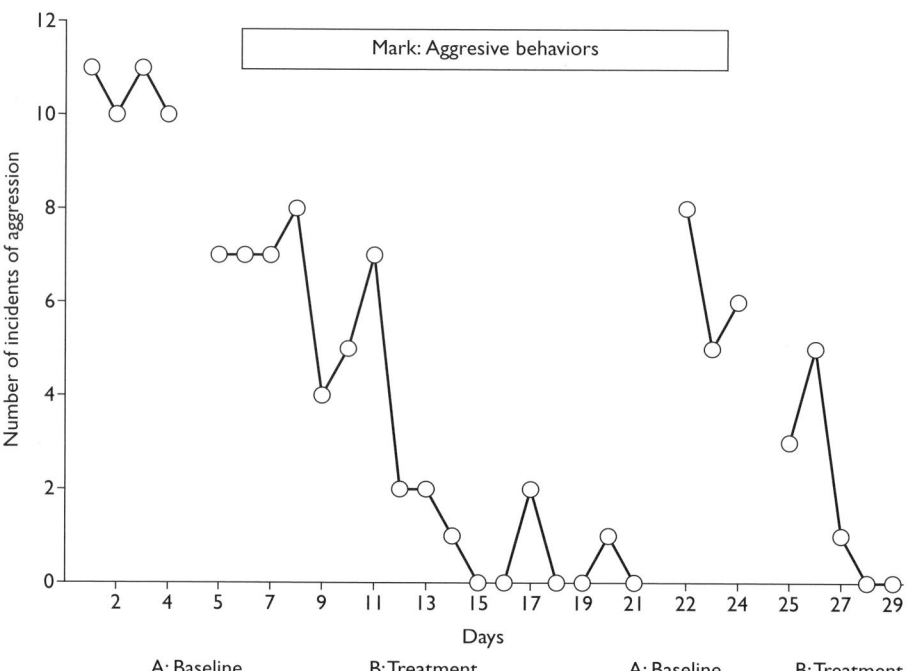

ratings dropped to 1.25 (slight problem) during the first intervention condition (B), increased to baseline level with removal of the interventions/supports, and then returned to acceptably low levels with return to the intervention condition. Average percentage of work completed by Mark remained at approximately 70% for all four conditions. However, the ranges were much smaller during the treatment conditions (66–100%; 68–92%) than during baseline conditions (0–90%; 20–80%), indicating that the intervention had the effect of eliminating the bad days during which Mark completed very little work.

Mark completed the school year with few incidents of problem behaviors. End-of-the-year interviews with the next year's teachers indicated that Mark continued to demonstrate academic, social, and behavioral gains. He was able to participate in most of the classroom routines (although he needed more intensive reading and language instruction, requiring his participation in a remedial program separate from his peers), continued to use the picture routines throughout the day, enjoyed peer friendships, and, when angry or upset, was able to use his escape communication strategy with minimal prompting. His teacher recommended placement in a typical third-grade classroom without paraprofessional support for the following year.

Eight years following the implementation of the intervention, the principal of Mark's high school reported that Mark did not demonstrate any behavioral or mental health difficulties. Physical disabilities persisted, necessitating environmental accommodations (e.g., using an elevator between floors of the school, leaving his classes five minutes early, attending adapted physical education) and he remained classified as a student with TBI. In addition to the environmental supports, Mark received consultative special education services to ensure that he was able to keep pace with the instruction and to assist with writing. With these supports in place, Mark participated in the general curriculum. Eight years after the initiation of the photo advance organizer, Mark continued to use a daily routine planner and homework checklist. The principal reported that the organizers were Mark's idea, and that he had offered a solid rationale based on his awareness of his organizational weakness.

## Case Illustration: Adolescent

Feeney and Ylvisaker[28] presented three successful single-subject experiments involving older adolescents who were severely injured several years earlier as young adolescents. All appeared to be progressing adequately in the early months after their return home from inpatient rehabilitation, but later evidenced severely challenging behaviors that escalated over the high school years. In all three cases, behaviors included physical aggression. In each case, there was reason to believe that the escalation of challenging behaviors was associated with gradually increasing academic demands and expectations for independent work, which the students were unable to meet.

Jim was an 18-year-old man who had been injured at age 15 in an automobile–bicycle accident. Records indicated probable widespread diffuse damage, including bilateral frontal lobe injury. He received treatment in an acute care hospital for two months, followed by six months of inpatient rehabilitation. Prior to his injury, Jim was an above average student with above average athletic ability. School records suggested some difficulties with teachers, including an indication of "adolescent behavior" (e.g., verbally challenging teachers, refusing to participate in class activities). He was a popular student and had never been suspended. He lived at home with a mother, stepfather and four siblings.

Jim's injury resulted in residual motor disability that included left hemiplegia, making walking difficult. He could not resume his athletic pursuits. Three years post-injury, his speech continued to be mildly labored. Cognitive problems included significantly slowed processing, necessitating teaching and testing modifications. Disorganization was manifested in difficulty organizing written work. Ultimately, Jim simply refused to attempt written assignments (which he dismissed as a "worthless waste of time"). When specifically directed to complete an assignment, Jim routinely refused and frequently threatened physical assault. However, he would complete assignments of equal or greater difficulty when he initiated the work. One year post-injury, Jim's Full Scale WAIS-R IQ was 92 (Performance, 85; Verbal, 94). Although there was no pre-injury IQ score on record, teachers and other school clinicians asserted that this result was substantially lower than estimated pre-injury IQ.

Jim returned to school at the end of his sophomore year. Demands were light and no behavior problems emerged. However, from the beginning of his junior year, Jim was judged to be noncompliant. Challenging behaviors included physical assault, which included hitting, slapping, and kicking peers and, later, teachers. In November of that year he was expelled from school and sent to a special education center for vocational training and Graduate Equivalency Diploma preparation. In this restrictive placement, noncompliance and physical aggression escalated. He was frequently truant and often refused to work when he was in school. The experimental intervention began at the mid-point of that year in that vocational program.

The intervention included tasks at the same level of difficulty and delivered by the same educational staff as at baseline (with some support from a behavioral consultant). Five substantive changes were made in the intervention regimen, consistent with the theory and practice of positive cognitive, behavioral, communication, and executive function supports:

- *Daily Routine: Negotiation and Choice:* Jim's daily routine was task analyzed collaboratively by instructional staff, the consultant, and Jim. Decisions about the minimum amount of work that needed to be completed (in order to accomplish the stated goals) and the sequencing of the routine were negotiated between Jim and the instructional staff. In some cases, the sequence of activities was nonnegotiable (e.g., lunch, certain classes). However, the goal of negotiation was to ensure that Jim was engaged in planning and decision making, and also to ensure successful performance.

- *Positive Behavioral Momentum:* An attempt was made to place a student-preferred or relatively easy activity before every mandated or stressful activity.

- *Organizational Supports:* Jim was provided with photograph cues that showed him engaged in his routines so that he could stay organized and on task without nagging. He was asked to identify the parts of each activity that were best indicators of the specific behaviors needed to complete an activity. Then a photo was taken of Jim (and possibly others as well) engaged in those elements of the routine. In some cases, a photo of the activity materials was a sufficient cue (e.g., a picture of his math book). The photos were both advance organizers and an ongoing reference. All photos were held in a small binder, easily toted (and readily hidden) in a fanny pack or sweatshirt pocket. There was no principle guiding the number of photos given, although Jim never had more than 20 for each school day.

- *Goal–Plan–Do–Review Framework for Routines:* The instructional staff ensured verbal rehearsal of the goal and plan at the beginning of every element of the routine and a review of performance after completion of every element. Both rehearsal and review were as simple and conversational as possible (e.g., "Let's figure out what you have to do next, Jim?" "So how'd it go, Jim? Did the plan work?"). The review included recording what worked and what did not work for Jim.

- *Positive Communication from Support Staff:* Because of Jim's consistently negative responses to what he perceived to be nagging and scolding (perceived by staff to be "helpful verbal cues" and "informative feedback"), staff were trained to interact with him in a respectful and nonjudgmental manner.

Figure 9.2 presents the systematic reduction of aggressive behavior in response to the intervention. At baseline, Jim averaged more than 30 episodes of aggression per school day. This was reduced to zero with the intensive, support-oriented intervention (B condition). The C condition in this changing treatments design differed from the B condition only in that written cues were substituted for photograph cues. The written cues included an organized presentation of the tasks that needed to be completed and clear criteria for success. Rehearsal and review continued as in the B condition. In both the B and C conditions, staff did not place explicit time demands (e.g., requiring that a certain amount of work be done by a specified time). It was known that this type of demand resulted in oppositional behavior.

Finally, to verify causal efficacy of the interventions and to underscore the need for ongoing support, there was a return to baseline (A). This included

**Figure 9.2**
Frequency of aggressive behaviors during baseline and treatment conditions: Jim

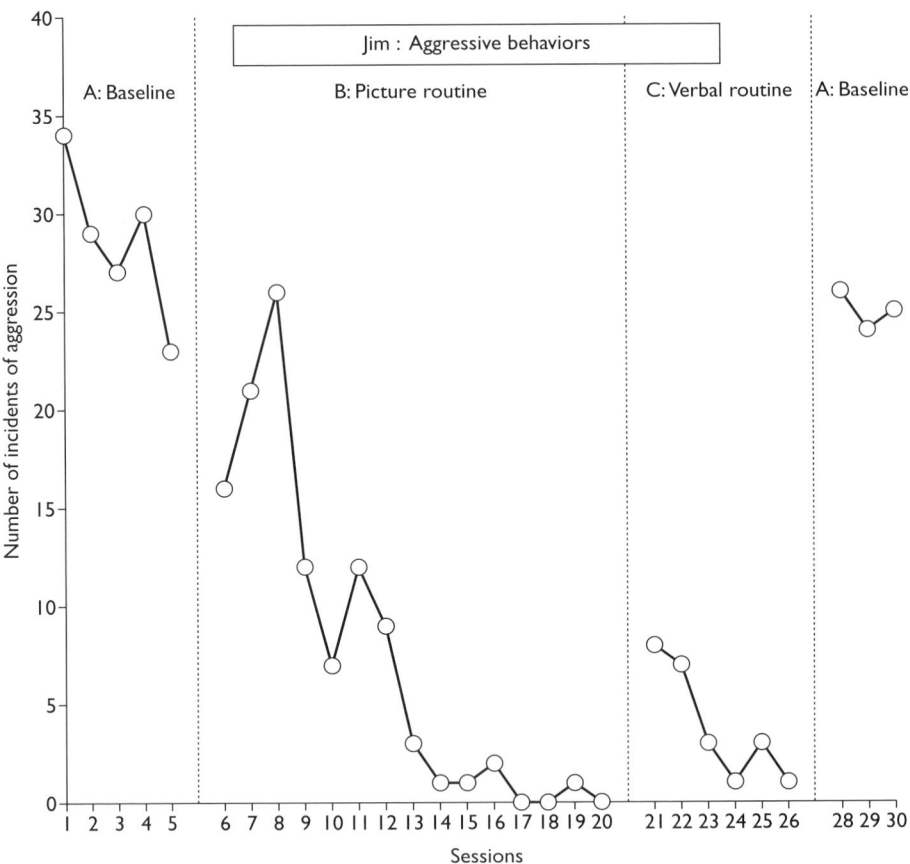

periodic, nonspecific reminders with no photograph or written cues and no verbal rehearsal or review. Once it was established that Jim needed the C condition supports (i.e., due to renewed escalation of aggression), they were reimplemented.

Intensity of aggressive episodes followed a similar pattern. Aggressive episodes were rated as very disruptive during both of the A conditions, but as only a minor problem during the two intervention conditions (B and C). Furthermore, Jim completed very little assigned work during the baseline condition (slightly over 20% on average). During the intervention conditions, this increased to over 80% on average, with at least 70% of his work completed every day. Withdrawal of intervention produced a reduction to near baseline levels.

At the completion of the study, staff returned to the level of support provided during the C condition. Jim received his high school diploma and subsequently obtained employment in an auto repair center doing oil and tire changes. Jim was assisted by a work case manager/job coach in obtaining the job and establishing satisfactory performance at the job site. Verbal routines were established with the supervisor. The job coach remained in place for one month, with systematic fading. The routines were gradually faded to rehearsal prior to the work day, with the supervisor giving work slips for work to be completed in sequence. For example, the work slips may have been placed one on top of the other in the order they were to be completed. When finished, the slip was placed in the "done" box and Jim moved onto the next slip. His boss reported that he was happy with Jim's performance and continued to give him increased responsibility when Jim asked for it.

## Generalization

Generalization of treatment gains has long been the Achilles heel of behavioral and other interventions. In the two cases presented in this section, as in all of our work with individuals with challenging behavior, interventions and supports have been implemented within the routines of everyday life, that is, wherever the challenging behaviors exist. This is consistent with the "point of participation" focus for intervention promoted by leaders in the field of behavioral psychology,[53] academic strategy intervention,[54] and social skills intervention.[55]

*We have moved from "train and hope it generalizes" to "train for generalization (and hope it generalizes)" to "train and generalize to simulated conditions of use" to, finally, recognizing generalization for the powerless explanatory fiction that it is and skipping it by training in the context of use in the first place.[53]*

## Evidence

A review of the effectiveness of behavioral (nonpharmacologic) interventions for individuals with behavior disorders after TBI is currently underway, sponsored by the Academy of Neurologic Communication Disorders and Sciences. The authors identified 50 studies reported in the research literature, involving 177 participants. All but 5 of the studies were single-subject experiments or case studies and only one was a randomized controlled study[47]; 14 of the studies (63 participants), including Wade and colleagues' RCT,[47] used children or adolescents as participants. Of the 50 studies, only one (5 participants; stress inoculation procedures) reported no meaningful improvements on at least one behavioral measure. Thus evidence exists to support behavioral interventions as a guideline for clinical practice in serving both children and adults with TBI.

However, due to the extraordinary variability within the participants and interventions delivered, specific practice standards cannot yet be derived. Nevertheless, a clear clinical trend was observed in the direction of increasing use of the Positive Behavior Supports framework for intervention. Of the studies published in the 1980s, 7 used "traditional" ABA contingency management procedures, 2 combined ABA/PBS, and none strictly PBS; in the 1990s: 13 traditional ABA, 11 combined, 4 PBS; in the 2000s: 2 traditional ABA, 5 combined, 9 PBS. The PBS framework has also been increasingly used in serving individuals with developmental disabilities[56] and has a growing evidence base with that population.[57]

# Social Skills Intervention

Many reviews of outcome following pediatric and adult TBI have highlighted the important role of social competence in successful reintegration into school, family and social networks, and the frequency with which these competencies are impaired.[58] For students with and without identified disability,

> the ability to interact successfully with peers and significant adults is one of the most important aspects of students' development. The degree to which students are able to establish and maintain satisfactory interpersonal relationships, gain peer acceptance, establish and maintain friendships, and terminate negative or pernicious interpersonal relationships defines social competence and predicts adequate long-term psychological and social adjustment.[59]

Even if followed by good neurological outcome, severe TBI is known to threaten social relationships and increase social isolation over time.[60] To date, no studies have specifically documented the number of genuine friends maintained after pediatric TBI, although experienced clinicians have documented a decrease in meaningful friendships.[61] Even animal studies have shown that bilateral frontal and temporal lobe lesions (common in TBI) reduce social perception and result in group exclusion.[62]

As we use the term, social skills include both general competencies and specific goal-directed, situationally appropriate, verbal and nonverbal behaviors. Individuals use such skills to affect the responses of others, achieve acceptance by peers, family members, and teachers, and meet the demands of school and community. Socially skilled individuals are capable of affecting others positively and with the intended effect, and of being affected positively by others as they intend. Adequate social skills increase the likelihood of reciprocal friendships and a satisfying social life.

Although theoretically distinguishable, social skills and behavioral self-regulation overlap in practice. Both Mark and Jim, described in the behavior management section of this chapter, used behaviors that would be identified as socially unskilled. However, they were classified as having a behavior disorder because their difficulties had little to do with not knowing the relevant social rules, roles, and routines, and more to do with difficulty regulating their behavior with that knowledge, combined with oppositionality.

The relationship between social skills, peer acceptance (enabling the child to have adequate opportunities for satisfying interaction) and friendship (i.e., symmetrical, emotionally committed relationships) is reciprocal. Children who are rejected by their peers often exhibit depression, loneliness, negative self-concept, anxiety, low academic achievement, and higher truancy and drop-out rates.[63] Students with acquired brain injury predictably attempt to reconnect with their preinjury friends and peers. However, physical, cognitive, and personality changes often result in a gradual loss of friends and increasing isolation. Reduced social opportunities may then further jeopardize social interactive success, leading to a downward social spiral.

Table 9.2 lists supports that may be needed for students with social interaction difficulties. This framework, developed by Wiig and colleagues,[64] divides a continuum of needs and associated supports into four general categories: beginner, advanced beginner, competent, and expert. Of particular value in this framework is the distinction between knowledge and performance. Frontal lobe impairment has long been associated with a dissociation between knowing what to do on specific occasions and actually doing it. From a neuropsychological perspective, failure to act on one's social knowledge may be a result of impulsiveness, impaired initiation, weak social perception, slow processing, anxiety, or retrieval problems, all of which are associated with frontal lobe impairment. Because of this dissociation, individuals with brain injury may be at a higher level in the column headed "Knowledge", but at a lower level in the other three columns. That is, the student may have relatively extreme self-regulatory weakness and therefore need relatively intense supports despite excellent declarative and procedural knowledge of social rules, roles, and routines acquired before the injury.

Traditionally, social skills interventions have focused on the acquisition of declarative knowledge ("This is what I should do in this situation") and procedural knowledge ("This is how I do it") of specific social behaviors or competencies. Typically the skills are taught in a social skills training setting, using coached role-playing procedures (e.g., scripting, modeling, prompting, cuing, reinforcing). Several training programs have been developed within this traditional paradigm, generally for students with developmental disabilities or emotional/behavioral disorders. Ylvisaker and colleagues[65] described procedures used in many of these training programs.

Students who lack declarative and procedural knowledge of relevant social skills or competencies need explicit instruction. However, even applied to students with congenital disability who presumably need such instruction, the traditional model of social skills training has not been supported by evidence reviews. Gresham and colleagues[59] reviewed narrative reviews and meta-analyses of the extensive social skills intervention research literature and concluded that "SST [social skills training] has not produced large, socially important, long-term, or generalized changes in the social competence of students with high-incidence disabilities". Specifically, they described two meta-analyses. The first included 99 studies of SST applied to students with emotional and behavioral disturbance, with a small mean effect size of 0.20. The second included 53 studies of SST applied to students

**Table 9.2**
**Supports for Students with Social Skills Deficits**

**S-MAP for Social Skills**

| Performance Level | Knowledge | Performance | Competing Behaviors | Environmental Supports |
|---|---|---|---|---|
| **Expert**<br>**4**<br>**Minimal deviation from competent social behavior** | • Knows what skills are expected in familiar and unfamiliar situations<br>• Knows how to perform expected skills in familiar and unfamiliar situations | • Uses appropriate skills with no supporting prompts, cues, or structure<br>• Uses appropriate skills in stressful and/or novel situations<br>• Avoids all use of inappropriate behaviors | • Identifies internal states and uses coping strategies to manage them<br>• Is aware of and controls internalizing behaviors<br>• Is aware of and controls externalizing behaviors | • Does not need a behavior plan<br>• Does not need environmental modifications<br>• Does not need a personal assistant or small group setting<br>• Uses appropriate skills without antecedent supports or planned contingencies |
| **Competent**<br>**3**<br>**A few deviations** | • Knows what skill is expected in familiar situations<br>• Knows how to perform expected skills in familiar situations | • Uses appropriate skills in familiar or controlled environments<br>• Uses appropriate skills in stressful situations with supports<br>• Uses appropriate skills in real-life situations that have been practiced<br>• Uses appropriate skills in most practice situations | • Uses coping strategies in response to a few identified internal states<br>• Is aware of and controls internalizing behaviors in practiced situations<br>• Is aware of and controls externalizing behaviors in practiced situations | • Needs a limited behavior plan<br>• Needs environmental modifications or other antecedent supports in unfamiliar situations<br>• Needs presetting and/or coaching in special situations<br>• Needs a personal assistant or small group setting in special situations |

| | | | |
|---|---|---|---|
| **Advanced beginner 2** **Several deviations** | • Recognizes what skill is expected in practice situations<br>• Recognizes appropriate use of skill in practice situations | • Uses inappropriate behaviors in unfamiliar or uncontrolled situations<br>• Uses inappropriate skill sometimes in stressful situations with supports<br>• Uses appropriate skills only with cues or prompts<br>• Uses appropriate skills in many practice situations | • Identifies some internal states but inconsistently uses coping strategies to manage them<br>• Controls internalizing behaviors during practice situations<br>• Controls externalizing behaviors during practice situations | • Needs a limited behavior plan<br>• Needs some environmental modifications or other antecedent supports<br>• Needs presetting and coaching in many situations<br>• Needs a personal assistant or small group setting for some situations<br>• Needs planned contingencies applied to some behaviors |
| **Beginner 1** **Many major deviations** | • Does not know what skill is expected in situations<br>• Does not know how to perform the expected skills | • Uses behavior inappropriate to most situations regardless of cues or prompts<br>• Uses inappropriate skills in stressful situations regardless of supports<br>• Refuses to use an appropriate skill that is within repertoire<br>• Uses inappropriate skill in familiar, practiced situations | • Has difficulty identifying internal states<br>• Has difficulty recognizing internalizing behaviors<br>• Has difficulty recognizing externalizing behaviors | • Needs behavior plan in all situations<br>• Needs some environmental modifications and other antecedent supports throughout the day<br>• Needs presetting and coaching throughout the day<br>• Needs a personal assistant or small group setting throughout the day<br>• Needs planned contingencies applied to behavior throughout the day |

Modified with permission from Wiig E, Larsen V, Olson J. S-MAPS: rubrics for curriculum-based assessment and intervention. Eau Claire, WI: Thinking Publications, 2004:66–67.

with learning disabilities, with a similarly small mean effect size of 0.21. Barkley's review of the literature on decontextualized social skills training similarly concludes that this approach has minimal demonstrated effectiveness with students who are impulsive as a result of ADHD.[55] In general, meta-analyses and narrative reviews of experiments with several populations using decontextualized social skills training suggest minimal effect on real-world behavior, peer social skills ratings, and maintenance of new social behaviors over extended periods of time.

It is reasonable to conclude that traditional decontextualized SST would be even less effective for students who retain pretraumatically acquired declarative and procedural knowledge of social rules, roles, and routines, but have difficulty applying that knowledge without support in social situations. Our experience with many children and adolescents with social interaction difficulties after brain injury suggests that the following components of intervention/support are particularly important:

- knowledgeable, understanding, and competent communication partners who therefore do not misinterpret and react punitively to neurologically based awkward behaviors that result from impulsiveness, failure to initiate, misreading of social cues, anxiety, and the like
- selection of highly specific and personally important skills for context-sensitive training
- extensive practice of social behaviors in the situations in which they are required, with satisfying natural and logical consequences for successful performance
- situational coaching that includes advance cues (presetting) prior to potentially problematic interactions
- situational training specifically designed to improve social perception and the ability to interpret the behavior of others
- situational training specifically designed to improve self-monitoring of stress levels so that students can remove themselves from stressful situations as needed
- application of the Goal–Plan–Do–Review format to social interaction so that the students understand that the goal is their social success, not "social appropriateness" understood abstractly as some authority figure's goal
- counseling specifically designed to help the student develop a personally compelling sense of self that includes positive social interaction as a component.

To overcome the resistance that many students with TBI experience when faced with this effort, we often frame their process as a project that will result in insights and perhaps in a product that can help other students. Thus the student with brain injury is engaged as a collaborator in a helping project, while at the same time addressing social issues of personal concern. Table 9.2 outlines supports that may be necessary in school settings.

## Illustrations

Mark and Jim, the case illustrations from the behavior intervention section of this chapter, were similar to many students with TBI in the following ways. They possessed adequate declarative and procedural knowledge of appropriate social behaviors, at least in familiar situations; they had considerable difficulty reading social cues; they processed information rather slowly, which contributed to social awkwardness; they were impulsive and had low frustration tolerance; Jim experienced anxiety, Mark experienced considerable sadness, and both externalized their response to these emotions; and they reacted negatively to any interaction that they considered critical or disrespectful. In addition, both were accustomed to effortless social success before their injuries and were therefore frustrated by their social failures.

In the previous section, we presented their interventions as behavior management, but these students could have been selected as case illustrations in the social skills section as well. From a social interaction perspective, their intervention included.

- organizing their environments to reduce anxiety and increase success
- training everyday communication partners to use cues and feedback that had been negotiated in advance and were considered respectful by the students
- training the students to use negotiated scripts when they needed help or a break
- presetting the students with social scripts and providing contextualized coaching
- framing their social activities within the same goal–plan–do–review schema that was used for academic tasks.

## Educational intervention

Many studies have reported persistent cognitive impairments after pediatric TBI. With respect to educational disability, Boyer and Edwards[66] found that, although 35% of their cohort had pre-existing education-related impairments, over 60% were either in special education programs or were receiving no educational program one year post-injury. Ewing-Cobbs and colleagues[67] found that 79% of the children and adolescents with severe TBI either had repeated a grade or had special education programs at a two-year follow-up. Nelson and Kelly[68] evaluated 17 students with severe TBI four to five years post-injury. Although they restricted their study to students in mainstream schools, they identified a variety of deficits in memory and learning that affect educational progress. Taylor and colleagues[46] followed 53 students with severe TBI and compared them with orthopaedic controls. The students with TBI had poorer outcomes on measures of mathematics and writing, and on teacher reports of academic functioning. Superficial academic measures, such as word decoding, showed fewer deficits. (Reading comprehension was not assessed.) Academic and behavioral outcome was influenced by the family's psychosocial status. Students from disadvantaged families continued to deteriorate in academic performance over the four years of the study.

Ylvisaker and colleagues[69] described six major themes that have evolved over the years since TBI became a special education category in the United States in 1990.

*Theme #1: Incidence and Prevalence of Persistent Disability*
Although TBI in childhood is a high-incidence medical event, persisting educational disability associated with TBI is generally considered a low frequency phenomenon. The primary reasons for this judgment are that systems are not in place to count children with education-relevant disability associated with TBI and many of these students have needs that are unrecognized by the educational system. For example, in 1997–98, the US Office of Special Education Programs reported that only one fifth of 1% of special education students (11,895) were included in the TBI category. However, an extrapolation from well documented epidemiological surveys would predict a dramatically larger number of students with TBI in need of services.

Diagnostic classification does not ensure appropriateness of services and supports. Nevertheless development and implementation of procedures to identify education-related needs and create appropriate interventions and supports for students with TBI should be an important goal for professionals who serve these children.

*Theme #2: TBI as an Educational Disability*
Although there exists enormous diversity within the population of students with TBI, there are also central tendencies that need to be accounted for in educational planning. Common consequences of childhood TBI and their educational implications are outlined in Table 9.3.

*Theme #3: Assessment*
There is too much diversity within the population of students with TBI to create assessment batteries specific to this etiology. However, successful interpretation of educational test results for these students presupposes understanding that a child may evidence reasonable levels of knowledge and academic skill (based on relatively intact preinjury acquisitions stored in posterior areas of the brain) despite substantial difficulty acquiring new knowledge and skill, and effectively regulating behavior in unstructured or stressful contexts (due to relatively compromised prefrontal and limbic regions). For a variety of reasons, the ecological validity of standardized office-bound assessments has been questioned.[22,39,40-43] Thus testing must be complemented by real-world observation of performance under a variety of conditions and disciplined real-world experiments (e.g., diagnostic teaching) to create effective intervention and support plans.

**Table 9.3**
**Common consequences of TBI in children and their educational implications**

*Neurologic recovery:* Often children experience prolonged and unpredictable improvement based on several dynamics of neurologic recovery.

**Implications:**
- Educational systems need to be flexible and programs highly individualized.
- Frequent review and modification of the student's placement and program may be required, a practice not consistent with the tradition of annual reviews.

*Evolving ability profiles:* In some cases, the student's disability increases over time, possibly related to a type of brain injury that has its first noticeable consequences at a later developmental stage or to the dynamics of the student's adjustment.

**Implications:**
- Long-term monitoring systems must be implemented, even if the student is not receiving special education services (e.g., using Section 504 of the Rehabilitation Act).
- School staff need to be alert to the possibility that disability may gradually increase over time so that intervention can be implemented as promptly as possible.

*Disability related to vulnerable parts of the brain:* Theoretically any part of the brain can be involved in TBI. However, closed head injury is frequently associated with damage to the frontal lobes and anterior and medial temporal lobes, with relative sparing of posterior regions.

1. **Challenges related to frontal lobe injury** include reduced awareness of strengths and limitations; disinhibited thinking and behavior; weak initiation; relatively weak control over cognitive processes, like attention; disorganized thinking and acting; relatively weak planning, problem solving, and strategic behavior; relatively weak learning from consequences; relatively weak effortful learning and retrieval; difficulty holding several thoughts in mind at one time; inflexibility; perseveration; inconsistent behavior and academic performance; concrete thinking and difficulty generalizing; relatively weak social perception and awkward social behavior.

   **Implications:**
   - Impairment may be difficult to assess. Many of these impairments are consistent with good performance on psychological, neuropsychological, and psychoeducational testing. Therefore necessary services and supports may not appear to be justified based on testing.
   - Disability may be misinterpreted (e.g., neurological disinhibition as a psychiatric disorder), with inappropriate services a possible consequence.
   - Traditional teaching and behavior management that emphasizes manipulation of consequences may be ineffective.
   - Long-term, contextualized coaching in "executive functions" may be necessary.

2. **Needs related to temporal lobe (including limbic system) injury** may include weak learning (new learning) relative to the existing knowledge base acquired before the injury and weak emotional/behavioral regulation.

   **Implications:**
   - The student may need much more repetition than would seem necessary.
   - The student may need substantial antecedent support for behavioral self-regulation.

3. **Needs related to widespread microscopic damage** include relatively slowed processes.

   **Implication:**
   - The student may need reduced assignments, evaluation of work based on quality, not quantity, and time accommodations.

4. **Strengths related to relative sparing of posterior parts** of the brain may include retention of much pre-injury knowledge and skill, and basic motor and sensory functions.

   **Implication:**
   - Assessments must go far beyond testing academic knowledge and skill (acquired before the injury) and sensorimotor functions.

*Psychoreactive phenomena:* The evolution of emotional consequences after a life-altering injury is unpredictable, but may include reactions that profoundly influence educational performance. At one stage or another after the injury, some children become depressed and withdrawn, others angry and defiant, and others overly desirous of pleasing, resulting in social vulnerability.

**Implications:**
- Schools should monitor students' mental health and social relationships after an injury, and provide counseling and support when indicated.

Reproduced with permission from Ylvisaker M, Todis B, Glang A, Urbanczyk B, Franklin C, DePompei R et al. Educating students with TBI: themes and recommendations. J Head Trauma Rehabil 2001; 16(1):76–93.

*Theme #4: Interventions and Supports in Educational Settings*
Just as diversity in the population renders a "TBI Battery" untenable, it also eliminates the possibility of a "TBI Curriculum". However, there are interventions and supports that have been shown to be effective for students with specific educational impairments that are shared with many students with TBI. These evidence-based strategies are listed in Table 9.4 along with characteristics of many students with TBI that suggest the usefulness of the strategies for these students. Table 9.5 describes more general approaches that have been found useful for students with disabilities similar in relevant respects to many students with TBI.

*Theme #5: Training and Support for Staff Working with Students with TBI in School Settings*
Together, the authors have consulted several hundred schools serving students with TBI. Both general and special educators routinely acknowledge the need for help when they begin to serve these students. Our experience, supported by considerable research in staff training, is that educators need more than training sessions outside of their context of practice. To have an impact as classroom practices and ultimately on student performance, training and support for educators must:

- relate in practical ways to their everyday interaction with students
- be ongoing
- involve specific teacher assignments and intervention experiments, with concrete feedback, including collaborative problem solving
- be broadly consistent with the school's culture and existing constraints on teachers' time, and meet the objectives of those seeking help
- ultimately result in improvements in the student's performance.

Practical consultation, or "coaching", includes collaborative design of dynamic assessment procedures to identify critical obstacles to student success, followed by intervention proposals that include explanation of theory, modeling of skills, practice in simulated and natural settings, objective feedback, and ongoing hands-on situational coaching for application. It is also helpful when consultants videotape themselves interacting with the student so that staff can watch and micro-analyze the procedures implemented by a specialist.

*Theme #6: Intervention and Support for Families*
Taylor and colleagues[44–46] have shown that following brain injury, the outcome for the child and the family are reciprocally related. The better the family adjustment, the better the child's outcome; and the better the child's outcome, the better the family's adjustment. Furthermore, Braga and colleagues[70] found that serving children indirectly by providing intensive education and support for families results in superior outcomes compared with traditional clinical services. Therefore, family-centered services and supports should be considered a critical component of educational interventions for

**Table 9.4**
**Research-based instructional strategies related to characteristics of many students with TBI**

| TBI characteristic | Instructional strategy | Description |
|---|---|---|
| • Fluctuating attention<br>• Decreased speed of processing | Pacing of tasks adjusted to familiarity of the routine and processing abilities (e.g., slow processors may benefit from rapid pacing within familiar teaching routines). | Delivering material in small increments and requiring responses at a rate consistent with a student's processing speed increases acquisition of new material. |
| • Memory impairment (associated with need for errorless learning)<br>• High rates of failure | High rates of success and avoidance of errors. | Acquisition and retention of new information tends to increase with high rates of success. |
| • Organizational impairment<br>• Inefficient learning | Task analysis, clear and explicit instructions, and advance organizational support. | Careful organization of learning tasks, including systematic sequencing of teaching targets and advance organizational support, increases success; graphic organizers facilitate successful performance of complex tasks (e.g., reading comprehension, writing). |
| • Inefficient learning<br>• Inconsistency | Frequent practice and review (including cumulative review). | Acquisition and retention of new information is increased with frequent review. |
| • Inefficient feedback loops<br>• Implicit learning of errors | Errorless learning combined with corrective feedback when errors occur. | Students with severe memory and learning problems benefit from errorless learning. When errors occur, learning is enhanced when those errors are followed by non-judgmental corrective feedback. |
| • Possibility of gaps in the knowledge base | Teaching to mastery. | Learning is enhanced with mastery at the acquisition phase. |
| • Frequent failure of transfer<br>• Concrete thinking and learning | Facilitation of transfer/generalization. | Generalizable strategies and general case teaching (wide range of examples and settings) increase generalization. |
| • Inconsistency<br>• Unpredictable recovery<br>• Unusual scatter of skills and knowledge | Ongoing situational assessment. | Adjustment of teaching based on ongoing assessment of students' progress facilitates learning. |
| • Difficulty with social interaction | Coached support in context. | Presetting and ongoing context-sensitive coaching by peer experts and staff. |
| • Unusual profiles<br>• Unpredictable recovery | Flexibility in curricular modification. | Modifying the curriculum facilitates learning in special populations. |

Modified with permission from Ylvisaker M, Todis B, Glang A, Urbanczyk B, Franklin C, DePompei R, et al. Educating students with TBI: themes and recommendations. J Head Trauma Rehabil 2001; 16(1):76–93.

children with brain injury. In addition, training in procedures for collaborating respectfully and effectively with families[71] should be included in staff development programs.

**Table 9.5**
**Integrated approaches to educational, behavioral, and social intervention that have a research base and are applicable to many students with TBI**

| TBI characteristic | Approach | Description |
|---|---|---|
| • New learning needs<br>• Impaired strategic behavior<br>• Impaired organizational functioning | Metacognitive/strategy intervention | Organized curricula designed to facilitate a strategic approach to difficult academic tasks, including organizational strategies; validated for adolescents with and without specific learning disabilities.[72–73] |
| • Decreased self-awareness<br>• Denial of deficits | Self-awareness/attribution training | Facilitation of students' understanding of their role in learning; validated for students with learning difficulties.[74] |
| • Weak self-regulation related to frontal lobe injury<br>• Disinhibited and potentially aggressive behavior | Contextualized cognitive behavior modification | Facilitation of self-control and regulation of behavior in natural social contexts; validated with adolescents with ADHD and aggressive behavior.[75] |
| • Impulsive behavior<br>• Reduced emotional control<br>• Inefficient learning from consequences<br>• History of failure<br>• Defiant behavior<br>• Initiation impairment<br>• Working memory impairment | Positive, antecedent-focused behavior supports | Approach to behavior management that focuses primarily on the antecedents of behavior (in a broad sense); validated in developmental disabilities and with some TBI subpopulations.[57,28–29] |
| • Frequent loss of friends<br>• Social isolation<br>• Weak social skills | Contextualized coaching of social interaction; development of positive roles and routines; assertiveness training; circle of friends | A set of procedures designed to support students' social life and ongoing social development; validated in developmental disabilities,[76] students with emotional disturbance[77] and TBI.[78] |

Modified with permission from Ylvisaker M, Todis B, Glang A, Urbanczyk B, Franklin C, DePompei R, et al. Educating students with TBI: themes and recommendations. J Head Trauma Rehabil 2001; 16(1):76–93.

## Illustrations

As was the case with social interaction, Mark and Jim had educational needs that were similar to many students with TBI.

- They both appeared to retain much of their pretrauma learning (but with gaps), thus presenting profiles of knowledge and ability that belied their significant organizational and learning impairments.
- They both required more intensive than expected organizational supports to stay focused and complete even moderately complex tasks (e.g., reading/writing for Mark; writing and complex vocational tasks for Jim).

- They processed new information slowly and reacted negatively to time pressure.
- They were inconsistent in their performance from day to day.
- They had an impulsive learning style, often saying their first poorly considered response and then reacting negatively to feedback or criticism.
- They had significant difficulties with abstractions and integration of information from multiple sources.
- Their learning was most efficient within the context of familiar routines of interaction and instruction.
- Both were accustomed to relatively effortless learning before their injuries, making effortful learning emotionally burdensome. They both reacted negatively to failure.

From an educational perspective, the key components of instruction and educational intervention were directly associated with this list of needs.

- Traditional standardized assessments were invalid, requiring ongoing contextualized assessments to understand the students needs and create effective support plans.
- Both students used individualized graphic advance organizers effectively for organizationally demanding tasks.
- Time pressure (e.g., "You must independently complete this work in 20 minutes") was eliminated.
- To deal with day-to-day inconsistency, staff were oriented to its neurological basis and trained to apply supports flexibly; the students were trained to report their level of physical or emotional distress to staff.
- The Goal–Plan–Do–Review routine helped the students inhibit impulsive responses.
- To address weakness in abstract thinking, staff ensured that lessons had ample concrete illustrations.
- Teaching/learning interactions were positively scripted and routinized.
- To address the students' emotional reactions to failure, teaching/learning routines were organized to be as free of errors as possible; positive momentum was built before difficult tasks; the students were taught escape communication to use when stress mounted; and they participated in decision making about their educational programs.

# Serving Students with Brain Injury: A Continuum of Needs and Supports

The ultimate goal of rehabilitative and educational interventions is to enable students to be as successful and independent as possible in natural and minimally restrictive environments. In this chapter, we have presented and illustrated a support-oriented approach to achieving this goal for students with behavioral, social, and educational disabilities after brain injury. We close with a general discussion of the concept of a continuum of supports. This continuum was developed to communicate the notion that every effort is made to create and implement supports so that students are able to regulate their behavior as independently as possible while also acquiring the knowledge and skills needed to be socially and academically successful. The continuum also reflects the reality that supports need to be provided flexibly (i.e., increased or decreased, depending on existing stressors, familiarity or novelty of tasks and settings, and the like) and that some kinds of support may be needed indefinitely. Finally, we use this continuum to communicate to staff and families that levels of support should be determined on the basis of objective criteria. Ideally these criteria are negotiated early in the process of developing support programs so that a reduction in supports is not seen by the family or others as improperly motivated.

Although a wide variety of supports might be useful for an individual student, we have found it helpful to organize these supports along two primary dimensions: environmental supports and staff supports. The environmental support continuum provides a framework for understanding the kinds of environmental modifications needed to ensure that the student is able to maintain positive behaviors and social interactions while also achieving academic goals. "Specialized supports" describes circumstances in which the student participates in routine activities in an environment specifically designed for those activities (e.g., a specialized classroom setting for most routine activities). "Modified supports" describes circumstances in which the student requires environmental adjustments for specific activities (e.g., receiving math instruction in a resource room; eating lunch with a small group of lunch buddies rather than in the cafeteria). "Adapted supports" describes circumstances in which typical environments are adapted to increase the probability of success (e.g., creating a specific place in a classroom for the student to go when anxious or upset). "Typical supports" describes circumstances in which the student is able to learn and maintain positive interactions with the supports that are available to any person in that environment (e.g., homework help).

The staff support continuum provides a framework for understanding the kinds of personnel and prompting supports that a student needs in order to maintain successful interactions and behavioral control, while also achieving academic goals. "Intensive staff supports" describes situations in which a staff person is available to support the student directly and constantly (e.g., when the student first returns to school and is unfamiliar with the routine and tasks; when the student demonstrates challenging behaviors that create a health and safety risk). "Specific staff supports" describes specific situations requiring direct prompting from staff to ensure that the student is able to participate in the activity (e.g., the student understands and can navigate the general routine, but is unable to master specific elements of the routine independently). "Periodic staff supports" describes situations in which the student is learning new routines or attacking novel tasks, and requires specific, time-limited support to ensure optimal participation. "Independence" describes circumstances in which additional staff assistance is not needed (e.g., the student is able to manage the majority of the academic, social, and behavioral demands without difficulty).

The supports mentioned in the previous sections of this chapter (i.e., behavioral supports, social interaction supports, and cognitive-academic supports) fit easily within this meta-support framework, which can be used to help staff and family members understand social, environmental, and educational modifications and negotiate changes in these modifications over time. For example, during the initial stages of intervention, Mark received intensive staff supports (e.g., a one-to-one aide) in an adapted environment. He participated in a majority of the typical classroom routines, but had an area he could retreat to when angry or upset. He also received modified instruction in the typical classroom environment. As he became more successful behaviorally and socially, his level of staff support became specific (i.e., the aide stayed with him when learning new things or in crowded environments, but withdrew when he was engaged in familiar activities) and his environment was increasingly typical (i.e., his need for retreat decreased and he was increasingly able to manage the typical classroom instructions). At the end of the following school year (nearly two years after the intervention) his program included periodic staff supports (i.e., he had a shared aide) that occurred primarily in a typical classroom routine.

During the initial stages of intervention, Jim received specific staff supports (i.e., he checked in and checked out with educational staff at the beginning of the day and before starting tasks, and he received support during activities that were difficult and resulted in increased likelihood that he would have behavioral difficulties) in a specialized environment (he was in a special education program in a specialized setting). As he became increasingly successful socially and behaviorally, he received periodic staff support in the specialized environment. He remained at this level of support for the duration of his schooling.

Mark and Jim illustrate the process of moving to less intensive supports on both domains of the continuum, based on pre-established criteria. They are also emblematic of the reality that for many children with neurologic disabilities, some supports may be needed indefinitely.

# References

1.  Max JE, Robin DA, Lingren SD et al. Traumatic brain injury in children and adolescents: psychiatric problems at two years. J Am Acad Child Adolesc Psychiatry 1997; 36:1278–1285.

2.  Costeff H, Grosswasser Z, Landman Y, Brenner T. Survivors of severe traumatic brain injury in childhood: I, late residual disability. Scand J Rehabil Med 1985; 12(Suppl):10–15.

3.  Andrews TK, Rose FD, Johnson DA. Social and behavioral effects of traumatic brain injury in children. Brain Inj 1998; 12:133–138.

4.  Bloom DR, Levin HS, Ewing-Cobbs L et al. Lifetime and novel psychiatric problems after pediatric traumatic brain injury. J Am Acad Child Adolesc Psychiatry 2001; 40:572–579.

5.  Brown G, Chadwick O, Shaffer D, Rutter M, Traub M. A prospective study of children with head injuries: III, psychiatric sequelae. Psychol Med 1981; 11:63–78.

6.  Fletcher JM, Levin HS, Lachar D et al. Behavioral outcomes after pediatric closed head injury: relationships with age, severity, and lesion size. J Child Neurol 1996; 11:283–290.

7.  Kinsella G, Ong B, Murtagh D, Prior M, Sawyer M. The role of the family for behavioral outcome in children and adolescents following traumatic brain injury. J Consult Clin Psychol 1999; 67:116–123.

8.  Asarnow RF, Satz P, Light R, Zaucha K, Lewis R, McCleary C. The UCLA study of mild closed injury in children and adolescents. In: Broman S, Michel ME, editors. Traumatic head injury in children. New York: Oxford University Press, 1995: 117–146.

9.  Light R, Asarnow R, Satz P, Zaucha K, McCleary C, Lewis R. Mild closed-head injury in children and adolescents: behavior problems and academic outcomes. J Consult Clin Psychol 1998; 66:1023–1029.

10. Schwartz L, Taylor HG, Drotar D, Yeates KO, Wade SL, Stancin T. Long-term behavior problems following pediatric traumatic brain injury: prevalence, predictors, and correlates. J Pediatr Psychol 2003; 28:251–263.

11. Yeates KO. Closed-head injury. In: Yeates KO, Ris MD, Taylor HG, editors. Pediatric neuropsychology: research, theory, and practice. New York: Guilford Press, 2000: 92–116.

12. Anderson V, Moore C. Age as a predictor of outcome following pediatric head injury: a longitudinal perspective. Child Neuropsychol 1995; 1:187–202.

13. Hebb DO. The effects of early experience on problem solving at maturity. Am Psychol 1947; 2:737–745.

14. Levin HS, Culhane KA, Mendelsohn D et al. Cognition in relation to magnetic resonance imaging in head-injured children and adolescents. Arch Neurol 1993; 50:897–905.

15. Michaud LJ, Rivara FP, Jaffe KM, Fay G, Dailey J. Traumatic brain injury as a risk factor for behavioral disorders in children. Arch Phys Med Rehabil 1993; 74:368–375.

16. Taylor HG, Alden J. Age-related differences in outcomes following childhood brain insults: an introduction and overview. J Int Neuropsychol Soc 1997; 3(6):555–567.

17. Woodward H, Winterhalter K, Donders J, Hackbarth R, Kuldanek A, Sanfilippo D. Prediction of neurobehavioral outcome 1–5 years post pediatric traumatic head injury. J Head Trauma Rehabil 1999; 14:351–359.

18.    Scheibel RS, Levin HS. Frontal lobe dysfunction following closed head injury in children and adults. In: Krasnegor NA, Lyon GR, Goldman-Rakic PS, editors. Development of the prefrontal cortex: evolution, neurobiology, and behavior. Baltimore, MD: Paul H Brookes, 1997:241–263.

19.    Kolb B. Brain plasticity and behavior. Mahwah, NJ: Lawrence Erlbaum, 1995.

20.    Koskiniemi M, Kyykka T, Nybo T, Jarho L. Long term outcome after severe brain injury in preschoolers is worse than expected. Arch Pediatr Adolesc Med 1995; 149:249–254.

21.    Eslinger PJ, Biddle KR. Adolescent neuropsychological development after early right prefrontal cortex damage. Dev Neuropsychol 2000; 18(3):297–329.

22.    Anderson SW, Damasio H, Tranel D, Damasio AR. Long-term sequelae of prefrontal cortex damage acquired in early childhood. Dev Neuropsychol 2000; 18(3):281–296.

23.    Marlowe WB. Consequences of frontal lobe injury in the developing child. J Clin Exp Neuropsychol 1989; 12:105–112.

24.    Marlowe WB. The impact of a right prefrontal lesion on the developing brain. Brain Cogn 1992; 20:205–213.

25.    Mateer CA, Williams D. Effects of frontal lobe injury in childhood. Dev Neuropsychol 1991; 7:359–376.

26.    Williams D, Mateer CA. Developmental impact of frontal lobe injury in middle childhood. Brain Cogn 1992; 20:196–204.

27.    Eslinger PJ, Biddle KR, Grattan LM. Cognitive and social development in children with prefrontal cortex lesions. In: Krasnegor NA, Lyon GR, Goldman-Rakic PS, editors. Development of the prefrontal cortex: evolution, neurobiology, and behavior. Baltimore, MD: Paul H Brookes, 1997:295–335.

28.    Feeney T, Ylvisaker M. Choice and routine: antecedent behavioral interventions for adolescents with severe traumatic brain injury. J Head Trauma Rehabil 1995; 10(3):67–82.

29.    Feeney T, Ylvisaker M. Context-sensitive behavioral supports for young children with TBI: short-term effects and long-term outcome. J Head Trauma Rehabil 2003; 18(1):33–51.

30.    Ylvisaker M, Feeney T. Traumatic brain injury in adolescence: assessment and reintegration. Semin Speech Lang 1995; 16(1):32–44.

31.    Ylvisaker M, Feeney T. Collaborative brain injury intervention: positive everyday routines. San Diego, CA: Singular, 1998.

32.    Max JE, Roberts MA, Koele SL et al. Cognitive outcome in children and adolescents following severe traumatic brain injury: influence of psychosocial, psychiatric, and injury-related variables. J Clin Exp Neuropsychol 1999; 5:58–68.

33.    Anderson VA, Catroppa C, Haritou F et al. Predictors of acute child and family outcome following traumatic brain injury in children. Pediatr Neurosurg 2001; 34:138–148.

34.    Yeates KO, Taylor HG, Drotar D et al. Pre-injury family environment as a determinant of recovery from traumatic brain injuries in school-age children. J Int Neuropsychol Soc 1997; 3:617–630.

35.    Biddle KR, McCabe A, Bliss LS. Narrative skills following traumatic brain injury in children and adults. J Commun Disord 1996; 29(6):447–470.

36. Chapman SB. Cognitive-communication abilities in children with closed head injury. Am J Speech Lang Pathol 1997; 6:50–58.

37. Dennis M, Barnes M. Comparison of literal, inferential, and intentional text comprehension in children with mild or severe closed head injury. J Head Trauma Rehabil 2001; 16:456–468.

38. Burgess PW, Shallice T. Response suppression, initiation, and strategy use following frontal lobe lesion. Neuropsychologia 1996; 34:263–273.

39. Eslinger PJ, Grattan LM, Damasio H, Damasio AR. Developmental consequences of childhood frontal lobe damage. Arch Neurol 1992; 49:764–769.

40. Hanton G, Bartha M, Levin H. Metacognition following pediatric brain injury: a preliminary study. Dev Neuropsychol 2000; 18:383–398.

41. Koelfen W, Freund M, Dinter D, Schmidt B, Koenig S, Schultze C. Long-term follow-up of children with head injuries classified as "good recovery" using the Glasgow Outcome Scale: neurological, neuropsychological, and magnetic resonance imaging results. Eur J Pediatr 1997; 156:230–235.

42. Varney NR, Menefee L. Psychosocial and executive deficits following closed head injury: implications for orbital frontal cortex. J Head Trauma Rehabil 1993; 8:32–44.

43. Wilson, BA. Ecological validity of neuropsychological assessment: do neuropsychological indices predict performance in everyday activities. Appl Prev Psychol 1993; 2:209–215.

44. Taylor HG, Yeates KO, Wade SL, Drotar D, Klein S, Stancin T. Influences on first-year recovery from traumatic brain injury in children. Neuropsychology 1999; 13:76–89.

45. Taylor HG, Yeates KO, Wade SL, Drotar D, Stancin T, Burant C. Bidirectional child–family influences on outcomes of traumatic brain injury in children. J Int Neuropsychol Soc 2001; 7:755–767.

46. Taylor HG, Yeates KO, Wade SL, Drotar D, Stancin T, Minich N. A prospective study of short- and long-term outcomes after traumatic brain injury in children: behavior and achievement. Neuropsychology 2002; 16(1):15–27.

47. Wade SL, Michaud L, Maines T. Putting the pieces together: preliminary efficacy of a family problem-solving intervention for children with traumatic brain injury. J Head Trauma Rehabil. In press 2005.

48. Damasio AR. Descartes' error: emotion, reason, and the human brain. New York: Avon, 1994.

49. Rolls ET. The orbitofrontal cortex and reward. Cereb Cortex 2000; 10(3):284–294.

50. Schlund MW. Effects of acquired brain injury on adaptive choice and the role of reduced sensitivity to contingencies. Brain Inj 2002; 16:527–535.

51. Evans JJ, Wilson BA, Schuri U et al. A comparison of "errorless" and "trial-and-error" learning methods for teaching individuals with acquired memory deficits. Neuropsychol Rehabil 2000; 10(1):67–101.

52. Aman MG, Singh NN. Aberrant behavior checklist. East Aurora, NY: Slosson Educational, 1994.

53. Risley T. Get a life: positive behavioral intervention for challenging behavior through life arrangement and life coaching. In: Koegel L, Koegel R, Dunlap G, editors. Positive behavioral support: including people with difficult behavior in the community. Baltimore, MD: Paul H Brookes, 1996:425–438.

54.     Resnick LB. Education and learning to think. Washington, DC: National Academy Press, 1987.

55.     Barkley RA. Adolescents with attention-deficit/hyperactivity disorder: an overview of empirically based treatments. J Psychiatr Pract 2004; 10(1):39–56.

56.     Koegel LK, Koegel RL, Dunlap G, editors. Positive behavioral support: including people with difficult behavior in the community. Baltimore, MD: Paul H Brookes, 1996:403–423.

57.     Carr EG, Horner RH, Turnbull AP et al. Positive behavior support for people with developmental disabilities: a research synthesis. Washington, DC: American Association of Mental Retardation, 1999.

58.     McDonald S. Traumatic brain and psychosocial function: let's get social. Brain Impairment 2003; 4:36–47.

59.     Gresham FM, Sugai G, Horner RH. Interpreting outcomes of social skills training for students with high-incidence disabilities. Except Child 2001; 67(3):331–344.

60.     Kozloff R. Network of social support and the outcome from severe head injury. J Head Trauma Rehabil 1987; 2(3):14–23.

61.     Ylvisaker M, Adelson D, Braga LW et al. Rehabilitation and ongoing support after pediatric TBI: twenty years of progress. J Head Trauma Rehabil 2005; 20(1):95–109.

62.     Franzen EA, Myers RE. Neural control of social behavior: prefrontal and anterior temporal cortex. Neuropsychologia 1973; 11:141–157.

63.     Rubin KH, Bukowski W, Parker J. Peer interactions, relationships, and groups. In: Eisenberg N, editor. Handbook of child psychology: social, emotional, and personality development. 5th ed. New York: John Wiley & Sons, 1998:619–700.

64.     Wiig E, Larsen V, Olson J. S-MAPS: rubrics for curriculum-based assessment and intervention. Eau Claire, WI: Thinking Publications, 2004.

65.     Ylvisaker M, Feeney T, Urbanczyk, B. Social skills following traumatic brain injury. Semin Speech Lang 1992; 13(4):308–321.

66.     Boyer MG, Edwards P. Outcome 1 to 3 years after severe traumatic brain injury in children and adolescents. Injury 1991; 22(4):315–320.

67.     Ewing-Cobbs L, Fletcher JM, Levin HS, Iovino I, Milner ME. Academic achievement and academic placement following traumatic brain injury in children and adolescents: a two-year longitudinal study. J Clin Exp Neuropsychol 1998; 20:769–781.

68.     Nelson JE, Kelly TP. Long-term outcome of learning and memory in children following severe closed head injury. Pediatr Rehabil 2002; 5(1):37–41.

69.     Ylvisaker M, Todis B, Glang A et al. Educating students with TBI: themes and recommendations. J Head Trauma Rehabil 2001; 16(1):76–93.

70.     Braga LW, Campos da Paz A, Ylvisaker M. Direct clinician-delivered versus indirect family-supported rehabilitation of children with traumatic brain injury: a randomized controlled trial. Brain Inj 2005; 19(10):819–831.

71.     Ylvisaker M, Feeney T. Everyday people as supports: developing competencies through collaboration. In: Ylvisaker M, editor. Traumatic brain injury rehabilitation: children and adolescents. Revised ed. Boston: Butterworth-Heinemann, 1998:429–464.

72.     Schumaker JB, Deshler DD. Validation of learning strategy interventions for students with learning disabilities: results of a programmatic research effort. In: Wong BYL, editor. Contemporary intervention research in learning disabilities: an international perspective. New York: Springer-Verlag, 1992.

73.     Pressley M. Cognitive strategy instruction that really improves children's academic performance. Cambridge, MA: Brookline Books, 1995.

74.     Borkowski JG, Chan KS, Muthukrishna N. A process-oriented model of metacognition: links between motivation and executive functioning. In: Shraw G, Impara J, editors. Issues in measurement of metacognition. Lincoln, NB: University of Nebraska Press, 2000.

75.     Robinson TR, Smith SW, Miller MD, Brownell MT. Cognitive behavior modification of hyperactivity-impulsivity and aggression: a meta-analysis of school-based studies. J Educ Psychol 1999; 91:195–203.

76.     Forest M, Lusthaus E. Promoting educational equality for all students: circles and maps. In: Stainback S, Stainback W, Forest M, editors. Educating all students in the mainstream of regular education. Baltimore, MD: Paul H Brookes, 1989:43–57.

77.     Goldstein AP. The prepared curriculum: teaching prosocial competencies. Champaign, IL: Research Press, 1988.

78.     Glang A, Singer G, Todis B, editors. Children with acquired brain injury: the school's response. Baltimore, MD: Paul H Brookes,1997.

# 10 Needs, Beliefs, and Prognosis

*David A Johnson and David Rose*

*It is wisdom to consider the end of things before we embark, and to forecast consequences – L'Estrange[1]*

The importance of family functioning to recovery, rehabilitation and outcome after child brain injury has been repeatedly demonstrated by a number of authorities.[2-4] Paradoxically, these matters may receive scant attention in rehabilitation practice. One of the most important factors is the provision of accurate and meaningful information for family members on the child's condition, prognosis, and management. However, a wide range of research has shown prevalent misunderstanding and misinformation about recovery from brain injury in children and adults, both in professional and lay groups alike. Consequently, the accuracy, reliability, and utility of information given to families may be in doubt.

In this chapter we consider the importance of information, beliefs, and prognosis for the family of a child with brain injury. We suggest that improved education, communication, and collaboration between families, clinicians, and scientists are essential to reducing the burden of care, improving recovery and development, and securing a better quality of life for both child and family

## The Need for Information

Rehabilitation services for adult brain injury survivors are relatively well established in many countries, and the family's burden and rehabilitative role generally acknowledged.[5] Evidence of recovery, rehabilitation, and long-term outcome has been extensively documented. Nonetheless, a high level of unmet need continues to be reported and "Calls for health services to respond to the needs of carers continue to be made ...."[6] In their follow-up of adults with brain injury, four to six months after discharge from inpatient rehabilitation, McPherson et al.[6] found that carers wanted more information on recovery and management. Further, the need for many carers was unrelated to either injury severity or level of functional deficit. Thus, even with established rehabilitation services there is a continuing need for information to assist the family in community care and support of the brain-injured person.

Appropriate rehabilitation services for children who suffer brain injury are often absent, or relatively limited in scale, compared to provision for adults. This lack of provision is unlikely to reflect the absence of need, given the generally greater vulnerability of the developing brain to the effects of injury. Rather, it is suggested that misinformed prognosis, reflecting widespread misconceptions about recovery after damage to the immature brain, is a key factor.[7] The rehabilitation needs of the brain-injured child should be substantially greater than those of an adult counterpart, because of the greater vulnerability of the developing brain and the longer time scale for recovery and development. Hence, there is a lengthy period in which the adverse effects of brain damage upon development and behavior may be manifest. The child and parents are at risk of encountering a greater range and multiplicity of impairments, delays and deficits, often appearing gradually and over many years after the original injury. Consequently, the stresses and needs of a brain-injured child's family are likely to be greater in all respects, than those for the brain-injured adult. Unfortunately, families typically receive inadequate information, help and support,[8] in spite of their abundant needs.

There is considerable misunderstanding and consequently misinformed action among families of children with brain injury. Examples include a father's belief that his very severely head injured daughter simply needed to leave hospital and return home in order to recover, to the equally obstructive grandfather's opinion that his grandson's brain would heal itself and repair the damage gradually over time and hence there was no need for help in or out of school. Such individuals typically refuse to accept information or guidance on the child's condition and needs, and decline any follow-up. Any interference by hospital or community agencies is not tolerated, irrespective of the child's true needs and prognosis. Such families are deaf to information that the child's progress will be hampered unnecessarily. It is concerning to note the findings in one study that parents were found to lack a solid understanding of their child's condition, even at three years after injury.[9] As suggested by Gouvier et al.[10;11] "Families who cling to incorrect beliefs ... are not likely to create an environment that is consistent with promoting optimal recovery."

Follow-up studies of children with acquired brain injury have consistently identified a core of unmet needs of parents, involving information on condition and prognosis.[12] Noting the similarities with adult studies, Armstrong and Kerns[9] concluded:

*"... regardless of the age of the patient, family members of all traumatic brain injury patients continue to report a high proportion of needs following the first year post injury ... all parents place special emphasis on receiving honest answers and understandable explanations from professionals ..."*

Investigating children with brain injury secondary to cardiac surgery, Menezes and Shinebourne[13] illustrate the importance of providing the parents with a realistic prognosis. The authors found that parents *"wanted practical support, information and honesty about the future ... Above all they wanted to be offered a realistic view of the future"*. Families may have no concerns with the child's acute care, when the knowledge and skill base, as well as the burden of responsibility, is clearly with hospital staff. However, when the child is discharged from hospital and the burden shifts to the community and support is in limited supply, or not immediately available, an increasing number of concerns are likely to surface. Aitken et al.[14] found that, *"Several parents recalled that they did not know what questions to ask at time of discharge and were poorly prepared to cope with the needs of their children and families after returning home"*. Given the combination of parents' obvious inexperience with brain injury, their emotional distress, and the probable lack of precise information and guidance given by the hospital, Aitken et al.'s[14] findings are not unexpected. The unpreparedness of the families at that early stage creates a substantial handicap for any attempt at managing the children's problems and meeting their needs thereafter. Lack of information increases the risks of misunderstanding of post-traumatic impairments and disabilities, which makes it difficult for the problems to be managed effectively and, in turn, creates further stress upon the carers and greater strain upon family relationships.

The specific needs identified in these studies focus on the provision of information and support. Parents see the need to remain hopeful about the future, they want to know that their child can and will get better, but they also want to be involved in their child's care. That requires that they know what to do, how to do it, and when and how to ask for help. Parents are aware of the need for communication with professionals when the problems arise and not just at routine follow-up. Related needs included provision of social support, including shared experiences with other parents, a greater level of understanding and acceptance of child's problems and consequent parental burden by the school, community, and extended family.

The situation is likely to be considerably more difficult for the grandparents of the very young child who suffers non-accidental brain injury. Typically, grandparents are placed suddenly as temporary or adoptive carers in place of the perpetrators, the child's parents. The grandparents have to contend with the significant psychological impact of the event, the fact that their own son or daughter has seriously and often repeatedly assaulted their infant grandchild. The grandparents may well benefit from their past experience as parents but they are likely to need far more information and support than their younger counterparts. They may more easily become isolated from their elderly peers and lack many social supports. While the early years of infancy and preschool may create relatively straightforward care needs, there will be very real concerns about the ability of elderly grandparents to cope with the demands of a school-age child with growing cognitive and behavioral disability. For the more severely injured child with profound physical and mental disability, the grandparents become more acutely aware of their own increasing physical disability as they age, and the growing child's long-term needs. For a baby injured at 3 weeks of age, the consequent changes in brain state and behavior during childhood, adolescence, and early adult years mean that the grandparents lack the physical and psychological capacities with which to cope, even if they survive that long.

# The problem of prognosis

*"In discussing the course of therapy, we are concerned not only about the content and quality of the therapy service, including expertise, but also about what has been called truth-telling about the nature and prognosis of the child's condition . . ."[15]*

*"Inaccurate knowledge among health professionals could have serious consequences in terms of treatment and recovery . . ."[11]*

If a need for information is acknowledged, a critical question becomes its quality. Providing incomplete, ill-formed or unduly optimistic information may be counterproductive. Middleton[16] suggested many parents may have been given early and perhaps erroneous predictions that a child with a very severe injury is likely to be a vegetable, or that after a good physical recovery the child's cognition and behavior will be equally as good. Middleton[16] suggested that,

*". . . This knowledge may come from professionals who treated children in the acute phase of their injury and rarely see them beyond a year post injury; popular myths gleaned from television or newspaper articles; or an in depth search of the internet for literature, which may vary in . . . its quality. It is easy to see how parents and children may be confused and find it difficult to hear other professionals offering alternative explanations and likely prognoses"*

Conflicting information creates an unhealthy state of dissonance and hinders rehabilitation and development.

Examples of problematic prognoses and misinformation are readily found in practice.

*Case 1: A 3-year-old boy was a pedestrian struck by a car. He sustained very severe head injury and consequent brain damage. The neurosurgeon's prognosis informed: "The Clinical findings at this time suggest that he had so-called 'diffuse axonal injury'. This means that there was evidence of neuronal damage most probably at the brain stem level but as one would expect in a boy of this age, his nervous system has made a complete recovery from this injury and I don't think that there are any long-term sequelae (aged 4 years 7 months) that could now attribute specifically to a head injury . . .".*

*Case 2: At 2 months old a female child suffered multiple injuries, including very severe head injury with right parietal skull fracture and brain damage. It was recorded that the major injury was neurological. Investigations revealed bifrontal subdural haematomas, with left to right shift, right frontal lobe haemorrhage, and widespread haemorrhagic intracerebral contusions to the frontal, temporal and deep regions of the brain. Subsequently, behavioral difficulties and sleep disturbance were attributed to diet or age, rather than brain injury. At 5 years old, the pediatrician prognosticated: ". . . at the present time there is no evidence that [she] will in the future suffer any consequences from the head injury. The overwhelming probability is that she will not". Aged 6 years, the child's teacher reported to the school nurse, who in turn informed mother, that the child had some difficulty concentrating. School had no information about the brain damage. The doctors had told mother that her daughter had made a good recovery. The problems persisted throughout the first few years of school but she was considered not to have any significant learning difficulties that required formal recognition. Neuropsychological assessment at 10 years old revealed low general intellectual ability, with specific impairments in cognition and behavior entirely consistent with the effects of the early brain injury.*

*Case 3: A news bulletin reported a government minister's thanks to a local hospital who had treated his nephew with very severe head injury. The report informed that the 15-year-old boy had spent 10 days in coma following the accident a year ago, but that he had now made a full recovery. The report quoted a nurse, who had treated the boy initially, ". . . we don't always hear how people get on after they leave hospital . . .". Her colleague was also quoted, ". . . it's good to know he's a normal wee boy again, running about and doing what wee boys do . . .".*

Some authors consider that the nature of child brain injury makes prognosis almost impossible Thus, Savage et al.[17] suggested that, *"The very nature of a TBI . . . the ongoing developmental processes of brain maturation, along with the changing cognitive challenges during the child's education, complicate prognostic challenges even further . . ."*. It is difficult but not impossible and we should not evade our professional responsibility in understanding the complexities and communicating them to the family. As Plum and Posner[18] suggested, *"The scientific, philosophic and emotional uncertainties attending predictions of outcome from human illness can intimidate even experienced physicians. Nevertheless the problem must be faced"*. Professionals may also be anxious about giving a realistic prognosis and thereby destroying the parents' hope for their child to recover and be normal again. However, parents and carers need clear and reliable information, and understanding of their circumstances, if they are to best help the child after leaving hospital. Is there too much concern with the individual's feelings and not enough with clinical reality or, indeed, the individual's rights? Is there an attempt at overdressing acute medicine or medical skills, to the extent that the technical advances since the 1950s, which ensure that many more lives are saved now, somehow acquire miraculous effects that transcend both acute clinical care and the biological capacity of the immature brain to ensure optimal development, good outcome and quality of life in adulthood. Thus, acute medicine or therapeutics becomes omnipotent. In a discussion of prognosis Galen[19;20] informs that the doctor *"...should incline to the bright side when possible..."*. In that sense, the prognosticator may adopt a role of protector against bad news, perhaps believing that there are things with which the parents should not be worried just yet.[20] Having had the acute stress of the child surviving a life-threatening condition, the immediacy of which prevents any preparation at coping, to inform parents that there is more bad news to come but not for a few more years yet, may be considered by some as going too far, or creating unnecessary burdens for a family already stressed.

Clinical experience and research, however, suggests that the fundamental problem of prognosis is a lack of professional knowledge and understanding of the critical factors in recovery and outcome, notably those of age at insult and biological vulnerability, development and time since injury, and measurement of outcome. Central to this is the evident confusion about age and recovery, essentially that children either do or do not recover better from brain injury than adults.[21] The statement usually attributed to Hans Teuber illustrates the "younger is better" view, *"If I am to have brain damage I'd best have it early rather than late in life"*.[22] The notion of younger is better is usually referred to as the "Kennard Principle". However, there is no evidence that Kennard ever postulated such a simplistic view.[23] Nonetheless, investigations of professional beliefs in this field have found strong adherence to the notion that younger age predicts better recovery.

The opposing view, that children do not achieve a good recovery after brain injury because of their age and stage of development, is illustrated by Sir Thomas Crisp English,[24] a London surgeon, who lectured in 1904:

> *"It is usually stated that children recover remarkably well from injuries to the head but my experience has not borne out this statement ... The seriousness of severe head injuries in children seems to lie in their occurrence at a time when the higher intellectual faculties are being developed ... It would be logical to expect that injuries to the brain in children would be even more likely to result in some permanent impairment, for its structure is more delicate and its development more complex than in any other region."*

Furthermore, the long-term perspective on recovery, disability, and hence rehabilitation need has been well documented in the clinical literature. An early paper by Strecker and Ebaugh[25] reported the neuropsychiatric consequences of head injury in children, stating:

> *"The serious deferred results of head injury in adults are even more pronounced in children. Here they attain vital clinical and social significance, since the physical, neurologic, psychiatric and psychologic findings bear a close relation to school progress, delinquency, criminality and future adjustability in general"*

More recent evidence confirms that concern with long-term development and outcome.[26-29]

In what appears to have been the first attempt to evaluate professional beliefs associated with age and outcome from brain injury, Hart and Faust[30] concluded: ". . . although the Kennard Principle suffers from over simplicity and obsolescence, it remains alive and well in the minds of many practitioners involved in clinical neuropsychology". Using a variant of the Hart and Faust study, Rose and colleagues[31-34] have conducted a series of investigations into professionals' beliefs about age and recovery and extended the application of Hart and Faust's conclusion. With the exception of educational psychologists (see below) Rose's group found that all professions surveyed, including neurosurgeons, neurologists, neuropsychologists, general practitioners, nurses, physiotherapists, occupational therapists, speech therapists, and lawyers, predicted better recovery in younger, than older, cases.[35] Interestingly, no significant relationships were found between the time since qualifying and the case predicted outcome, which suggests no significant change in the content of professional education. Findings from a series of pilot studies with students and staff in UK medical schools (Johnson, unpublished data) support the view that there is a lack of knowledge about the age and recovery from brain injury. For example, although students who had received neuroscience teaching tended to have more accurate beliefs about age and recovery from brain injury, they still tended to believe that young age is advantageous to recovery (McLeod and Johnson, unpublished data). This suggests that evidence against the Kennard Principle is not being given sufficient prominence in the medical curriculum. Consequently, a critically important opportunity is being missed, at a cost to the care and outcome of the medical students' future patients. As suggested by Duerson et al.[36] misconceptions may be carried by students into professional educational programmes and subsequently interfere with the establishment of knowledge-based effective rehabilitation services.

In their study of educational psychologists' beliefs Rose's group[31] found that young children with brain injury were consistently rated as needing more support, and for longer, than adolescents. The authors suggested that the apparently greater awareness of educational psychologists may be due to their training, which ". . . *particularly emphasises the importance of children successfully passing through stages of cognitive development and the long-term consequences of difficulties arising at any of these developmental stages*". However, that is not consistent with clinical experience or findings from other studies, which suggest that educational psychologists do not have adequate training, knowledge, contact or experience with head-injured children.[37-39] One study[40] investigated school psychologists' knowledge of traumatic brain injury (TBI). Well over half (65%) reported no training about head-injured children. A generally low level of knowledge about brain injury was found, with only 27% respondents correctly identifying the effects of age and injury, and only 30% the effects of age and cognitive outcome. The authors concluded:

*"...it is apparent that educators need a broad based knowledge of head injury ... Yet information about traumatic head injury is not included in the training of most professionals who deal with these children in the schools."*

It appears therefore that professional education and hence understanding of recovery from child brain injury is seriously defective. This creates an inexpert population of presumed experts from whom parents will seek information on guidance. Professional opinion on age and recovery from brain injury may be little better than lay beliefs.

## The Bases of Prognosis

Good doctors use both individual clinical expertise and the best available external evidence, and neither alone is enough.[41]

The importance of prognosis was recognised early in medicine. Thus, Hippocrates[42] wrote:

*"It appears to me a most excellent thing for the physician to cultivate Prognosis; for by foreseeing and foretelling, in the presence of the sick, the present, the past, and the future, and explaining the omissions which patients have been guilty of, he will be the more readily believed to be acquainted with the circumstances of the sick; so that men will have confidence to intrust themselves to such a physician. And he will manage the cure best who has foreseen what is to happen from the present state of matters".*

Similarly, William Farr,[43] considered to be the father of modern epidemiology, suggested:

*"Every medical man should be well versed in prognosis. It will enable him to take into consideration the subsequent phases of the malady, and rescue him from the system of expediency, where every symptom is treated as an isolate fact, and, according to the urgency of immediate circumstances, without regard to the subsequent states through which the patient must inevitably pass; while diseases often require to be treated, in the early stages, for phenomena not developed, and only acquiring intensity at a future period ... An accurate prognosis in such cases gives the physician the advantages a general possesses, well informed beforehand of the enemy's forces, plans of battle and order of attack".*

That analogy suggests the importance of being forewarned and forearmed in the anticipation and treatment of the effects of aberrant post-traumatic development, particularly at times of major neurodevelopmental change, such as puberty and sexual awareness.

Prognosis should be an exact process of prediction based upon established knowledge and experience of a series of factors associated with the specified condition. It requires a symbiotic relationship between the two critical factors in clinical practice, knowledge, and experience. Knowledge should encompass both clinical and experimental science, how the literature informs of the acute and long-term consequences of early injury.[24;29;44-45] Experience should encompass the target population at time stages relevant to the prognosis given, e.g. a neurosurgeon's experience and expertise is likely to be focused upon acute recovery and short-term follow-up, rather than many years after injury. Similarly, an educational psychologist is unlikely to have experience of the long-term educational and employment outcome of adults injured as children.

Unfortunately, the literature on recovery and outcome from brain injury in childhood yields a body of inconsistent information. In their attempt to establish the facts, clinicians are confronted by conflicting information. For example,

> *"It is now recognised that traumatic brain injury is an event that will alter the entire subsequent developmental trajectory for a child. As a child injured in the early years of life attempts to acquire new skills, the apparently subtle deficits in new learning . . . may compound over the years into a significant late morbidity".*[46]

Alternatively, "Despite some contradictions, most literature supports children faring better than adults who have severe brain injury".[47] How do busy clinicians decide which conclusion to adopt? It is reasonable to suggest that they should possess the requisite knowledge to critically evaluate such papers. Conversely, one may suggest that, at least in the latter example of professional guidelines on management, the critical analysis had already been conducted and publication assured the reader of established and reliable information. Unfortunately, this cannot be assumed to be the case. The AANS[47] guidelines rely upon studies using inadequate and inappropriate measures, notably the Glasgow Outcome Scale, a global measure developed for adults, and generally short-term follow-up without controlling for age. Use of such measures

> *". . . may underestimate the severity of disability when applied to young children. The extent of cognitive and functional impairment may be underestimated without direct assessment of cognitive function and adaptive behaviour. Long term follow up of children . . . is particularly important since young children may demonstrate deficits at older ages that were not evident at the time of the injury. Careful longitudinal follow up emphasizing family functioning, cognitive development and psychological development is crucial to planning appropriate interventions".*[48]

Thus, inadequate measures, and uncritical analysis and reporting, yield inappropriate and unreliable information for prognosis and hence treatment.

The apparently confusing literature may create uncertainties for clinicians, or they may simply ignore it and rely upon experience alone when advising parents of a child's prognosis. Does the acute care doctor, therefore, err on the side of caution and predict a "Favourable Outcome"[49] in the knowledge that this will cover severe motor or cognitive disability, moderate disability or a good recovery, while not explaining the terms and wide range of possibilities precisely? Is the prediction simply for an imprecise "Good Recovery", or a "Good Recovery B"* on the basis that the available information (e.g. CT scan) implies, rather than proves, that the child has made a complete recovery?[50] It may be considered by some that the best course of action is to say little, offer general encouragement and hope for the best. In any event, the parents are left with less than the necessary information with which to manage the subsequent years of aberrant development.

# The Public's Need for Information

Brain damage, in its various guises, is commonplace. Although the true prevalence of acquired neurological disability in the community is unknown it is reasonable that the public would have some contact with, or close knowledge of, an adult or child with cerebral insult of some sort. For example, Gouvier et al.[10] found that 55% of their sample had some personal experience with head injury or stroke. Unfortunately, it seems that personal experience may not lead to any better knowledge and understanding of the problems.

Initial research of lay opinion on the effects of brain damage appears to have arisen from a growing awareness of the ever-increasing burden placed upon families after brain injury and the lack of effective communication or help from hospital or other agencies. Parents and families have the major role in helping the brain-injured person's social interaction and adjustment within the community and in providing for their long-term care. They are likely to seek help and support from relatives and friends. The parents and child, as well as siblings, will come into frequent contact with other lay people in the local community, from whom understanding and support is essential. Successful integration into the community is a long-term goal for the brain-injured child but it may be hampered by a variety of factors, including cognitive and behavior changes that others find difficult to understand or cope with. The reactions of others to a child's impulsive or explosive behavior in a shop, for example, can greatly influence the parent's management of the child, the future use of community resources and, of course, the parent's emotional state. Yet, it is unlikely that many parents will have been provided with information in advance on what to expect, when and how to manage such problems, or whom to call for help. The so-called hidden disability of brain damage is particularly important for children and others' understanding of their behavior.

---

* "Good Recovery B" implies that the information available is that the child has made a complete recovery with no detectable sequelae from the head injury: Crouchman et al.[50]

There are no established public education programmes about the effects of acquired brain injury. The level of knowledge and understanding about brain injury generally in the community has been found to be poor. Thus, Willer et al.[51] suggested: *"One possible contribution to the coping difficulties experienced by individuals with brain injuries and their families is the substantial level of misconception about the nature of brain injury among the general public"*. There appear to be no major geographical or population differences in beliefs,[10;52] suggesting there is a universal experience of brain injury that transcends individual cultures.[53]

A limited number of studies have explored public conceptions about head injury, brain damage, and recovery. In the USA[10] and Canada[51] a significant portion of the general population, sampled from shopping mall users, were found to hold common misconceptions about brain injury. For example, Gouvier et al.[10] found that 31 per cent of respondents

*"believed that most people with brain damage look and act retarded, and 26% were unaware that emotional problems following head injury were related to brain damage."*

Also of note was their finding that

*"Nearly half believed that the recovery process is complete as soon as the person feels "back to normal", and the majority believed that 100% recovery from severe head injury was possible."*

In a recent replication of those earlier studies, Guilmette et al.[52] found no significant improvement in the level of knowledge about moderate to severe brain injury. In comparing lay and non-expert heath professionals Swift and Wilson[11] concluded that both groups

*". . . do not fully appreciate the long-term nature of brain injury [and] people are substantially unaware of the diversity of problems that brain injury can cause, particularly cognitive and behavioural effects."*

Further, that such *"Inaccurate knowledge among health professionals could have serious consequences in terms of treatment and recovery"*.

## Sources of Information

*"In religion and politics people's beliefs and convictions are in almost every case gotten at second-hand, and without examination, from authorities who have not themselves examined the questions at issue but have taken them at second-hand from other non-examiners, whose opinions about them were not worth a brass farthing"*.[54]

The identified misconceptions may stem from a variety of sources. In the shopping mall sample of Gouvier et al.[10] the frequent sources of information about head injury were television talk shows (42%), personal discussion with professionals (42%), discussions with friends (38%), television news programmes (33%) and daily newspapers (33%). However, in spite of this diversity of resources, Gouvier et al. noted that

> "...a majority of respondents with personal experience had discussed head injuries with professionals, yet still had the same misconceptions as those without experience, [which] raises some questions about the adequacy of education provided by health care providers".

Media coverage of neurological disorders has increased in the UK, particularly with individual victims working in television and more general medical science programmes. There have been few reports of recovery from child head injury, perhaps out of a greater sensitivity for the child's privacy, or the belief that children make a good or complete recovery in any event. However, media coverage of high profile cases suggests that ignorance or misunderstanding of the consequences of early neurological insult prevails. Thus, in a case of a child who suffered extensive head and brain injuries, the treating pediatrician was reported in a national newspaper as saying "We expect her intelligence to be preserved ... I reserve judgement about a complete recovery" (*The Times*, 26 August 1996). Similarly, the child's father was "looking forward to getting her back completely to normal as soon as possible" (*Daily Telegraph*, 27 May 1997). There was no discussion of any family factors, extended rehabilitation, aberrant psychosocial development or family need. The media are at best likely to give inconsistent information and may reinforce myths and misconceptions. Whatever the source of the reported information, the media are more likely than not to be an unreliable source of information for public education on brain injury. As Guilmette and Paglia [52] suggest, the

> "... potentially negative consequences, medical and legal, of such misinformation make it all the more vital to educate the general public and TBI survivors and their families in order to foster an environment more conducive to support TBI survivors".

## Provision of Information

Parents are a child's primary carers but they have other, many and varied, responsibilities to all of their children, to themselves as partners and to the extended family, as well as employers and other formal commitments. At various times parents have to adopt specific and unfamiliar roles on behalf of the child, for which they have no experience and little professional support. They must act as communicators and liaise with professionals in hospital, education and the community, as well as more diverse agencies such as lawyers. These multiple roles create significant levels of stress and strain, often chronic and cumulative, adversely affecting the parents' mental and physical health, personal relationships and quality of life.[55–56] Stressed carers of any age are unlikely to be able to provide optimal environments to help recovery of the brain-injured child. Elderly grandparents are likely to be more vulnerable at least physically, but the strains of trying to cope with a disruptive, withdrawn or otherwise maladaptive youngster may become disproportionately greater for them. Consequently, the importance of considering parental stress after child brain injury should be self-evident and a primary goal for intervention.[57–58]

Providing information about child development helps parents to respond appropriately to their children. Informed parents are better equipped to problem solve, more confident of their decisions, and more likely to respond appropriately to their children's needs. It can help to reduce feelings of anxiety, stress, isolation, and rejection. The need for active, rather than passive, dissemination of information has been acknowledged.[6;14] Simply providing information without appropriate help and support, however, may be counterproductive, increasing anxiety and depressive symptoms.[59] There should be proactive engagement of the family in rehabilitation. A recent study by Melnyk et al.[60] offers some guidance. The authors report improved outcomes in the parents of critically ill young children following their participation in an educational-behavioral intervention programme – Creating Opportunities for Parent Empowerment (COPE). That intervention

> "...focussed on increasing 1) parents' knowledge and understanding of the behaviours and emotions young children typically display during and after hospitalisation and 2) direct parent participation in their children's emotional and physical care".

The findings suggest that if parents are better able to understand the nature of the child's condition, difficulties and needs then they experience less stress, anxiety and depression. However, one of the unique problems for families of brain-injured children is their long-term need for information. Unless the child is seen routinely throughout the remaining period of maturation how will the parents and child be alerted to the risks in sufficient time to prevent problems, or minimise their impact and facilitate everyone's optimal adaptation. Who prompts the parents to ask the necessary questions if there is no routine follow-up or rehabilitation?

Critics may argue that the degree of uncertainty in the individual case warrants caution and provision of restricted information. But that may lead to a false sense of security. Would any one of us be satisfied with having received less than full information if our children failed in school because of cognitive difficulties that had a significant impact upon their learning but did not affect their general ability or IQ and hence created no recognised need in the eyes of the educators? Similarly, if one's daughter, injured at 10 years old, became pregnant a few years later or contracted a sexually transmitted disease, as a result of her disinhibited attempts to gain friends, and particularly a boyfriend who would love and care for her, so that she could be accepted just like the other girls, rather than rejected by them? To what extent should parents be informed of the neurologically turbulent period of adolescence? Should the potential risks of endocrine change, brain growth and sexual behavior be explained, especially for females? If not, why not? There is no justifiable reason for withholding information if there is a recognisable and avoidable risk. Why should parents have to wait until the maladaptive behavior is established before help is provided? Information, engagement, and follow-up could prevent considerable psychosocial adversity for child and family.

The type and level of information needed will vary, relative to the child's age and stage of development, the nature and severity of injury, premorbid characteristics and the environments in which the child is placed. The main topics include coping with stress for the parents, nature and severity of injury, consequences for development, general management of the child within the confines of the brain injury, present strengths and weaknesses, present and anticipated future treatment, educational resources and programmes, how and what information to provide for other agencies and, not least, children's legal rights. Suggestions about the content of general educational programs should be tailored by consideration of the various misconceptions identified.[11;35]

## The Need for Change

There can be no doubt that parents and families of children with brain injury have substantial unmet needs. In order to address those needs, to improve the child's progress in the long-term and reduce the mental and physical burdens of care upon families, fundamental changes are necessary in professional and public education and the dissemination of information. The need for change greatly exceeds the provision of information booklets by support groups, useful though they are. It is the core of information and its providers that have to change. The primary sources of information, hospital doctors, nurses, therapists, and teachers, have to become consistent, reliable and long-term providers of accurate and meaningful information, advice, and support. It is our ethical and legal responsibility to the child. The clinical process of prognosis after child brain injury must be thoroughly reviewed and the full range of evidence evaluated. Similarly, the teaching content of professional education and training in development and neuroscience, clinical and experimental, should be reevaluated to ensure all professional groups are fully cognisant of the critical issues determining recovery and outcome from child brain injury. Kessler[61] suggested that clinical judgment, the weighing of all factors in diagnosis, seems to be disappearing and questions if "...*education of residents is faltering under the weight and preoccupation with surgery as the only phase of our armamentarium worth teaching*?" Professional thinking has to evolve beyond acute critical care to encompass the family as a dynamic and long-term positive influence upon the child's condition and prognosis. There is a growing population of children, becoming progressively disabled or handicapped adults.[62] The population of disabled individuals is as great a threat to social and economic stability as is the ageing population generally.

Such changes to professional education will take time, even if the principal faults are readily accepted. Neurorehabilitation still suffers from a Cinderella image in rehabilitation medicine,[63] and is, as yet, far from the headline grabbing, action-packed life-saving adventures of *ER/Casualty/Trauma* and the like television programmes. Interim measures are necessary. Clarification of terms and consistency of use is fundamental to effective communication,[64] whether it is in the media, or between any combination of hospital, home, school, community pediatrics and social services. Journals publishing outcome studies should ensure that only valid and appropriate measures are used.[65] Families and support groups should become more proactive in disseminating their information widely and frequently to all professionals, public and media. Those professionals who persist with the notion that a child will make a complete recovery from brain damage should be challenged to produce the scientific evidence upon which they rely and to critically evaluate its method. The provision of information to parents on a child's condition and prognosis has very long-term and wide-ranging implications. It is our ethical and moral responsibility to ensure that families receive accurate and meaningful information at all times.

# References

1.  L'Estrange Sir Roger (1616–1704). Webster's Revised Unabridged Dictionary. 1913.

2.  Braga LW, Campos da Paz Jr. A. Neuropsychological pediatric rehabilitation. In: Christensen AL, Uzzell B, editors. International handbook of neuropsychological rehabilitation. New York: Kluwer Academic/Plenum, 2000: 283–295.

3.  Sohlberg MM, McLaughlin KA, Todis B, Larsen J, Glang A. What does it take to collaborate with families affected by brain injury? A preliminary model. J Head Trauma Rehabil 2001; 16(5):498–511.

4.  Wade SL, Taylor HG, Drotar D, Stancin T, Yeates KO, Minich NM. A prospective study of long-term caregiver and family adaptation following brain injury in children. J Head Trauma Rehabil 2002; 17(2):96–111.

5.  Lezak MD. Brain damage is a family affair. J Clin Exp Neuropsychol 1988; 10(1):111–123.

6.  McPherson KM, McNaughton H, Pentland B. Information needs of families when one member has a severe brain injury. Int J Rehabil Res 2000; 23(4):295–301.

7.  Johnson DA, Rose D. Prognosis, rehabilitation and outcome after inflicted brain injury in children – a case of professional developmental delay. Pediatr Rehabil 2004; 7(3):185–193.

8.   Waaland PK, Burns C, Cockrell J. Evaluation of needs of high- and low-income families following pae-
     diatric traumatic brain injury. Brain Inj 1993; 7(2):135–146.

9.   Armstrong K, Kerns KA. The assessment of parent needs following paediatric traumatic brain injury.
     Pediatr Rehabil 2002; 5(3):149–160.

10.  Gouvier WD, Prestholdt PH, Warner MS. A survey of common misconceptions about head injury and
     recovery. Arch Clin Neuropsychol 1988; 3(4):331–343.

11.  Swift TL, Wilson SL. Misconceptions about brain injury among the general public and non-expert
     health professionals: an exploratory study. Brain Inj 2001; 15(2):149–165.

12.  Hawley CA, Ward AB, Magnay AR, Long J. Parental stress and burden following traumatic brain
     injury amongst children and adolescents. Brain Inj 2003; 17(1):1–23.

13.  Menezes AM, Shinebourne EA. Severe brain injury after cardiac surgery in children: consequences for
     the family and the need for assistance. Heart 1998; 80(3):286–291.

14.  Aitken ME, Mele N, Barrett KW. Recovery of injured children: parent perspectives on family needs.
     Arch Phys Med Rehabil 2004; 85(4):567–573.

15.  Flett PJ, Stoffell BF. Ethical issues in paediatric rehabilitation. J Paediatr Child Health 2003;
     39(3):219–223.

16.  Middleton JA. Practitioner review: psychological sequelae of head injury in children and adolescents. J
     Child Psychol Psychiatry 2001; 42(2):165–180.

17.  Savage RC, DePompei R, Tyler J, Lash M. Pediatric traumatic brain injury: a review of pertinent
     issues. Pediatr Rehabil 2005; 8(2):92–103.

18.  Plum F, Posner JB. The diagnosis of stupor and coma. 3rd ed. Philadelphia: Davis, 1982.

19.  Galen. On prognosis. In: Nutton V, editor. Corpus medicorum graecorum. Berlin: Akademie Verlag,
     1979.

20.  Forrester J. Postal diagnosis: breaking the bad news in the 17th century. BMJ 1995;
     311(7021):1694–1696.

21.  Fabian AA. Prognosis in head injuries in children. J Nerv Ment Dis 1956; 12:428–431.

22.  Schneider GE. Is it really better to have your brain lesion early? A revision of the "Kennard principle".
     Neuropsychologia 1979; 17(6):557–583.

23.  Finger S, Almli CR. Margareth Kennard and her "principle" in historical perspective. In: Finger S,
     LeVere TE, Almli CR, Stein DG, editors. Brain injury and recovery: theoretical and controversial
     issues. New York: Plenum, 1988: 117–132.

24.  English TC. The after-effects of head injury: Lecture 1. Lancet 1904; 20:485–489.

25.  Strecker EA, Ebaugh FG. Neuropsychiatric sequelae of cerebral trauma in children. Arch Neurol Psy-
     chiatry 1924; 12:443–453.

26.  Grattan LM, Eslinger PJ. Frontal lobe damage in children and adults: a comparative review. Dev Neu-
     ropsychol 1991; 7(3):283–326.

27.     Johnson DA, Almli CR. Age brain damage and performance. In: Finger S, editor. Recovery from brain damage: research in theory. New York: Plenum, 1978: 115–132.

28.     Koskiniemi M, Kyykka T, Nybo T, Jarho L. Long-term outcome after severe brain injury in preschoolers is worse than expected. Arch Pediatr Adolesc Med 1995; 149(3):249–254.

29.     Sherwin ED, O'Shanick GJ. The trauma of paediatric and adolescent brain injury: issues and implications for rehabilitation specialists. Brain Inj 2000; 14(3):267–284.

30.     Hart K, Faust D. Prediction of the effects of mild head injury: a message about the Kennard Principle. J Clin Psychol 1988; 44(5):780–782.

31.     Brooks BM, Rose FD, Johnson DA, Andrews TK, Gulamali R. Support for children following traumatic brain injury: the views of educational psychologists. Disabil Rehabil 2003; 25(1):51–56.

32.     Johnson DA, Rose FD, Brooks BM, Eyers S. Age and recovery from brain injury: legal opinions, clinical beliefs and experimental evidence. Pediatr Rehabil 2003; 6(2):103–109.

33.     Siddiqui UN, Rose FD, Attree EA. Recovery from brain damage: views of general practitioners on the importance of age at the time of injury. Med Sci Res 2005; 24:237–238.

34.     Webb C, Rose FD, Johnson DA, Attree EA. Age and recovery from brain injury: clinical opinions and experimental evidence. Brain Inj 1996; 10(4):303–310.

35.     Hux K, Rogers T, Mongar K. Common perceptions about strokes. J Community Health 2000; 25(1):47–65.

36.     Duerson MC, Thomas JW, Chang J, Stevens CB. Medical students' knowledge and misconceptions about aging: responses to Palmore's Facts on Aging Quizzes. Gerontologist 1992; 32(2):171–174.

37.     Farmer JE, Johnson G. Misconceptions about traumatic brain injury among educators and rehabilitation staff. Personal communication 2003.

38.     Hawley CA, Ward AB, Magnay AR, Long J. Children's brain injury: a postal follow-up of 525 children from one health region in the UK. Brain Inj 2002; 16(11):969–985.

39.     Johnson DA, Munro S, Snodgrass C, Pentland B. Return to education after head injury in children: identifying needs. Health Bull 1998; 56(6):899–904.

40.     Mira MP, Meck NE, Tyler JS. School psychologists' knowledge of traumatic head injury: implications for training. Diagnostique 1988; 13(2–4):174–180.

41.     Sackett DL, Rosenberg WM, Gray JA, Haynes RB, Richardson WS. Evidence based medicine: what it is and what it isn't. BMJ 1996; 312(7023):71–72.

42.     Hippocrates. The book of prognostics. London, 1849.

43.     Farr W. On prognosis (British Medical Almanack 1838). Soz Praventivmed 2003; 48(5):219–224.

44.     Adelson PD, Dixon CE, Kochanek PM. Long-term dysfunction following diffuse traumatic brain injury in the immature rat. J Neurotrauma 2000; 17(4):273–282.

45.     Kennard MA, Fulton JF. Age and reorganisation of central nervous system. Mt Sinai J Med 1942; 9:594–606.

46.     Forsyth RJ, Wong CP, Kelly TP et al. Cognitive and adaptive outcomes and age at insult effects after non-traumatic coma. Arch Dis Child 2001; 84(3):200–204.

47.     The Brain Trauma Foundation. The American Association of Neurological Surgeons: The Joint Section on Neurotrauma and Critical Care. Age. J Neurotrauma 2000; 17(6–7):573–581.

48.     Ewing-Cobbs L, Duhaime AC, Fletcher JM. Inflicted and non-inflicted traumatic brain injury in infants and preschoolers. J Head Trauma Rehabil 1995; 10(5):13–24.

49.     Pillai S, Praharaj SS, Mohanty A, Kolluri VR. Prognostic factors in children with severe diffuse brain injuries: a study of 74 patients. Pediatr Neurosurg 2001; 34(2):98–103.

50.     Crouchman M, Rossiter L, Colaco T, Forsyth R. A practical outcome scale for paediatric head injury. Arch Dis Child 2001; 84(2):120–124.

51.     Willer B, Johnson WE, Rempel RG, Linn R. A note concerning misconceptions of the general public about brain injury. Arch Clin Neuropsychol 1993; 8(5):461–465.

52.     Guilmette TJ, Paglia MF. The public's misconception about traumatic brain injury: a follow up survey. Arch Clin Neuropsychol 2004; 19(2):183–189.

53.     Simpson G, Mohr R, Redman A. Cultural variations in the understanding of traumatic brain injury and brain injury rehabilitation. Brain Inj 2000; 14(2):125–140.

54.     Twain M. The autobiography of Mark Twain. London: Chatto & Windus, 1960.

55.     Montgomery V, Oliver R, Reisner A, Fallat ME. The effect of severe traumatic brain injury on the family. J Trauma 2002; 52(6):1121–1124.

56.     Wade SL, Stancin T, Taylor HG, Drotar D, Yeates KO, Minich NM. Interpersonal stressors and resources as predictors of parental adaptation following pediatric traumatic injury. J Consult Clin Psychol 2004; 72(5):776–784.

57.     Perrott SB, Taylor HG, Montes JL. Neuropsychological sequelae, familial stress, and environmental adaptation following pediatric head injury. Dev Neuropsychol 1991; 7(1):69–86.

58.     Sokol DK, Ferguson CF, Pitcher GA, Huster GA, Fitzhugh-Bell K, Luerssen TG. Behavioural adjustment and parental stress associated with closed head injury in children. Brain Inj 1996; 10(6):439–451.

59.     Springer JA, Farmer JE, Bouman DE. Common misconceptions about traumatic brain injury among family members of rehabilitation patients. J Head Trauma Rehabil 1997; 12:41–50.

60.     Melnyk BM, Alpert-Gillis L, Feinstein NF et al. Creating opportunities for parent empowerment: program effects on the mental health/coping outcomes of critically ill young children and their mothers. Pediatrics 2004; 113(6):e597–e607.

61.     Kessler LA. In a high tech age, is clinical judgment a lost art form? Surg Neurol 1999; 52(1):22–23.

62.     Dennis M, Spiegler BJ, Hetherington R. New survivors for the new millennium: cognitive risk and reserve in adults with childhood brain insults. Brain Cogn 2000; 42(1):102–105.

63.     Pinto KS, Rocha AP, Coutinho AC, Goncalves DM, Beraldo PS. Is rehabilitation the Cinderella of health, education and social services for children? Pediatr Rehabil 2005; 8(1):33–43.

64.     Almli CR, Finger S. Toward a definition of recovery of function. In: Finger S, LeVere TE, Almli CR, Stein DG, editors. Brain injury and recovery: theoretical and controversial issues. New York: Plenum, 1988: 1–13.

65.     Fletcher JM, Ewing-Cobbs L, Francis DJ, Levin HS. Variability in outcome after traumatic brain injury in children: a developmental perspective. In: Broman SH, Michel ME, editors. Traumatic head injury in children. New York: Oxford University Press, 1995: 3–21.

# *Index*

Items in parenthesis refer to an activity and its number. These numbers correspond with the activity numbers in the CD-ROM.